ASSISTED FERTILIZATION AND NUCLEAR TRANSFER IN MAMMALS

CONTEMPORARY ENDOCRINOLOGY

P. Michael Conn, SERIES EDITOR

ASSISTED FERTILIZATION AND NUCLEAR TRANSFER IN MAMMALS

Edited by

DON P. WOLF, PhD

and

MARY ZELINSKI-WOOTEN, PhD

Oregon Regional Primate Research Center,
Beaverton, OR

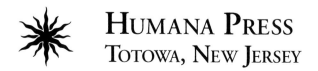

HUMANA PRESS
TOTOWA, NEW JERSEY

© 2001 Humana Press Inc.
999 Riverview Drive, Suite 208
Totowa, New Jersey 07512

For additional copies, pricing for bulk purchases, and/or information about other Humana titles,
contact Humana at the above address or at any of the following numbers: Tel: 973-256-1699;
Fax: 973-256-8341; E-mail: humana@humanapr.com; Website: http://humanapress.com

Cover design by Patricia F. Cleary

All articles, comments, opinions, conclusions, or recommendations are those of the author(s), and do not necessarily reflect
the views of the publisher.

This publication is printed on acid-free paper. ∞
ANSI Z39.48-1984 (American National Standards Institute)
Permanence of Paper for Printed Library Materials.

Printed in the United States of America. 10 9 8 7 6 5 4 3 2 1

Library of Congress Ctaloging -in-Publication Data

Assisted fertilization and nuclear transfer in mammals / edited by Don P. Wolf and Mary Zelinski-Wooten.
       p. ; cm. --(Contemporary endocrinology)
    Includes bibliographical references and index.
    ISBN 0-89603-663-4 (alk. paper)
    1. Reproductive technology. 2. Cell nuclei--Transplantation. 3. Fertilization in vitro. 4.
  Fertilization in vitro, Human. 5. Mammals--Reproduction. I. Wolf, Don P. II.
  Zelinski-Wooten, Mary. III. Contemporary endocrinology (Totowa, N.J.)
    [DNLM: 1. Reproduction Techniques. 2. Embryo Transfer--methods. 3. Fertilization in
  Vitro--methods. 4. Insemination, Artificial--methods. 5. Mammals--embryology. WQ
  208 A848 2001]
    QP252.A87 2001
    571.8'19--dc21   00-053979

PREFACE

The fields of assisted reproducton and nuclear transfer, while often controversial in their relatively brief lifetimes, have been and continue to be exceedingly dynamic. In *Assisted Fertilization and Nuclear Transfer in Mammals*, we have treated these subjects as a continuum because assisted sexual reproduction provides the technical groundwork for asexual reproduction by nuclear transfer and because both cytoplasmic and nuclear transfer protocols are in assisted reproductive technology (ART) clinical trial programs in this country. The basic reproductive physiology underlying these technological achievements holds the key to understanding the events comprising fertilization and early mammalian development, while providing treatment modalities for most cases of infertility. Our current efforts, detailed here, are predicated historically on the discovery in the late 1950s that sperm must undergo a process called capacitation before fertilizing an oocyte and, thereafter, on the development of strategies to recover and fertilize viable oocytes. Application in humans, pioneered by Patrick Steptoe and Robert Edwards in Cambridge, England, culminated in 1978 with the birth of Louise Brown, which was followed by explosive growth in the clinical use of this technology that was encouraged by the high interest level of the infertility community. At present, the clinical ARTs are available worldwide with over 300 programs in the US alone; according to the American Society of Reproductive Medicine in 1995, 11,315 women gave birth to children conceived by some form of ART. At the clinical level, we might trace this technological revolution from sperm isolation, cryopreservation, and capacitation, to in vitro fertilization, embryo cryopreservation, intracytoplasmic sperm injection, and extended embryo culture to the latest hot topics of in vitro oocyte maturation, oocyte cryopreservation, and cytoplasmic and nuclear transfer.

With regard to nuclear transfer in mammals, relatively undifferentiated embryonic cells have been used successfully as a source of the donor nucleus in a number of species beginning in the early 1980s and leading to application in the rhesus monkey in 1997. The revolutionary announcement in 1997 of somatic cell cloning by Ian Wilmut, Keith Campbell, and colleagues at the Roslyn Institute in Scotland opened the possibility that existing individuals could be reproduced asexually, and indeed that groups of genetically similar animals could be produced this way. In response to this discovery, the past two years has seen intense interest in the field, with confirmation of somatic cell cloning in other species and an ongoing debate concerning potential application in humans.

The present volume, *Assisted Fertilization and Nuclear Transfer in Mammals*, is by design unique, for instead of writing principally for the ART practitioner, we have written for a greater audience including students, practitioners of the clinical ARTs, our colleagues responsible for animal care, and research scientists. Our objectives include: The provision of an historical perspective on the development and application of these technologies in animals that in many, but not all, instances preceded clinical application; the treatment of subjects from both a basic scientist's and a practicing clinician's perspective in an effort to encourage communication between these sometimes diverse groups; and the inclusion of updates on several of the more dynamic clinical areas, such as gamete and embyro cryopreservation, intracytoplasmic sperm injection, and oocyte in vitro maturation. In all cases, detailed bibliographies have been encouraged in an effort to provide historical continuity for the student or for those desirous of additional insights and reading.

We would like to express appreciation to the distinguished authors who accepted our invitation to participate in this project, to Humana Press, and to Dr. P. Michael Conn, the series editor, for their confidence in our ability to organize and complete this project. We also thank Julianne White for her excellent editorial assistance.

Don P. Wolf
Mary Zelinski-Wooten

CONTENTS

Part II. Nuclear Transfer

CONTRIBUTORS

DOUGLAS J. AUSTIN, *Women's Care Fertility Center, Eugene, OR*

CATHERINE BOYD, *Jones Institute for Reproductive Medicine, Eastern Virginia School of Medicine, Norfolk, VA*

BENJAMIN G. BRACKETT, *Department of Physiology and Pharmacology, College of Veterinary Medicine, University of Georgia, Athens, GA*

THOMAS D. BUNCH, *Animal, Dairy, and Veterinary Sciences Department, Utah State University, Logan, UT*

KENNETH A. BURRY, *University Fertility Consultants, Oregon Health Sciences University, Portland, OR*

WILLIAM BYRD, *Southwestern Medical School, University of Texas-Dallas, Dallas, TX*

ROBERT H. FOOTE, *Department of Animal Science, Cornell University, Ithaca, NY*

MARSHA. J. GORRILL, *University Fertility Consultants, Oregon Health Sciences University, Portland, OR*

PAUL F. KAPLAN, *Women's Care Fertility Center, Eugene, OR*

SUSAN E. LANZENDORF, *Jones Institute for Reproductive Medicine, Eastern Virginia School of Medicine, Norfolk, VA*

JOSEPH E. MARTIN, *Fertility Center of San Antonio, San Antonio, TX*

SHOUKHRAT MITALIPOV, *Oregon Regional Primate Research Center, Beaverton, OR*

NADIA OUHIBI, *University Fertility Consultants, Oregon Health Sciences University, Portland, OR*

PHILIP E. PATTON, *University Fertility Consultants, Oregon Health Sciences University, Portland, OR*

ROGER A. PIERSON, *Department of Obstetrics, Gynecology and Reproductive Sciences, College of Medicine, Royal University Hospital, Saskatoon, Canada*

THOMAS B. POOLE, *Fertility Center of San Antonio, San Antonio, TX*

RANDALL S. PRATHER, *Animal Sciences Unit, Animal Science Research Center, Columbia, MO*

WILLIAM F. RALL, *Special Breeding and Species Preservation, Veterinary Resources Program, Office of Research Services, National Institutes of Health, Bethesda, MD*

WILLIAM A. REED, *Animal, Dairy, and Veterinary Sciences Department, Utah State University, Logan, UT*

JAMES M. ROBL, *Veterinary and Animal Science Department, University of Massachusetts, Amherst, MA*

JEFFREY B. RUSSELL, *Center for Human Reproduction, Newark, DE*

GARY D. SMITH, *Department of Obstetrics and Gynecology, University of Michigan, Ann Arbor, MI*

JAMES A. THOMSON, *Wisconsin Regional Primate Research Center, Madison, WI*

KENNETH L. WHITE, *Animal, Dairy, and Veterinary Sciences Department, Utah State University, Logan, UT*

DON P. WOLF, *Oregon Regional Primate Research Center, Beaverton, OR*

MARY B. ZELINSKI-WOOTEN, *Oregon Regional Primate Research Center, Beaverton, OR*

I   Assisted Fertilization

1

Developments in Animal Reproductive Biotechnology

Robert H. Foote, BS, MS, PHD

CONTENTS

INTRODUCTION

There have been an extraordinary series of exciting developments in knowledge of and technology applied to animal reproduction at the gamete, embryo, and whole animal level during the past 50 years. These developments include artificial insemination (AI), freezing (*see* Chapter 10) and sexing of sperm, superovulation, estrous cycle regulation, recovery of embryos developed in vivo, embryo freezing (*see* Chapter 10) and sexing, and embryo transfer (*see* Chapter 9). In addition, recovery of oocytes for in vitro maturation (IVM) (*see* Chapters 3, 4, and 16), in vitro fertilization (IVF) (*see* Chapter 2), and in vitro culture (IVC) (*see* Chapter 8) have led to new experimental approaches, advancing knowledge and ability to assist with problems in reproduction.

All of these biotechnologies utilize sperm and oocytes and/or the products of fertilization at some stage. Thus, all involve sexual reproduction. Also, the accumulated technologies in animal reproduction and breeding have helped to achieve asexual reproduction in mammals by cloning (*see* Chapters 13–17).

Artificial breeding was the first step on the stairs that helped to build the pathway to other biotechnologies. Application of AI has been the most powerful tool in human history utilized to improve the genetics of livestock and to control venereal diseases. Hundreds of millions of cows have been inseminated artificially. This has provided an unprecedented opportunity to conduct multiple studies on fertility of males and females and their gametes to increase our understanding of reproductive biology, to utilize this knowledge to enhance animal reproduction, and to advance reproductive biotechnolo-

From: *Contemporary Endocrinology: Assisted Fertilization and Nuclear Transfer in Mammals*
Edited by: D. P. Wolf and M. Zelinski-Wooten © Humana Press Inc., Totowa, NJ

3

gies. Many of the discoveries with cattle, such as freezing of bull sperm, have led to adoption of procedures for effective freezing of many types of cells and tissues in other species, including human cells.

Also, experimental results provided valid estimates of the variances that were needed to design new, more efficient experiments *(1,2)*. Unless this is done, time, money, and animals are wasted.

In this chapter, we will capture several of these discoveries and show how they have been woven into the fabric of the modern quilt of biotechnology. Cattle will be our chief model because AI and several other biotechnologies have been most intensively researched and exploited in the bovine species, and this story is not well known outside of agriculture.

EARLY HISTORY

The process of sexual reproduction and mammalian development has fascinated human beings throughout recorded history. Aristotle and other great thinkers in early history set forth various views based upon assumptions and dogma current at the time of their writings. Many myths surrounded the fascinating subjects of sex determination and the origin of new individuals. Interesting as those myths are, the history of events outlined here start with documented work that advanced both the science and the art of animal reproduction and biotechnology. Several major advances in the field are listed in Table 1. It is interesting to note that each of these landmark reports usually were published by one author *(3–10)*. Compare this with the numerous authors of today's biotechnology reports.

The rapid advances in science and technology have occurred primarily in the last half of the 20th century. However, these would not have happened without the foundations of testicular and ovarian organization laid down by the discovery of sperm and ova, and the description of the young embryo (Table 1). More historical details can be found in Bodemer *(11)*, Corner *(12)*, and Setchell *(13)*, and more recent work in Betteridge *(14)*, Biggers *(15)*, and Foote *(16,17)*. A priceless source of documented background information on sex and hormones is in Young *(18)*. The routine manipulation of gonadal function by gonadotropic hormones could not have occurred without the foundations of the pituitary-gonadal relationships established in the late 1920s and 1930s with animals.

MALE

Testis Characteristics and Testicular Biopsy

Details of testicular organization, cell types, their association and duration of spermatogenesis in the bovine are described and extensively referenced by Ortavant et al. in Johnson et al. *(19)*, which also includes references to studies on the testis of many species (see references to Clermont, Ortavant, Roosen Runge, Swierstra, and others in ref. *19*). These studies permitted accurate histopathologic evaluation of the testis of subfertile males, as well as calculation of the expected daily sperm production by normal testes per unit of time *(20; see* also Amann in ref. *19)*. These studies were models for more recent studies in men.

Testis size can be accurately estimated from length and width or scrotal circumference measurements *(20,21)*. This estimated size is highly correlated with testicular weight *(22)*, and both are highly correlated with potential sperm production *(23; see* also Amann in ref. *19)*. Thus, if semen collections contain few sperm obtained from a male with

Table 1
Selected Landmarks in Gamete and Embryo Discoveries and Manipulation[a]

Sex	Year	Description of the event
Male	1668	de Graaf published details of testis structure.
	1677	Leeuwenhoek and Ham discovered spermatozoa.
	1780	Spallanzani successfully inseminated a bitch.
	1799	Hunter inseminated a woman artificially.
	1841	Kölliker established that sperm come from the testis.
	1871	Von Ebner observed that testicular cells were in stages.
	1899	Ivanov organized AI in Russia, followed by Japan; by 1939 AI spread westward to the USA.
	1940	Phillips and Lardy reported the value of egg yolk for preserving bull sperm, Salisbury et al. devised yolk-citrate in 1941, and in 1963 Davis et al. published Tris-buffered yolk, the most widely used semen extender worldwide.
	1949	Polge et al. froze bull sperm successfully using glycerol.
	1951	Austin, and also Chang reported capacitation of sperm.
	1982	Gledhill et al. reported sexing of sperm based on DNA content.
	1970s	Sperm are used with other biotechnologies (IVF, etc.).
	1998	Wakayama and Yanagimachi produced offspring using freeze-dried sperm.
Female (and fertilization)		
	1672	de Graaf described the Graafian follicle.
	1827	von Baer described a real mammalian ovum.
	1840	Barry described blastocyst formation in the rabbit.
	1891	Heape performed embryo transfer in the rabbit.
	1929	Pincus superovulated rabbits and did embryo transfer.
	1943	Casida et al., superovulated cattle following a Russian report.
	1951	Willett et al., produced the first calf from embryo transfer.
	1959	Chang reported successful IVF and reported a series of contraceptive experiments starting in 1953, and leading to the Pincus pill.
	1960s	Estrous cycle regulation was established.
	1970s	Embryo transfer nonsurgically in cattle was commercialized.
	1972	Whittingham et al. froze mouse embryos.
	1978	Steptoe and Edwards performed human IVF and embryo transfer.
	1980s	Embryos were micromanipulated in various ways.
	1997	Wilmut et al. reported cloning Dolly from adult cells.

[a] See refs 3–18 for further reading.

normal-sized testes, either the semen collection conditions are poor or testicular pathology is present. Furthermore, testis size is highly inherited (21). Also, testis firmness is associated with semen quality and fertility (20,21). All these features are important in animal breeding and AI. The quality and quantity of sperm output largely determines the number of females that can be inseminated and the number of progeny produced by genetically superior sires. Extensive data obtained on testicular function, semen quality, and fertility in animals may provide lessons relevant to problems of infertility in man. Have there been changes with time? We have not been able to detect them, but the bulls lead a favored life in the clean country air.

Other aspects of testicular function can be measured without surgery (24). In addition, testicular biopsy procedures have been tested thoroughly in animals, and have implications for human medicine, where, for example, testicular biopsies are used frequently to obtain sperm for human IVF (*see* Chapter 7). Testicular biopsy can be performed repeatedly, along with semen collection, to monitor a male's reproductive potential *(20,21,25)*. Testicular biopsy is especially valuable in toxicity studies, where effects during exposure to an agent and during recovery can be monitored sequentially. However, the biopsy should be taken very carefully so as to avoid superficial blood vessels. Otherwise considerable damage can be done to localized areas of the testis. This precaution is seldom mentioned and followup is seldom reported in medical literature.

Artificial Insemination and Sperm Manipulation, Particularly in Cattle

Overviews of the development of AI in domestic animals, as well as in nondomestic animals *(33)*, have been published *(8,16,21,26–32)*, The need to select superior males, to make efficient use of them, and to maintain high pregnancy rates in low-cost agricultural programs has stimulated research into all aspects of domestic animal reproduction, particularly in cattle. The rapid spread of AI worldwide attests to the success of the program. Furthermore, public acceptance of AI laid the foundation for the scientific pursuit and practical opportunity to apply new technologies for the benefit of society. Therefore, AI is treated in some detail, starting with semen collection followed by semen evaluation, extension, and insemination. For brevity, only a few original papers will be cited directly.

Semen Collection

Providing the proper surroundings, sexual preparation, and semen collection equipment *(16,23,34–38)* facilitated obtaining the most sperm of the highest quality possible consistently at each semen collection. Applying this carefully controlled research resulted in doubling *(39)* the sperm harvested per bull. These studies reveal that the environment at the time donor semen is collected can markedly affect semen quality. This fact is relevant to the collection of semen samples in man, and indicates that collection of a series of semen samples is important, especially if the first one is of low quality.

Semen Evaluation

Semen quality was carefully evaluated, using the classical tests of sperm concentration, motility, and morphology *(20,21,40)*, and many other tests *(41–44)*, including the bull sperm swelling test *(45,46)*, which was adapted for human sperm *(47)* under the name "hypoosmotic swelling test (HOS)." The test for bull sperm was correlated with fertility, based on tens of thousands of inseminations. The large quantity of animal sperm available facilitated running multiple tests and doing biochemical analyses *(28,48)* to assess sperm function.

Initially, computer-assisted sperm analysis (CASA) was developed primarily for the human sperm market *(49)*, although early work had been done with bull sperm *(50)*. More recently, we assisted in developing equipment for CASA capable of measuring motion characteristics of stained and unstained sperm *(51–54)*. The CASA has added a valuable tool in the armament of sperm cell analysis. Flow cytometry, following staining of sperm with a variety of fluorescent dyes, also is useful in evaluating the quality of sperm by measuring the integrity of both the plasma and mitochondrial membranes in fresh and cryopreserved sperm *(55,56)*.

In vitro tests of sperm fertilizing ability are another useful way to evaluate semen quality. The first IVF report was in 1951, as Chang *(57)* noted in reviewing his life's work. Hamster oocytes *(21)* for testing fertilizing ability of bull sperm have been replaced with bovine oocytes. The latter are available in large numbers from live or slaughtered cattle *(59,60)*. Literally millions of bovine oocytes *(59)* have been used to test sperm capacitation *(3,4)* and oocyte maturation systems with improvement in IVF. These in vitro systems, especially competitive fertilization studies *(61,62)*, have yielded results that are highly correlated with fertility obtained in large breeding trials (*see* Davis and Foote, in ref. *21*). The IVF system has been successfully applied to produce bovine embryos commercially *(63)*, but the programs are small compared to the multimillion dollar human IVF programs.

Fertilization following microinjection of sperm from sterile or subfertile bulls *(64,65)* indicates that caution should be followed in using intracytoplasmic sperm injection (ICSI) routinely in human IVF programs, at least without counseling (*see* Chapter 7). Four bulls used in artificial insemination had fertility rates (estimated by no return of the cows to subsequent service) of 75, 69, 42, and 0%, and when used for routine IVF *(65)* had fertilization rates of 80, 54, 1, and 2%, respectively. When ICSI was used the corresponding values were 39, 22, 21, and 34%. The bull with the 42% fertility rate in artificial insemination had few surviving progeny, and detailed karyotyping revealed that chromosomal defects of this sire were found in some of the progeny. This sire was removed from service and all past users of the semen were notified of the problem. The ICSI study revealed that bulls with defective sperm that were incapable of normal fertility in vivo produced fertilization rates with ICSI equivalent to the most fertile sire. A chromosomal defect was inherited.

A potential application in commercial AI of an in vitro sperm procedure is to treat part of an ejaculate of semen with in vitro capacitation procedures *(67,68)*. This fraction could be combined with the control portion of the ejaculate for insemination. Because the time of ovulation is not known in each cow inseminated, such treated sperm might increase the window of opportunity for sperm to be conditioned for maximal fertilization of freshly ovulated oocytes and those ovulated a few hours later. Microencapsulation of sperm *(69)* also may accomplish the objective of making sperm available for a longer period. Furthermore, some capsules might be formed that would also delay release of sperm.

Semen Processing and Preservation

The initial development and rapid expansion of AI in cattle was based upon the discovery of the beneficial effects of egg yolk *(70,71)* and later, heated milk *(72)*. Both protected bull sperm so that they could be cooled to and stored at 5°C without coldshock, thus preventing a marked reduction in fertility *(73)* by cooling. Of great benefit was the addition of antibiotics to extended semen *(74,75)*. This increased fertility of some bulls by more than 20%. Venereal diseases of cattle were eliminated by AI. The use of antibiotics in extended semen was worth hundreds of millions of dollars to the animal industry worldwide. Eventually, the commercial AI stations developed specific-pathogen free bull studs, but antibiotics continue to be used for insurance.

The Cornell University (CUE) self-carbonating egg yolk extender *(21)* maintained high sperm survival at 5°C and fertility levels exceeded 70% following a single insemination. This extender was modified by researchers in New Zealand to "Caprogen", where liquid semen is still used. A tris-buffered egg yolk extender *(76)* containing glycerol provided excellent protection for sperm in liquid and frozen semen. Today it is the most widely used extender to preserve frozen semen in many species. Catalase additions to semen extender are beneficial to sperm stored at room temperature, unless they are maintained under anaerobic conditions. Bull sperm are sensitive to oxidative damage

(21), as are human sperm *(77,78)*. In the presence of light and oxygen, DNA can be damaged *(79)*. Also, at ambient temperatures egg yolk can be reduced to 1% (v/v) compared with 20% egg yolk used at 5°C and −196°C *(31)*. These semen extenders have been adapted for preserving human sperm, but useful information on animal models is often overlooked by the medical field *(80,81)*.

Freezing and Packaging Semen

The discovery of the protective effects of glycerol on sperm *(82)* revolutionized the field of cryobiology (*see* Chapter 10). Fortunately, glycerol was an excellent cryoprotectant for bull sperm, and it provided a model for other species and other cell types *(83)*. However, there is still a need to reduce sperm mortality during freezing *(84,85)*, as frozen-thawed sperm are less fertile *(86)*. Freezing sperm shortens the capacitation time in some species *(21,59)*, and this may be associated with membrane damage during freezing.

The application of frozen semen for commercial artificial insemination was made possible, in part, by the marked improvement in thermal characteristics of liquid nitrogen tanks for storing sperm at −196°C. The inefficient insulated tanks previously available were greatly improved by Linde Company (New York, NY) as a result of a major private grant by Rockefeller Prentice so that his company, American Breeders Service, (DeForest, WI), could market semen worldwide. The world of cryobiology followed this development with bull sperm.

Another revolution in the processing of semen was the development of straws by Instruments de Médecine Vétérinaire (IMV; L'Aigle, France) *(87)* for packaging semen. Billions of straws (0.25 mL and 0.50 mL capacity) have been produced since these replaced glass ampules. The cost of developing the straw system was covered by the cattle AI market, and now the straw is used for cryopreservation of human and animal sperm and other types of cells.

Insemination Procedures and Results

Development of the nonsurgical intrauterine insemination procedure for cattle by Danish workers greatly reduced the number of sperm required per insemination *(21,31)*. When 4–5 million fresh or frozen-thawed motile sperm are inseminated, essentially normal high fertility is maintained in cattle *(21,88)*, and 500,000 sperm inseminated reduces fertility to about 40%. With rabbits properly inseminated intravaginally, 50,000 total (about 35,000 motile) sperm inseminated result in normal fertility and birthrates. With the high extension rate of bull sperm (usually at least 1:50), so that an ejaculate of semen is used to inseminate several hundred cows, no problems result from inclusion of minute quantities of seminal plasma inseminated into the uterus.

Because of the opportunity to inseminate tens of thousands of cows in controlled experiments *(88)*, fertility can be used to evaluate quantitatively tests of semen quality *(21,53)* and many aspects of the AI operation *(89,90)*. In the report by Foote and Kaproth *(88)*, results were based on 88,486 inseminations. Large numbers of inseminations are required for accuracy because of the statistical noise due to the binomial variation of a pregnancy being 0 or 1. When 25 inseminations result in 60% pregnancies, the estimated fertility, with 95% confidence limits, is 40–80%. Obviously, the estimate based on a small sample may not be accurate.

When there are thousands of inseminations, measures of semen quality may not be correlated with fertility unless the tests of semen quality also are replicated. In unpublished studies (Foote, Cornell University), the correlation between the estimated percentage of motile sperm and fertility was greatly increased from 0.25 to 0.66 when the motility estimates of several observers were averaged over triplicate subsamples and compared with single estimates. When the percentage of motile sperm is accurately determined under physiologic conditions, and sperm concentration is known, so that the number of progressively motile normal sperm inseminated can be calculated, this number is one of the best indications of the potential fertility of that semen. These are tests that can be conducted in any andrology laboratory.

Conclusions on Cattle AI

The AI of cattle did more than improve cattle genetically, control venereal disease, and increase understanding of reproductive physiology. The liquid semen and then the frozen semen success story converted some of the doubting public into supporters and users, as early development of AI was accompanied by ill-founded criticisms, and speculations. This was the beginning of the reproductive biology revolution. The public recognized that scientists in laboratories could really make things work practically. This big step in AI paved the way to building other reproductive technologies, such as estrous cycle regulation, embryo manipulation, and embryo transfer.

AI in Other Species

Artificial insemination with frozen boar sperm has been less successful than in cattle because freezing boar sperm reduces fertility and litter size (91). However, swine AI is spreading worldwide because of the ease with which farmers do their own insemination, and the development of rapid transit making extended liquid semen available soon after semen collection.

The biotechnology of AI has been widely applied to sheep and goats (92,93), certain breeds of horses (91), foxes, dogs (21,33,94,95), endangered species (33,96), and poultry (97). In turkeys, 100% are inseminated artificially. We have used AI in rabbits for many years (21) as an excellent laboratory model for many aspects of reproduction in domestic animals and humans. Also, rabbits are one of the best models for risk assessment involving male reproductive toxicants (98) because of their testicular sensitivity to toxicants and ease of collecting semen for evaluating sperm quality and fertility.

Frozen-thawed sperm have more difficulty in penetrating the cervix compared with unfrozen (fresh) sperm. Many more frozen-thawed sperm are required with intracervical than with intrauterine insemination, and fertility is reduced (93,99). Therefore, the use of frozen semen is limited in species where it is difficult to pass the inseminating catheter through the cervix. The response of sperm from various species to different freezing protocols has been reviewed by Watson (100).

Because of the interest in utilizing special genetic lines of mice as models for various diseases, much emphasis has been placed on cryopreservation of mouse sperm (101). Recently, freeze-dried mouse sperm maintained the ability to fertilize oocytes by microinjection and produced live offspring (102).

Sexing of Sperm

The development of laminar flow cell sorters (103–105) has made it possible to separate sperm from many species, based on the DNA content of sperm containing an X vs Y chromosome. Separation is over 90% accurate (106). This can be accomplished at the astounding speed of several thousand sperm per second. This rate of separation is sufficient for IVF and for limited types of insemination in vivo *(107)*. However, it is too slow for separating the billions of sperm in an ejaculate of bull semen for routine AI. Also, there is some damage to sperm during the high-speed trip at about 60 miles per hour through the sorter, and a significant fraction of the cells pass through unsorted. The procedure is being used selectively with human sperm by one IVF group *(108)* in cases with sex-linked problems.

Sperm from many species have been "sexed," and the procedure could be used with endangered species to increase the number of females for more rapid expansion of the population. Fewer than 50% males would be needed for AI. However, widespread use of sex-separated sperm in animals will require more rapid separation of sperm, perhaps based on a principle other than the DNA content.

Sperm as a Vector for Gene Transfer

The sperm cell offers a simple method of getting DNA into an oocyte. Whether or not sperm can be impregnated with gene constructs and these be incorporated into the genome has been controversial, but it has been reported *(109,110)*.

FEMALE

Estrous Cycle Regulation and AI

Accompanying the development of AI was the need to either detect estrus accurately from behavioral signs of the female, or use electronic technology *(111,112)*, and to determine the best time to inseminate *(113)*. An alternative was to control ovulation time. Practical procedures had to be accurate, low cost, and with immediate interpretation. Extensive studies were conducted by many researchers *(17,114)*, using a variety of treatments, to regulate ovulation. The principle followed was to cause regression of the female's corpus luteum with prostaglandin $F_2\alpha$ or analogs, while maintaining the progesterone concentration with an implant containing progesterone. The progesterone implant was removed after the corpus luteum had regressed, and the sudden decline in progesterone was followed by a luteinizing hormone (LH) surge and ovulation. Additionally, gonadotropin releasing hormone (GnRH) or an analog often was included to assist in a controlled time of ovulation *(115)*. A fixed predetermined time to inseminate a group of animals is especially helpful for animals managed under range conditions, where corralling animals individually for AI is impractical.

The principle of regulating the estrous cycle by preventing the LH surge through the administration of progesterone was the basis for the contraceptive "Pincus" pill for humans. Interesting reflections on the basic studies, with typical Chang humor, were recounted by Chang *(57)*.

EMBRYO PRODUCTION,
CULTURE, EVALUATION, AND MANIPULATION

Superovulation

In order to increase a superior cow's genetic contribution to the population, additional ova or embryos have been obtained for several decades by superovulation *(114,116,117)*. The blood FSH concentration is elevated by injecting follicle-stimulating hormone (FSH) twice daily over a period of 3–4 d and regressing the corpus luteum with prostaglandin $F_2\alpha$ or an analog. Artificial insemination is performed at the appropriate time. More sperm are required for successful AI in superovulated cows than in control cattle (99). The techniques developed have resulted in the collection of millions of bovine embryos nonsurgically from cows followed by transfer with nonsurgical procedures (118–121).

Embryo Evaluation

Evaluation has been based primarily upon morphologic appearance when embryos are viewed microscopically. This evaluation includes an appropriate stage of development for embryos of a particular age, normality of blastomeres with sharply defined membranes, degree of fragmentation, and other signs of degeneration (120). These tests can be applied quickly and simply without manipulation of the embryo, and so are suitable for clinical work. Other tests, such as dye exclusion, glucose uptake, enzyme activity, protein synthesis, and quantitative determination of the number of cells forming the trophectoderm vs the inner cell mass have been used in various research studies. At present, the appearance and rate of embryo cleavage and development into a blastocyst are probably the most reliable practical tests of the ability of an embryo to develop into normal young (120,122).

Embryo Culture

Embryo culture has become a tool of great importance, not only for the development of naturally formed zygotes and laboratory-produced embryos into blastocysts capable of becoming normal young (see Chapters 8 and 16), but also for their use in the production of transgenic animals and cloning (see Chapters 13–17). Despite remarkable advances (15,122), culture systems currently are not equal to the natural oviduct and uterus in promoting preimplantation development.

The complex environment surrounding the preimplantation embryo in the oviduct and uterus supplies substrates to meet energy needs, amino acids, vitamins, and other nutrients for growth and development; an appropriate ionic, gas, and pH environment; and various protective substances (see Chapter 8). In addition, the reproductive system provides a dynamic transfer system that facilitates rapid waste disposal.

Co-culture of embryos, usually with oviductal epithelial cells (122,123), was employed to simulate natural conditions and stimulate blastocyst development. Co-culture promoted blastocyst development, but this could be mediated either through adding beneficial components or by mitigating effects of undesireable components (21,122) of the culture system (see Chapter 8). The commonly used media for coculturing embryos was Ham's F10 and TC199. These media were designed for tissue culture, and it would be fortuitous if they were optimal for embryo culture. They no longer are as suitable for embryos as many media that have been developed specifically for embryo culture.

The early work on culturing mouse and rabbit embryos by Whitten, Brinster, Foote, and others has been reviewed by Biggers (15). Superovulation of the rabbit provided a large supply of oocytes and embryos (124). Our laboratory was the first 30 years ago to culture rabbit zygotes into hatched blastocysts without serum, but bovine serum albumin (BSA) was included (21). More recent studies on mice in Bigger's laboratory, and hamsters in Bavister's laboratory, have been discussed in detail by Bavister (122). In the past few years, we have modified KSOM, developed in Biggers' laboratory for mice, and other media to produce two completely defined culture systems with no serum or BSA for culturing rabbit zygotes to blastocysts *(21)*. The appropriate balance of inorganic ions, total osmotic pressure of the medium, concentration of glucose, and balance of amino acids were important in designing media devoid of macromolecules that promoted 90–100% development of zygotes into blastocysts *(21)*. Similarly, completely defined media for culturing cattle embryos produced in vitro have been developed *(21,122)*. A gas environment containing about 5% O_2 rather than the frequently used 95% air (about 19% O_2) was an important component, along with a compatible mixture of solutes. When using 95% air, addition of antioxidants, such as taurine or superoxide dismutase to the medium was beneficial *(21)*. These culture systems promote development of blastocysts in vitro that are capable of becoming normal young. This is an essential characteristic of a good culture system.

Embryo Freezing

Freezing of embryos *(125)* was patterned after the initial cryopreservation of mouse embryos by Whittingham et al. (*126; see* Chapter 10). Cryopreservation simplified the process of embryo transfer. Embryos could be collected at one time and place and be frozen. Then they could be shipped and a specified number thawed for use whenever and wherever there were recipients at the appropriate stage of their reproductive cycle to receive embryos. So, again, one step in reproductive technology led to another.

Embryo Sexing

Sexing of embryos *(127,128)* has become a relatively simple technique. Only one blastomere is required to obtain sufficient DNA for the test after amplifying it with the polymerase chain reaction (PCR). The sex is determined accurately. The blastocyst is not harmed by removing a single blastomere. Sexing of embryos offers a technique for AI organizations to obtain young bulls for progeny testing, and the female embryos produce calves maintained in dairy herds.

Embryo Bisection

Embryo splitting is a relatively simple procedure *(129)* that has been thoroughly tested in cattle. The pregnancy rate is about 50% with half embryos compared to 60% with whole embryos. Split embryos also can be frozen with about a 10% reduction in pregnancy rate due to freezing.

Embryos Made in the Laboratory

Oocytes collected from the ovary with the aid of ultrasound imaging of the ovaries (*see* Chapter 2) require a good culture system following maturation in vitro (IVM) and fertilization in vitro with capacitated sperm (IVF). This practice is effective when used with adult cattle that fail to superovulate. Oocyte retrieval can be repeated weekly, including during pregnancy, without interrupting reproduction *(63)*.

Prepubertal calves can be ovulated *(130)* and oocytes fertilized in vivo. However, the in vivo ovarian aspiration technique, along with FSH to induce superfollicular development, makes possible collection of many oocytes from prepubertal calves *(131)* for in vitro production of blastocysts. This multiple ovulation-embryo transfer (MOET) program can provide more genetic information and speed up sire evaluation by reducing the generation interval in the conventional progeny test program *(132,138)*.

Oocytes collected from the ovaries of slaughtered cattle *(60)* also are capable of being matured and fertilized in vitro, cultured, and transferred to produce young. This has greatly facilitated studies advancing knowledge of the early changes in the zygote and embryo, along with requirements for development *(63,123,139)*.

TRANSFER OF EMBRYOS

All of the techniques for producing embryos in vivo following superovulation, or in vitro fertilization with or without microinjection, splitting, sexing, and so forth, eventually must include skillful transfer of the embryos to suitable recipients. So beyond the knowledge of molecular biology and skills with micromanipulation equipment, knowledge of the physiology and anatomy of the whole animal, and skill to place the embryos gently in their new home are vital to the final success of applying these reproductive biotechnologies (*see* Chapter 9).

Estrous cycle regulation was a big help in simplifying the transfer of fresh embryos. It is critical to have donors of embryos at the same stage of the reproductive cycle as the recipients. Otherwise the embryos transferred will not be compatible with the new environment *(120,125)*. A large group of random cycling recipients would be required to have a small percentage in synchrony with donors. This would be expensive. The group of recipients can be greatly reduced in size by regulating the cycles of the donors and recipients to be in synchrony.

In the initial development of cattle embryo transfer, young embryos were collected surgically by flushing the oviducts. The embryos were examined, and those judged to be normal were transferred surgically to oviducts, usually one per recipient on the side of the corpus luteum. The Japanese developed a nonsurgical procedure *(119)* to collect embryos that had been transported to the uterus, and these were transferred individually to a uterine horn of a recipient cow ipsilateral to the corpus luteum. Modifications of this procedure are used worldwide in cattle and horses. In horses, the embryo is placed in the large body of the uterus. During early development, the embryo puts on a spectacular display of movement that can be visualized with ultrasound equipment.

Surgical transfer of embryos, often with the aid of a laparoscope, is used in small animals such as sheep, goats, and swine, and many of the endangered species *(140,141)*. Recently Li et al. *(142)* reported moderate success using special equipment to assist in transcervical transfer of embryos in swine.

Kidder *(143)* and Kidder et al. *(144)* developed a small catheter assembly that could be guided through a ferret cervix, first located with the aid of fiber optics and a TV screen. The unit was suitable for transcervical passage for intrauterine insemination *(144)*, as well as for intrauterine recovery and transfer of embryos in the ferret. This is the first known report of successful nonsurgical embryo recovery and nonsurgical transfer of the same embryos in any carnivore. Nonsurgical procedures are especially important in propagating endangered species. An example of a litter of kits produced using these nonsurgical procedures is in Fig. 1.

CONCLUSIONS

Advances in genomic analysis and the application of reproductive technologies, including production of transgenic and cloned animals *(145–151; see* Chapters 13–17), are

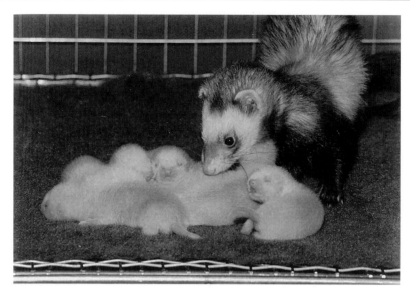

Fig. 1. Litter of 7 kits resulting from nonsurgical collection of blastocysts and nonsurgical transfer to the recipient mother shown. Adapted with permission from ref. *(143)*

moving forward at a pace that rivals the speed of our revolving planet. This would not have been possible without the foundations laid in the preceding years when the research tools available were much simpler *(21)*. To date, artificial breeding is still the most powerful animal reproductive biotechnology developed and applied, worldwide, with extraordinary improvement in genetics, disease control, and management of livestock. It is hoped that this chapter will assist readers in becoming more aware of how beneficial each step was—from AI to estrous cycle regulation and synchronization, gamete manipulation, and sexing and embryo culture of naturally produced and laboratory-made embryos—in helping researchers to climb the animal biotechnology stairway in search of knowledge and application to improve the quality of life. Today we are entering a new era with genetic engineering *(152)* and cloning *(153–158)* of transgenic animals to produce products of great value in human medicine. Many of these important developments preceded the implementation of electronic gateways, so the current generation of researchers may have missed some earlier fascinating discoveries that now are treated as commonplace. After all, the launch of a space vehicle would have been unbelievable 50 years ago, and now it is commonplace.

REFERENCES

1. Hafs HD, Bratton RW, Henderson CR, Foote RH. Estimation of some variance components of bovine semen criteria and their use in the design of experiments. J Dairy Sci 1958;41:96–104.
2. Seidel GE Jr, Foote RH. Variance components of semen criteria from bulls ejaculated frequently and their use in experimental design. J Dairy Sci 1973;56:399–405.
3. Austin CR. Observations on the penetration of sperm into the mammalian egg. Australian J Biol Sci 1951; Ser B 4:581–596.
4. Chang MC. Fertilizing capacity of spermatozoa deposited into the Fallopian tubes. Nature 1951;168:697.
5. Heape W. The artificial insemination of mammals and subsequent possible fertilization or impregnation of their ova. Proc Royal Soc London 1897;61:52–63.

6. Ivanoff EI. On the use of artificial insemination for zootechnical purposes in Russia. J Agr Sci 1922;12: 244–256.

7. Leeuwenhoek A. De natis è semine genitali animalculis. Royal Soc (London) Philos Trans 1678;12: 1040–1043.

8. Milovanov VK. Artificial Insemination of Livestock in the USSR (Translated by A. Birron, Z.S. Cole.) S. Monson, Jerusalem. Tech. Services, US Dept. Commerce, Washington, DC, 1964.

9. Nishikawa Y. Fifty years of artificial insemination of farm animals in Japan. English Bul 2. Kyoto University, Kyoto, 1962.

10. Spallanzani L. Dissertations relative to the natural history of animals and vegetables. (Translated by T. Beddoes in Dissertations Relative to the Natural History of Animals and Vegetables, Vol. 2.) J Murray, London, 1784, pp. 195–199.

11. Bodemer CW. The biology of the blastocyst in historical perspective. In: Blandau RJ, ed. The Biology of the Blastocyst. University of Chicago, Chicago, IL, 1971, pp. 1–25.

12. Corner GW. The discovery of the mammalian ovum. In: Lectures on the History of Medicine (Mayo Foundation). WB Saunders, Philadelphia, PA, 1933, pp. 401–426.

13. Setchell BP, ed. Male Reproduction. Van Nostrand Reinhold Co., New York, NY, 1984.

14. Betteridge KG. An historical look at embryo transfer. J Reprod Fertil 1981;62:1–13.

15. Biggers JD. Pioneering mammalian embryo culture. In: Bavister BD, ed. The Mammalian Preimplantation Embryo. Plenum, New York, NY, 1987, pp. 1–22.

16. Foote RH. Cryopreservation of spermatozoa and artificial insemination: past, present and future. J Androl 1982;3:85–100.

17. Foote RH. In vitro fertilization and embryo transfer in domestic animals: applications in animals and implications for humans. J Vitro Fert Embryo Transfer 1987;42:73–88.

18. Young WC, ed. Sex and Internal Secretions. Williams and Wilkins Co, Baltimore, MD, 1961.

19. Johnson AD, Gomes WR, VanDemark NL, eds. The Testis. Vols. I, II, III. Academic, New York, NY, 1970.

20. Foote RH. Research techniques to study reproductive physiology in the male. Techniques and Procedures in Animal Science Research, ASAP, Albany, NY, 1969, pp. 81–110.

21. Foote RH. Artificial Insemination to Cloning. Tracing 50 Years of Research. Published by the author, Ithaca, NY, 1998.

22. Coulter GH, Foote RH. Relationship of testicular weight to age and scrotal circumference of Holstein bulls. J Dairy Sci 1976;59:730–732.

23. Hahn J, Foote RH, Seidel GE Jr. Testicular growth and related sperm output in dairy bulls. J Anim Sci 1969;29:41–47.

24. Kastelic JP, Cook RB, Coulter GH, Wallins GL, Entz T. Environmental factors affecting measurement of bovine scrotal temperature with infrared thermography. Anim Reprod Sci 1996;41:153–159.

25. Hunt WL, Foote RH. Effect of repeated testicular biopsy on testis function and semen quality in dogs. J Androl 1997;18:740–744.

26. Courot M, ed. The Male in Farm Animal Reproduction. Martinus Nijhoff, Boston, MA, 1984.

27. Herman HA. Improving Cattle by the Millions. NAAB and the Development and Worldwide Application of Artificial Insemination. University of Missouri Press, Columbia, MD, 1981.

28. Mann T, Lutwak-Mann C. Male Reproductive Function and Semen. Springer-Verlag, Berlin, 1981.

29. Maule JP, ed. The Semen of Animals and Artificial Insemination. Commonwealth Agricultural Bureaux, Farnham Royal, Bucks, UK, 1962.

30. Perry EJ, ed. The Artificial Insemination of Farm Animals, 4th ed. Rutgers University Press, New Brunswick, NJ, 1968.

31. Salisbury GW, VanDemark NL, Lodge JR. Physiology of Reproduction and Artificial Insemination of Cattle, 2nd ed. WH Freeman Co., San Francisco, CA, 1978.

32. Sipher E, ed. The Gene Revolution. The History of Cooperative Artificial Breeding in New York and New England, 1938–1940. Eastern A. I. Cooperative, Inc., Ithaca, NY 1991.

33. Watson PF, ed. Artificial Breeding of Non-Domestic Animals. Zool Soc London Symp 43. Academic, London, 1978.

34. Bratton RW, Foote RH. Semen production and fertility of dairy bulls ejaculated either once or twice at intervals of either four or eight days. J Dairy Sci 1954;37:1439–1443.

35. Bratton RW, Musgrave S, Dunn HO, Foote RH. Causes and prevention of reproductive failures in dairy cattle. III. Influence of underfeeding and overfeeding from birth through 80 weeks of age on growth,

sexual development, semen production and fertility of Holstein bulls. Cornell Univ. Expt. Sta. Bull. No. 964, Ithaca, NY, 1961, pp. 1–24.

36. Collins WJ, Bratton RW, Henderson CR. The relationship of semen production to sexual excitement of dairy bulls. J Dairy Sci 1951;34: 224–227.

37. Hale EB, Almquist JO. Relation of sexual behavior to germ cell output in farm animals. J Dairy Sci (Suppl) 1960;43:145–169.

38. Salisbury GW, Willett EL. An artificial vagina for controlled temperature studies of bull semen. Cornell Vet 1940;30:25–29.

39. Hafs HD, Hoyt RS, Bratton RW. Libido, sperm characteristics, sperm output and fertility of mature dairy bulls ejaculated daily or weekly for thirty-two weeks. J Dairy Sci 1959;42:626–636.

40. den Daas N. Laboratory assessment of semen characteristics. Anim Repro Sci 1992;28:87–94.

41. Foote RH. Semen quality from the bull to the freezer: an assessment. Theriogenology 1975;3:219–235.

42. Pace MM. Fundamentals of assay of spermatozoa. 9th Intl Cong Anim Repro Artificial Insem, Graficas Orbe, Madrid, 1980, pp. 133–146.

43. Saacke RG, DeJarnette JM, Bame JH, Karabinus DS, Whitman SS. Can spermatozoa with abnormal heads gain access to the ovum in artificially inseminated super- and single-ovulating cattle? Theriogenology 1998;50:117–128.

44. Saacke RG, Nadir S, Nebel RL. Relationship of semen quality to sperm transport, fertilization, and embryo quality in ruminants. Theriogenology 1994;41:45–50.

45. Bredderman PJ, Foote RH. Volume of stressed bull spermatozoa and protoplasmic droplets, and the relationship of cell size to motility and fertility. J Anim Sci 1969;28:496–501.

46. Foote RH, Bredderman PJ. Sizing of aging bull spermatozoa with an electronic counter. J Dairy Sci 1969;52:117–120.

47. Jeyendran RS, Van der Ven HH, Perez-Pelaez M, Crabo G, Zaneveld LJD. Development of an assay to assess the functional integrity of the human sperm membrane and its relationship to other semen characteristics. J Reprod Fertil 1984;70:219–228.

48. Gatti JL, Chevrier C, Paquignon M, Dacheux, JL. External ionic conditions, internal pH and motility of ram and boar spermatozoa. J Reprod Fertil 1993;98:439–449.

49. Katz DG, Davis RO. Automatic analysis of human sperm motion. J Androl 1987;8:170–181.

50. Amann RP, Hammerstedt RH. Validation of a system for computerized measurements of spermatozoal velocity and percentage of motile sperm. Biol Reprod 1980;23:647–656.

51. Farrell PB, Foote RH, McArdle MM, Trouern-Trend VL, Tardif AL. Media and dilution procedures tested to minimize handling effects on human, rabbit, and bull sperm for computer-assisted sperm analysis (CASA). J Androl 1996;17:293–300.

52. Farrell PB, Foote RH, Zinaman MJ. Motility and other characteristics of human sperm can be measured by computer-assisted sperm analysis of samples stained with Hoechst 33342. Fertil Steril 1996;66:446–453.

53. Farrell PB, Presicce GA, Brockett CC, Foote RH. Quantification of bull sperm characteristics measured by CASA and the relationship to fertility. Theriogenology 1998;49:871–879.

54. Tardif AL, Farrell PB, Trouern-Trend V, Simkin ME, Foote RH. Use of Hoechst 33342 stain to evaluate live fresh and frozen bull sperm by computer assisted analysis. J Androl 1998;19:201–206.

55. Garner DL, Thomas CA, Joerg HW, DeJarnett JM, Marshall CE. Fluorometric assessments of mitochondrial function and viability in cryopreserved bovine spermatozoa. Biol Reprod 1997;57:1401–1406.

56. Thomas CA, Garner DL, DeJarnette JM, Marshall CE. Effect of cryopreservation on bovine sperm organelle function and viability as determined by flow cytometry. Biol Reprod 1998;58:786–793.

57. Chang MC. Experimental studies of mammalian spermatozoa and eggs. Biol Reprod 1971;4:3–15.

58. Chen Y, Li J, Simkin ME, Yang X, Foote RH. Fertility of fresh and frozen rabbit semen inseminated at different times is indicative of male differences in capacitation time. Biol Reprod 1989;41:848–853.

59. Gordon I. Laboratory Production of Cattle Embryos. CAB International, Wallingford, Oxon, UK, 1994.

60. Lu KH, Gordon I, Gallaher M, McGovern H. Pregnancy established in cattle by transfer of embryos derived from in vitro fertilization of oocytes matured in vitro. Vet Rec 1987;121:259–260.

61. Dziuk PJ. Review. Factors that influence the proportion of offspring sired by a male following heterospermic insemination. Anim Reprod Sci 1996;43:65–88.

62. Parrish JJ, Foote RH. Fertility differences among male rabbits determined by heterospermic insemination of fluorochrome-labeled spermatozoa. Biol Reprod 1985;33:940–949.

63. Hasler JF, Henderson WB, Hurtgen PJ, Jin ZQ, McCauley AD, Mower SA, et al. Production, freezing and transfer of bovine IVF embryos and subsequent calving results. Theriogenology 1995;43:141–152.

64. Heuwieser W, Yang X, Jiang S, Foote RH. Fertilization of bovine oocytes after microsurgical injection of spermatozoa. Theriogenology 1992;38:1–9.
65. Heuwieser W, Yang X, Jiang S, Foote R.H. A comparison between in vitro fertilization and microinjection of immobilized spermatozoa from bulls producing spermatozoa with defects. Mol Reprod Dev 1992;33:489–491.
66. Kovács A, Vallagomez DAF, Gustavsson I, Lindblad K, Foote RH, Howard TH. Synaptonemal complex analysis of a three-breakpoint translocation in a subfertile bull. Cytogenet Cell Genet 1992;61:195–201.
67. Ehrenwald E, Parks JE, Foote RH. Cholesterol efflux from bovine sperm: II. Effect of reducing sperm cholesterol on penetration of zona-free hamster and in vitro matured bovine ova. Gamete Res 1988;20:413–420.
68. Parrish JJ, Susko-Parrish JL, Winer MA, First NL. Capacitation of bovine sperm by heparin. Biol Reprod 1988;38:1171–1180.
69. Vishwanath R, Nebel RL, McMillan WH, Pitt CJ, MacMillan KL. Selected times of insemination with microencapsulated bovine spermatozoa affect pregnancy rate of synchronized heifers. Theriogenology 1997;48:369–376.
70. Phillips PH, Lardy HA. A yolk-buffer pabulum for the preservation of bull semen. J Dairy Sci 1940;23:399–404.
71. Salisbury GW, Fuller HK, Willett EL. Preservation of bovine spermatozoa in yolk- citrate diluent and field results from its use. J Dairy Sci 1941;24: 905–910.
72. O'Dell WT, Almquist JO. Freezing bovine semen. I. Techniques for freezing bovine spermatozoa in milk diluents. J Dairy Sci 1957;40:1534–1541.
73. Foote RH, Bratton RW. The fertility of bovine semen cooled with and without the addition of citrate-sulfanilamide-yolk extender. J Dairy Sci 1949;32:856–861.
74. Almquist JO, Glantz PJ, Shaffer HE. The effect of a combination of penicillin and streptomycin upon the livability and bacterial content of bovine semen. J Dairy Sci 1949;32:183–190.
75. Foote RH, Bratton RW. The fertility of bovine semen in extenders containing sulfanilamide, penicillin, streptomycin, and polymyxin. J Dairy Sci 1950;33:544–547.
76. Davis IS, Bratton RW, Foote RH. Livability of bovine spermatozoa at 5, −25, and −85°C in Tris-buffered and citrate-buffered yolk-glycerol extenders. J Dairy Sci 1963;46:333–336.
77. Aitken RJ, Clarkson JS. Significance of reactive oxygen species and antioxidants in defining the efficacy of sperm preparation techniques. J Androl 1988;9:367–376.
78. lvarez JG, Touchston JC, Blasco L, Storey BT. Spontaneous lipid peroxidation and production of hydrogen peroxide and superoxide in human spermatozoa: superoxide dismutase as major enzyme protectant against oxygen toxicity. J Androl 1987;8:338–348.
79. Paufler SK, Foote RH. Influence of light on nuclear size and deoxyribonucleic acid content of stored bovine spermatozoa. J Dairy Sci 1967;50:1475–1480.
80. David G, Price WS, eds. Human Artificial Insemination and Semen Preservation. Plenum, New York, NY, 1980.
81. Iizuka R. Artificial insemination: Progress and clinical application. In: Seppälä, M, Hamburger L, eds. Frontiers in Human Reproduction. Annals New York Acad Sci 1991;626:399–413.
82. Polge C, Smith AU, Parkes AS. Revival of spermatozoa after vitrification and dehydration at low temperatures. Nature 1949;164:666.
83. Graham EF. Fundamentals of the preservation of spermatozoa. In: Rinfret AP, Petricciani JC, eds. The Integrity of Frozen Spermatozoa. Proc Conf Natl Acad Sci, Washington, DC, 1978, pp. 4–44.
84. Liu Z, Foote RH. Osmotic effects on volume and motility of bull sperm exposed to membrane permeable and nonpermeable agents. Cryobiology 1998;37:207–218.
85. Liu Z, Foote RH, Brockett CC. Survival of bull sperm frozen at different rates in media varying in osmolarity. Cryobiology 1998;37:219–230.
86. Shannon P, Vishwanath R. The effect of optimal and suboptimal concentrations of sperm on the fertility of fresh and frozen bovine semen and a theoretical model to explain the fertility differences. Anim Reprod Sci 1995;39:1–10.
87. Cassou R. Instruments used in the techniques for artificial insemination of domestic animals. 10th Intl Congr Anim Reprod Artificial Insem, Congress, Urbana, IL, 1984;3:361–363.
88. Foote RH, Kaproth MT. Sperm numbers inseminated in dairy cattle and nonreturn rates revisited. J Dairy Sci 1997;80:3072–3076.
89. Everett RW, Bean B. Semen fertility: an evaluation system for artificial insemination sires, technicians, herds and systematic fixed effects. J Dairy Sci 1986;69:1630–1641.

90. Grossman M, Koops WJ, Den Daas JHG. Multiphasic analysis of reproductive efficiency of dairy bulls. J Dairy Sci 1996;78:2871–2876.

91. Iritani A. Problems of freezing spermatozoa of different species. 9th Intl Congr Anim Reprod Artificial Insem, Madrid, Congress 1980, pp. 115–131.

92. Amoah EA, Gelaye S. Biotechnological advances in goat reproduction. J Anim Sci 1997;75:578–585.

93. Evans G, Maxwell WMC. Salamon's Artificial Insemination of Sheep and Goats. Butterworths, Sydney, Australia, 1987.

94. Boucher JH, Foote RH, Kirk RW. The evaluation of semen quality in the dog and the effects of frequency of ejaculation upon semen quality, libido and depletion of sperm reserves. Cornell Vet 1958;48:67–86.

95. Farstad W. Semen cryopreservation in dogs and foxes. Anim Reprod Sci 1996;42:251–260.

96. Wildt DE, Pukazhenthi BS, Brown JL, Monfort S, Howard JG, Roth TL. Spermatology for understanding, managing and conserving rare species. Reprod Fertil Dev 1995;7:11–824.

97. Barbato GF, Cramer PG, Hammerstedt RH. A practical in vitro sperm-egg binding assay that detects subfertile males. Biol Reprod 1998;58:686–699.

98. Foote RH, Berndtson WE. The germinal cells. In: Scialli AR, Clegg ED, eds. Reversibility in Testicular Toxicity Assessmen. CRC Press, Boca Raton, FL, 1992, pp. 1–55.

99. Hawk HW, Conley HH, Wall RJ, Whitaker RO. Fertilization rates in superovulating cows after deposition of semen on the infundibulum, near the uterotubal junction or after insemination with high numbers of sperm. Theriogenology 1988;61:1131–1142.

100. Watson PF. Recent developments and concepts in the cryopreservation of spermatozoa and the assessment of their post-thawing function. Reprod Fertil Dev 1995;7:871–891.

101. Songsasen N, Leibo SP. Cryopreservation of mouse spermatozoa. 1. Effect of seeding on fertilizing ability of cryopreserved spermatozoa. Cryobiology 1997;35:240–254.

102. Wakayama T, Yanagimachi R. Development of normal mice from oocytes injected with freeze-dried spermatozoa. Nature Biotech 1998;16:634–641.

103. Amann RP, Seidel GE Jr, eds. Prospects for Sexing Mammalian Sperm. Colorado Associated University Press, Boulder, CO, 1982.

104. Cran G, Johnson LA, Miller NGA, Cochrane D, Polge C. Production of bovine calves following separation of X- and Y-chromosome bearing sperm and in vitro fertilization. Vet Rec 1993;132:40–41.

105. Gledhill BL. Cytometry of mammalian sperm. Gamete Res 1985;12:423–438.

106. Johnson LA. Gender preselection in domestic animals using flow cytometrically sorted sperm. J Anim Sci 1992;70(Suppl 2):8–18.

107. Seidel GE Jr, Allen CH, Johnson LA, Holland MD, Brink Z, Welch GR, et al. Uterine horn insemination of heifers with very low numbers of nonfrozen and sexed spermatozoa. Theriogenology 1997; 48:1255–1264.

108. Fugger EF, Black SH, Keyvanfar K, Schulman JD. Birth of normal daughters after MicroSort sperm separation and intrauterine insemination, in-vitro fertilization, or intracytoplasmic sperm injection. Hum Reprod 1998;13:2367–2370.

109. Maione B, Lavitrano M, Spadafora C, Kiessling AA. Sperm-mediated gene transfer in mice. Mol Reprod Dev 1998;50:406–409.

110. Sperandio S, Lulli V, Bacci ML, Forni M, Maione B, Spadafoa C, Lavitrano M. Sperm-mediated DNA transfer in bovine and swine species. Ann Biotech 1996;71:59–77.

111. Dransfield MBG, Nebel RL, Pearson RE, Warnick LD. Timing of insemination for dairy cows identified in estrus by a radiotelemetric estrus detection system. J Dairy Sci 1998;81:1874–1882.

112. Foote RH. Estrus detection and estrus detection aids. J Dairy Sci 1975;58: 248–256.

113. Trimberger GW. Breeding efficiency in dairy cattle from artificial insemination at various intervals before and after ovulation. Nebraska Agric Expt Sta Bull 153, 26. Lincoln, NE, 1948.

114. Hansel W, Convey EM. Physiology of the estrous cycle. J Anim Sci 1983;57(Suppl 2):404–424.

115. Pursley JR, Kosorok MR, Wiltbank MC. Reproductive management of lactating dairy cows using synchronization of estrus. J Dairy Sci 1997;80:301–306.

116. Elsden RP, Nelson LD, Seidel GE Jr. Superovulating cows with follicle stimulating hormone and pregnant mare's serum gonadotropin. Theriogenology 1978;9:17–26.

117. Rowson LEA. Methods of inducing multiple ovulations in cattle. J Endocrinol 1951;7:260–270.

118. Brackett BG, Seidel GE Jr, Seidel SM, eds. New Technologies in Animal Breeding. Academic, New York, NY, 1981.

119. Foote RH, Onuma H. Superovulation, ovum collection, culture and transfer. A review. J Dairy Sci 1971;53:1681–1692.

120. Hasler JF, McCauley AD, Lathrop WF, Foote RH. Effect of donor-embryo- recipient interactions on pregnancy rate in a large-scale bovine embryo transfer program. Theriogenology 1987;27:139–168.
121. Seidel GE Jr. Superovulation and embryo transfer in cattle. Science 1981;211:351–358.
122. Bavister BD. Culture of preimplantation embryos: facts and artifacts. Hum Reprod Update 1995;1: 91–48.
123. Suzuki H, Foote RH. Bovine oviductal epithelial cells (BOEC) and oviducts: I. For embryo culture. II. Using SEM for studying interactions with spermatozoa. Microscopy Res Tech 1995;31:519–530.
124. Kennelly JJ, Foote RH. Superovulatory response of pre- and post-pubertal rabbits to commercially available gonadotrophins. J Reprod Fert 1965;9:177–188.
125. Hasler JF. Current status and potential of embryo transfer and reproductive technology in dairy cattle. J Dairy Sci 1992;75:2857–2879.
126. Whittingham DG, Leibo SP, Mazur P. Survival of mouse embryos frozen to −196°C and −269°C. Science 1972;178:411–414.
127. Anderson GB. Identification of embryonic sex by detection of H-Y antigen. Theriogenology 1987;27: 81–98.
128. Kobayashi J, Sekimoto A, Uchida H, Wada T, Sasaki K, Sasada H, Umezu M, Sato E. Rapid detection of male-specific DNA sequence in bovine embryos using fluorescence in situ hybridization. Mol Reprod Dev 1998;51:390–394.
129. Williams TJ, Elsden RP, Seidel GE Jr. Pregnancy rates with bisected bovine embryos. Theriogenology 1984;22:521–531.
130. Onuma H, Foote RH. In vitro development of ova from prepuberal cattle. J Dairy Sci 1969;52:1085–1087.
131. Tervit HR. Laparoscopy/laparotomy oocyte recovery and juvenile breeding. Anim Reprod Sci 1996;42: 227–238.
132. Dekkers JCM, Shook GE. Genetic and economic evaluation of nucleus breeding schemes for commercial artificial insemination firms. J Dairy Sci 1990;73:1920–1937.
133. Foote RH, Henderson CR, Bratton RW. Testing bulls in artificial insemination centres for lethals, type and production. Proc 3rd Intern Congr Anim Reprod 1956;3:49–53.
134. Henderson CR. Selecting and sampling young sires. Proc. 7th Ann. Conf., Columbia, MO. Natl. Assoc. Artificial Breeders, 1954, pp. 93–103.
135. Lohuis MM. Potential benefits of bovine embryo-manipulation technologies to genetic improvement programmes. Theriogenology 1995;43:51–60.
136. Nicholas FN. Genetic improvement through reproductive technology. Anim Reprod Sci 1996;42:205–214.
137. Robertson A, Rendel JM. The use of progeny testing with artificial insemination in dairy cattle. J Genet 1950;50:21–31.
138. Van Vleck LD. Potential genetic impact of artificial insemination, sex selection, embryo transfer, cloning and selfing in dairy cattle. In: Brackett BC, Seidel GE Jr, Seidel SM, eds. New Technologies in Animal Breeding. Academic, New York, NY, 1981.
139. Yang X, Anderson GB. Manipulation of mammalian embryos: principle, progress and future possibilities. Theriogenology 1992;38:315–335.
140. Loskutoff NM, Bartels P, Meintjes M, Godke RA, Schiewe MC. Assisted reproductive technology in non-domestic ungulates: a model approach to preserving and managing genetic diversity. Theriogenology 1995;43:3–12.
141. Wildt E. Genetic resource banks for conserving wildlife species: justification, examples and becoming organized on a global basis. Anim Reprod Sci 1992;28:247–257.
142. Li J, Rieke A, Day BN, Prather RS. Technical note: porcine non-surgical embryo transfer. J Anim Sci 1996;74:2263–2268.
143. Kidder JD. Development of nonsurgical reproductive biotechnologies in domestic ferret and rabbit models and characterization of cell allocation to the preimplantation blastocyst of the domestic ferret. Ph.D. Dissertation, Cornell University, Ithaca, NY, 1998.
144. Kidder JD, Foote RH, Richmond ME. Transcervical artificial insemination in the domestic ferret (Mustela putorius furo). Zool Biol 1998;17:393–404.
145. Prather RS, Barnes FL, Sims MM, Robl JM, First NL. Nuclear transplantation in the bovine embryo: assessment of donor nuclei and recipient oocyte. Biol Reprod 1987;37:859–866.
146. Pursel VG, Pinkert CA, Miller KF, Boldt RL, Hammer RE. Genetic engineering of livestock. Science 1989;244:1281–1288.

147. Robl JM, Prather R, Barnes F, Eyestone W, Northey D, Gilligan B, First NL. Nuclear transplantation in bovine embryos. J Anim Sci 1987;64Z:642–647.

148. Stice SL, Robl JM, Ponce de Leon FA, Jerry J, Golaeke PG, Cibelli JB, Kane JJ. Cloning: new breakthroughs leading to commercial opportunities. Theriogenology 1998;49:129–138.

149. Wall RJ, Kerr DE, Bondioli KR. Transgenic dairy cattle: genetic engineering on a large scale. J Dairy Sci 1997;80:2213–2224.

150. Willadsen SM. Nuclear transplantation in sheep embryos. Nature (London) 1986;320:63–65.

151. Wilmut I, Schnieke AE, McWhir J, Kind AJ, Campbell KHS. Viable offspring derived from fetal and adult mammalian cells. Nature 1997;385:810–813.

152. Hammer RE, Pursel V, Rexroad CE Jr, Wall RJ, Boldt DJ, Ebert KM, et al. Production of transgenic rabbits, sheep and pigs by microinjection. Nature 1985;315:680–683.

153. Foote RH, Yang X. Cloning of bovine embryos. Reprod Dom Anim 1992;27:13–21.

154. Heyman Y, Renard JP. Cloning of domestic species. Anim Reprod Sci 1996;42:427–436.

155. Colman A. Somatic cell nuclear transfer in mammals: progress and applications. Cloning 2000;1: 185–200.

156. Foote RH. Development of reproductive biotechnologies in domestic animals from artificial insemination to cloning: a perspective. Cloning 1999;1:133–142.

157. Kubota C, Yamakuchi H, Todoroki J, et al. Six cloned calves produced from adult fibroblast cells after long-term culture. PNAS 2000;97:990–995.

158. Lanza RP, Cibelli J, Blackwell C, et al. Extension of cell life-span and telomere length in animals cloned from senescent somatic cells. Science 2000;288:665–669.

2

Advances in Animal
In Vitro Fertilization

Benjamin G. Brackett, DVM, PHD

CONTENTS

INTRODUCTION

Much progress of relevance to the union of mammalian gametes in laboratory conditions has been reported during the last half century. Early in this interval, it was realized that spermatozoa must undergo the process of capacitation and that conditions for gamete union must, at least crudely, resemble those found at the normal site of fertilization, i.e., within the oviduct. Today it is possible to initiate early embryonic development of just about any mammalian species by co-incubating homologous ova with treated spermatozoa. This review will trace the development of in vitro fertilization (IVF) technology through experimentation with several laboratory and domestic animals. Information regarding nonhuman primates appears in Chapter 16. A few of hundreds of possible examples from available literature reports will be mentioned to illustrate advances in this important area of biological science. Utilization of IVF for enhancing reproductive efficiency, especially for cattle, and in preservation of genetically valuable and endangered animal species promises to impact significantly on animal breeding strategies.

EARLY IVF IN LABORATORY ANIMALS

Rabbit

Independent reports in 1951 by Austin involving rats and rabbits *(1)* and by Chang in rabbits *(2)* described a need for sperm cells to undergo a physiological change—termed sperm capacitation *(3)*—in the female reproductive tract prior to penetrating an ovum.

From: *Contemporary Endocrinology: Assisted Fertilization and Nuclear Transfer in Mammals*
Edited by: D. P. Wolf and M. Zelinski-Wooten © Humana Press Inc., Totowa, NJ

Three years later, Thibault et al. *(4)* reported that sperm capacitation was an essential prerequisite to fertilization of rabbit ova in vitro. Whether sperm cells were inadvertently capacitated to achieve authentic fertilization in vitro as suggested by a dozen or so earlier descriptive accounts involving rabbit, guinea pig, mouse, and rat gametes seems doubtful (for review, *see* ref. *5*), with the possible exception of reports of Moricard and Bossu *(6)* and Smith *(7)*. Independently, these authors found pieces of oviduct to be beneficial to sperm penetration through the rabbit zona pellucida in vitro.

Indisputable criteria for achievement of rabbit IVF including birth of live young were reported in 1959 by M.C. Chang *(8)*. This work, a first in mammals, involved exposure of recently ovulated ova to sperm taken from uteri of mated does, and later, transfer of cleaved ova to oviducts of hormonally synchronous recipient does that delivered live offspring. Similarly, birth of live offspring was achieved following transfer of rabbit embryos derived from IVF in several additional reports in the ensuing decade *(9–11)*, and by 1970, IVF was documented by microcinematography *(12)*. In addition to tubal ova, soon it was possible to fertilize ova recovered from the ovarian surface just after ovulation *(13)* and taken from ovarian follicles just prior to ovulation *(14,15)*.

It was recognized early in serious efforts to achieve IVF that best results followed rapid handling of gametes at near body temperature prior to insemination. Paraffin or silicone oil covering of media and high relative humidity assisted in maintaining constant temperature by preventing evaporation. An oxygen tension of 8% to resemble that measured within the oviduct *(16,17)* and 5% CO_2 to maintain proper pH of a bicarbonate-containing medium were found compatible with IVF *(18)*. Thus, a simple defined medium consisting of a salt solution with crystalline bovine albumin, glucose, and bicarbonate to maintain a pH of 7.8 to resemble estrous oviductal fluid *(19)* at 38°C (rabbit body temperature) was found to consistently support sperm penetration of rabbit ova *(18)*. This, in turn, allowed conduct of controlled experiments to test various influences on the mammalian fertilization process *(5)*. Early work in the rabbit provided a background for facilitating extension of IVF technology to other mammalian species (e.g., cat, cow, goat, hamster, human, mouse, and so on). This work involved assessment of factors for their influence on proportions of ova that could be fertilized and other efforts to capacitate rabbit spermatozoa in vitro. Cleavage of resulting zygotes was consistently obtained following transfer into a serum-containing medium with a more neutral pH. From embryo culture experiments involving in vivo-derived zygotes and 2-cell embryos, it soon became clear that pyruvate was an important substrate for support of initial cleavage development *(20–22)*. The need for transfer of inseminated ova into another medium could be eliminated by addition of 10^{-5} M pyruvate to the defined medium, which already contained adequate concentrations of glucose and albumin to support later cleavage stages of preimplantation rabbit embryos *(23,24)*. This medium developed for rabbit IVF has been variously referred to as Defined Medium (DM) *(24)*, Brackett's medium *(25)*, and Brackett-Olphant (BO) medium *(26)*.

IVF provided an improvement over in vivo testing for sperm fertilizing ability. A clearer understanding of in vivo and in vitro influences on sperm could now be determined. In rabbits with surgically removed oviducts, spermatozoa were capacitated in uteri as demonstrated by fertilization of approx 90% of recently ovulated ova recovered from ovarian surfaces *(27)*. Optimal IVF results (90.6% fertilization) could also be duplicated after sperm capacitation for 17 h in uteri of hormonally treated does that had been ovariectomized and salpingectomized a month before. Hormonal treatments consisted of intramuscular injections of an estradiol preparation for 6 d with a single progestin treatment at the time of mating *(28)*. Larger doses of progestin (than used in these experiments) inhibit capacitation of sperm in the uterus *(29)*. That uterine fluids produced under appropriate hormonal influences could effect capacitation was further demonstrated by IVF after sperm treatments with uterine fluid recovered from intact gonadotropin-treated does near the time of ovulation *(30)*. Rabbit epididymal sperm are more easily capacitated than are ejaculated sperm cells that have been exposed to additional male accessory gland secretions *(31,32)*. An important component of the capacitation of ejaculated sperm was shown by an immunological approach to involve removal or alteration of sperm surface proteins concurrent with increasing intervals of residence in the female reproductive tract *(33)*. It was further demonstrated that a seminal plasma glycoprotein with a molecular weight of approx 115,000 could be used to reversibly decapacitate uterine capacitated sperm *(34)*.

In other experiments, IVF was employed to assess acquisition of sperm fertilizing ability after membrane-altering sperm treatments, e.g., with lysolecithin *(30)*, or Sendai virus *(35)*. Following earlier leads, efforts to remove or alter sperm surface antigens (e.g., removal of decapacitation factor) involved incubation in DM prepared with additional NaCl, i.e., high ionic strength (HIS) medium (380 mOsm/kg). This led, by 1975, to achievement of in vitro capacitation combined with IVF and embryo transfer to obtain offspring, a mammalian first for ejaculated spermatozoa *(24)*. Variability in performance of spermatozoa from different bucks was recognized along with retardation in development of fertilization and early cleavage stages. The latter suggested delayed sperm penetration of ova. Various facets of this work were soon repeated in other laboratories *(36–38)*. Improvement in proportions of ova fertilized and in more normal temporal development followed application of this approach for IVF with cauda epididymal spermatozoa *(32)*. With additional incubation of HIS- or DM-treated epididymal spermatozoa prior to in vitro insemination, sperm penetration was almost complete by 3.25 h after insemination *(38)*, temporally comparable to in vitro penetration by spermatozoa capacitated in vivo *(12)*. Contemporaneous reports from several laboratories pointed out that ejaculated rabbit spermatozoa capacitated in vitro were not entirely equivalent to in vivo capacitated spermatozoa in fertilizing ability *(39–41)*. However, with 12–22 h of preincubation after HIS treatment, in vitro capacitated (ejaculated) spermatozoa rapidly penetrated ova and initiated development that was temporally comparable to that following in vitro insemination with in vivo capacitated uterine spermatozoa *(42)*. The desirabililty of removing inseminated ova from spermatozoa as quickly as possible *(27)* was confirmed. By transferring oocytes into fresh DM 6 h after insemination, fertilization results improved from 44% (17 of 39 oocytes) to 85% (40 of 47 oocytes) and development to the 4-cell stage improved from 35% (6 of 17) to 78% (31 of 40). In these experiments averages of 57% total and 29% progressive motility scores were noted for spermatozoa at insemination. Evidence from IVF and in vivo fertilization in test does documented an approximation of in vitro capacitation and IVF with the normal in vivo processes when the ejaculated spermatozoa were incubated for additional intervals after HIS treatment *(42)*. In this work, 43 of 52 embryos (83%) resulting from IVF of follicular, surface, and tubal oocytes, collectively, reached morula or blastocyst stages *(42)* following culture for 78–142 h post-insemination in serum-supplemented Ham's F-10 *(43)*. The proportion of 4-cell stage embryos (resulting from fertilization with in vitro capacitated spermatozoa) that developed into normal offspring was comparable to embryo transfer results after IVF with in vivo capacitated spermatozoa in previous work *(15)*. Despite functional results, there is no assurance that mechanisms of such in vitro treatments duplicate those that normally occur in vivo.

Hamster

In 1963 and 1964, Yanagimachi and Chang *(44,45)* reported initial success in fertilizing rodent ova in vitro along with in vitro capacitation of hamster epididymal sperm. Hamster sperm heads and male pronuclei with tails of fertilizing spermatozoa were found within ooplasm after incubation of ova with epididymal sperm in Tyrode's solution under paraffin oil. Spermatozoa recovered from the uterus of females mated 4–5 h before fertilized 134 (64.7%) of 207 ova, uterine sperm recovered 0.5 h after mating fertilized 52 of 100 ova, and epididymal sperm fertilized 80 (44.4%) of 180 ova. Although more rapid penetration of ova correlated with uterine exposure of sperm recovered after mating their experiments with epididymal sperm marked initial success with in vitro capacitation and IVF in a single system. Yanagimachi *(46)* described microscopic observation of sperm penetration to include absence of the outer acrosome membrane before the spermatozoon began penetrating the zona pellucida. Penetration was at an angle to the zona surface and required 3–4 min. Then, in less than 2 s, the sperm head lay flat on the oolemma and, without further motility, the spermatozoon sank into the vitellus.

Barros and Austin *(47,48)* found a higher incidence of polyspermy after insemination (with epididymal spermatozoa) of follicular oocytes recovered just before ovulation than for tubal ova. Both follicular fluid and tubal fluid supported the hamster sperm acrosome reaction in vitro *(47)*. Follicular contents recovered 9–10 h after human chorionic gonadotropin (hCG) injection induced the acrosome reaction in 97% of epididymal spermatozoa, whereas follicular contents recovered 4 h after hCG induced the acrosome reaction in only 43% of epididymal spermatozoa, suggesting accumulation of an active agent in the follicle in the preovulatory phase. After epididymal sperm incubation for 3 h with Tyrode's supplemented with follicular fluid sperm penetration of ova usually occurred 30–50 min after insemination *(49)*. Capacitation took place most efficiently with hamster follicular fluid present, but mouse follicular fluid was found to be better in this regard than rat follicular fluid, whereas rabbit follicular fluid was totally ineffective *(49)*. Bovine follicular fluids also induced the hamster acrosome reaction *(50)*. Two fractions of this fluid were implicated in capacitation *(50)*, a dialyzable and heat stable (at 90°C) fraction with sperm-activating properties, and a nondialyzable and heat labile (at 90°C) fraction responsible for induction of the acrosome reaction. Similar activities were found in bovine serum. The large molecular weight fraction was identified as albumin *(51)*. Data on electrophoretic components of hamster uterine fluid indicated an increase in albumin at the appropriate time for a physiological role in preparing spermatozoa for fertilization *(52)*. Meizel et al. *(53)* recognized important influences of taurine and hypotaurine found in sperm and reproductive tract fluids on hamster sperm motility, capacitation, and the acrosome reaction in vitro.

Although 75% or more of inseminated ova could be fertilized routinely development beyond the 2-cell stage was not possible *(54)*. Development of "hamster embryo culture medium" (HECM), a modified Tyrode's solution with polyvinylalcohol (PVA), present to replace previously used protein supplements (e.g., bovine serum albumin [BSA]), and an atmosphere of 10% CO_2, 10% O_2, and 37.5°C supported development of in vivo-fertilized embryos to blastocysts *(55–57)*. Deletion of glucose, phosphate, and pyruvate, reduction of lactate; and addition of glutamine *(57,58)* were important changes. Almost 30 years after the first successful IVF in golden hamsters, Barnett and Bavister *(59)* reported that IVF hamster embryos could develop in chemically defined, protein-free culture medium (HECM-3 with hypotaurine added) into morulae and blastocysts, and produce normal offspring after transfer to recipients. Inclusion of hypotaurine was essential for in vitro support of development to at least the 8-cell stage. Twenty offspring represented successful term development of 5% of the 2-cell embryos transferred into oviducts and 17% of the 8-cell embryos transferred into uteri of recipients. In contrast to chemically defined zygote culture conditions, sperm preparation and IVF were in BSA-supplemented medium *(54)*. Capacitation of cauda epididymal spermatozoa involved a 3.0–3.5-h incubation in HECM-3 with 3 mg/mL BSA, 5 mM glucose and phenylephrine, hypotaurine, and epinephrine (PHE) sperm-motility factors. The IVF medium also contained PHE and lowered concentrations of glucose (0.5 mM) and BSA (0.3 mg/mL).

Mouse

In 1968, Whittingham reported in vitro development of 65 of 159 ova (40.9%) to the 2-cell stage by 24 h after in vitro insemination with spermatozoa recovered from the uterus 1–2 h post-coitus *(60)*. Proof of fertilization included development of some in vitro-fertilized ova to 17-d-old fetuses following embryo transfer. The medium employed was a slight modification of that developed by Whitten and Biggers *(61)* to culture mouse zygotes to the blastocyst stage. Thus, progress by 1968 promised an opportunity to obtain all stages of preimplantational development in simple defined conditions.

In 1970, Cross and Brinster *(62)* reported development of 15-d-old fetuses from 3/95 mouse embryos that resulted from in vitro oocyte maturation and IVF. In their experiments, immature follicular oocytes were obtained from donors treated with pregnant mare serum gonadotropin (PMSG now referred to as equine CG) 48 h previously and inseminated with spermatozoa recovered from the uterus after mating.

A need for mouse epididymal spermatozoa to undergo capacitation was evidenced by Iwamatsu and Chang *(63)*. In Tyrode's solution supplemented with heat-treated bovine follicular fluid, the proportion of ova penetrated by fresh epididymal sperm increased from 2% at 1 h to 79% at 8 h of insemination. By contrast, epididymal sperm pretreated by incubation for 3-4 h in the same medium penetrated 17% of ova by 20 min, and 90% by 2 h after in vitro insemination *(63)*. Using a modified Krebs-Ringer bicarbonate solution containing glucose, sodium pyruvate, bovine albumin, and antibiotics Toyoda et al. *(64)* demonstrated epididymal sperm penetration to begin about 1 h (22.8% of ova penetrated) and to be completed within 2 h (96.4% penetrated) after insemination of ova. When a 2-h sperm incubation preceded insemination of ova, more than half of the ova were penetrated within 30 min, and all ova were penetrated by 1 h after insemination. Also, the mean number of penetrating sperm cells per penetrated ovum was higher (3.1) after preincubation than that (1.6) after use of fresh epididymal spermatozoa. Use of epididymal spermatozoa after increasing intervals of preincubation from 3–7 min up to 120 min resulted in increasing proportions of ova that underwent sperm penetration and early development of the fertilization process (i.e., at telophase of the second maturation division with enlarged sperm heads in the vitellus) at 1 h after insemination. Thus, capacitation of mouse epididymal spermatozoa was shown to be a progressive change that could be completed within an hour in a defined medium without factors uniquely supplied by the female reproductive tract *(64,65)*.

Miyamoto and Chang *(66)* added lactate to this medium for epididymal sperm capacitation and, following transfer to recipient female mice, demonstrated comparable fetal development of 2-cell mouse ova after IVF (13%) as that after fertilization in vivo (16%). In the same year, 1972, Mukherjee reported fertile progeny from transfer of blastocysts resulting from IVF of in vitro matured oocytes *(67)*. In these experiments epididymal spermatozoa were capacitated by in vitro incubation for 4 h at 37°C with heat-inactivated (56°C for 30 min) human follicular and tubal fluid (1:2).

A maximum rate of sperm capacitation occurred by addition of 200 mM NaCl to the medium used by Toyoda et al. *(64,65)* and the mechanism involved removal of a decapacitation factor *(68)*. The protein fraction eluted from previously washed epididymal sperm effected by treatment with the HIS medium decapacitated salt-capacitated sperm, and this decapacitation could be reversed by an additional incubation in the high-salt capacitating medium. Additional advances, as those reported by Hoppe and Pitts *(69)* and Fraser and Drury *(70)*, contributed to routine procedures, making mouse IVF a most useful research tool *(71)*.

Rat

Miyamoto and Chang *(72)* determined the need for rat sperm capacitation with best IVF results obtained by using spermatozoa recovered from the uterus 10–11 h after mating. Naturally ovulated ova (45%) were more readily fertilized than were superovulated (22%). In 1974, Toyoda and Chang obtained live young after transfer of 2-cell embryos that developed after direct in vitro insemination with epididymal spermatozoa *(73)*. The IVF medium consisted of modified Krebs-Ringer bicarbonate solution supplemented with glucose, sodium pyruvate, sodium lactate, BSA, and antibiotics. The time required for sperm penetration was shortened by sperm preincubation for 5–6 h and inclusion of a high potassium to sodium ratio (0.32) and 2 mM db-cAMP for IVF *(73)*. Under these conditions, 90% of rat ova were penetrated within 3 h after in vitro insemination.

Guinea Pig

Yanagimachi *(74)* found the medium developed for culture of early mouse embryos by Biggers, Whitten, and Whittingham (BWW medium) *(75)* to be adequate for guinea pig IVF. The time required for sperm penetration of ova was shortened from 3–4 h to 1 h after incubating fresh epididymal spermatozoa in the culture medium for 12–18 h before in vitro insemination. A close correlation between the sperm acrosome reaction and the ability to fertilize, and the necessity for calcium ions for initiation of a physiologic acrosome reaction and consequently for successful fertilization, were also reported *(74)*.

Heterologous IVF Experimentation

In 1972, Yanagimachi *(76)* showed that in vitro capacitated guinea pig epididymal spermatozoa could penetrate hamster ova freed from their zonae pellucidae, although penetration through the zona was not possible. In the same year, Hanada and Chang *(77)* reported that rat and mouse spermatozoa were also capable of penetrating zona-free hamster ova. The zona-free hamster ovum model was advocated for evaluation of capacitation, acrosome reaction, and male pronuclear development in species whose ova are difficult to directly study for any reason, e.g., human *(78,79)*, and pig *(80)*.

Slavik et al. *(81)* reported observations on developmental ability of hybrid zygotes resulting from IVF of in vitro-matured bovine ova with ram sperm. Fertilization was successful in 83% of bovine oocytes inseminated with bull sperm (control) compared with 67% of bovine oocytes inseminated with ram sperm (hybrid embryos). In both cases, two normal pronuclei were seen and comparable development of hybrid and control embryos to the 8-cell stage resulted after transfer of 2-cell embryos to ewe oviducts. Inability of nuclei of hybrid embryos to make the maternal to embryonic genomic transition was indicated by remarkably lowered values in frequency and intensity of tritiated uridine incorporation associated with onset of RNA synthesis. The morphological observations were consistent with delay or inefficient reactivation of the embryonic genome in the hybrid embryos *(81)*.

CONTEMPORARY MOUSE IVF

The importance of laboratory mice, including transgenic and "knock-out" strains, in modern medical research has provided impetus to further development of IVF and related technologies for their efficient use. Improved culture systems for mouse embryo development *(82–85)* now provide new opportunities in murine reproduction. Much current interest surrounds cytoplasmic and nuclear transfers, new technologies that can build on advances achieved through ongoing efforts to develop IVF technology. With the advent of cloning by somatic cell nuclear transfer, *(see* Chapters 13–17) it may no longer be necessary to pursue the goal of using sperm cells as vectors for introducing foreign DNA into ova *(86)*. Incubating mouse epididymal spermatozoa with the nuclease inhibitor, aurintricarboxylic acid (ATA), enabled an increase in the yield of 2-cell IVF embryos *(87)*. Experimental results suggested the ATA acts by preserving sperm nuclei from induced or spontaneously occurring damage and/or by promoting events, apart from improved ability of sperm cells to penetrate, that trigger early embryogenesis *(87)*.

Contemporary mouse IVF with emphasis on the male gamete promises new avenues for research and for practical applications. Sasagawa et al. *(88)* demonstrated that round spermatids can fertilize following intracytoplasmic injection and artificial oocyte activation as by electrostimulation and oscillogen injection. Nuclei of primary spermatocytes have been injected into oocytes and found to undergo meiosis, form an embryo, and produce live young. It was suggested that this approach may become available as a treatment for patients with azoospermia due to maturation arrest (*88; see* Chapter 7). Mouse spermatozoa obtained from the epididymis from a dead animal as long as 24 h after death can be used to fertilize oocytes and the resulting zygotes can develop into live young *(89)*. The importance of more efficiently preserving valuable transgenic mouse lines has led to research emphasis on cryopreservation of sperm *(90–93)* and ova *(94)* that can later be used for embryo production via IVF. Live mice have resulted from cryopreserved embryos derived in vitro using cryopreserved ejaculated spermatozoa recovered from mated mice *(95)*. Normal offspring have resulted from mouse ova injected with spermatozoa cryopreserved with or without cryoprotection *(96)*.

Strain differences have proven to be crucial components in mouse IVF and superovulatory protocols *(97)*. Three strains commonly used in genetic engineering (ICR outbred, C57BL/6 inbred, and B6SJ1F1 hybrid) were superovulated by four different timing regimens before insemination, with spermatozoa from males of the same strain. There was a significant strain influence on IVF rate. Groups according to timing regimen, i.e., hours between PMSG (eCG) and hCG, and hours between hCG and oocyte collection, affected the proportion of fertilized ova obtained and the effect of these groups varied across mouse strain. Therefore, the treatment that produced the highest fertilization rate was related to and contingent upon the mouse strain. This work demonstrated that responses to standardized IVF protocols vary significantly; the efficiency of IVF procedures can be optimized within specific mouse strains by the timing of superovulatory regimens; absence of cumulus cells during IVF in this work did not adversely affect fertilization rate *(97)*.

Visconti et al. *(98)* reported that it is now possible to replace BSA with synthetic cyclodextrins in media to support signal transduction leading to sperm capacitation. Data presented further support the coupling of cholesterol efflux to the activation of membrane and transmembrane signaling events leading to the activation of a unique signaling pathway involving cross-talk between cAMP and tyrosine kinase second messenger systems; this defines a new mode of cellular signal transduction initiated by cholesterol release *(98)*.

Adham et al. *(99)* reported interesting experiments with mice carrying a mutation at the acrosin locus (Acr) generated through targeted disruption in embryonic stem cells and transmitted through germ lines of chimeric male and female mice. The homozygous Acr mutant males were fertile and yielded litters comparable in number and size to Acr+/+ mice. Incubation of ova with equally mixed sperm cells of Acr+/+ and Acr–/– mice resulted in fertilization only with Acr + sperm cells. Further investigation revealed that Acr– sperm cells penetrate ova more slowly than Acr + sperm and thereby have a selective disadvantage following competitive insemination *(99)*. This work serves to emphasize the redundancy of mechanisms for achievement of discrete links comprising the chain of reproductive events necessary for procreation.

The mouse model is useful in assessing contraceptive effects as illustrated by studies with murine recombinant (r) fertilization antigen (FA)-1 used to actively immunize female mice *(100)*. The FA-1 antigen is only found in sperm/testis. A significant reduction in fertility correlating with circulating antibody titers was completely reversible with passage of time. Anti-rFA-1 antibodies from immunized mice, but not immunoglobulins from PBS-treated control mice, significantly blocked murine sperm binding to the zona pellucida and IVF of murine oocytes. These findings suggest that rFA-1 is an exciting candidate for immunocontraception *(100)*.

Mouse breeding through several generations has been useful in reproductive toxicology for many years. Burruel et al. *(101)* followed up an earlier observation linking gamma-irradiation of male mice to reduction in IVF performance 6 wk later. In this experiment, after acute 137 Cs gamma-irradiation yielding an absorbed dose of 1.0 Gy, adult cycle day (CD)1 FO males were mated weekly with CD1 females. Males from F1 litters conceived 5 and 6 wk after paternal FO irradiation were allowed to mature. Their epididymal spermatozoa were evaluated for IVF using ova from unirradiated 8–12 wk-old CD1 females. For F1 males conceived 5 wk after paternal FO irradiation, the mean fertilization rate was similar to that of the control (i.e., 80.74 ± 15.74 SD%, n = 5, and 89.40 ± 10.94 SD%, n = 8, respectively). By contrast, the fertilization rate for spermatozoa from F1 males conceived 6 wk after paternal FO irradiation (56.14 ± 21.93 SD%, n = 5) was significantly less than the fertilization rate for control spermatozoa or for that of the F1 males conceived 5 wk after paternal FO irradiation. Apparently spermatozoa obtained 6 wk after paternal FO irradiation can transmit a decrease in fertilization rate to the F1 males as well as exhibit decreased fertilization rate themselves when tested directly by IVF *(101)*.

Follicular fluid at a dilution of 10^{-4} markedly increased the proportion of mouse sperm exhibiting high velocity and stimulated chemotactic behavior as determined by tracking on a chemotactic Zigmond chamber and recorded by videomicroscopy *(102)*. Highest sperm velocities and greater proportions of affected cells were seen with exposure to oviductal fluid. Chemotaxis was reported upon exposure of spermatozoa to oviductal fluid at dilutions of 10^{-3} and 10^{-5} and a possible sequential activity of oviductal and follicular fluids to direct spermatozoa toward ova was suggested *(102)*. Sperm-ovum chemotaxis requires further study (under rigorous conditions that can be confirmed in several appropriate laboratories) in mice and in other species. Identification of specific factors involved could prove to be very useful.

Two IVF experiments, one with zona pellucida intact and the other involving zona-free ova, were used to assess effects of a monoclonal antibody mMN9 against equatorin, a protein located at the equatorial segment of the acrosome *(103)*. The mMN9 antibody did not affect sperm motility, zona binding, or zona penetration, but it significantly inhibited fertilization. At 5 h after insemination nearly half of the unfertilized zona-intact oocytes had accumulated sperm in the perivitelline space, and by electron microscopy many unreleased cortical granules were seen beneath the oolemma indicating no sperm-oocyte fusion. Confocal laser-scanning light microscopy with indirect immunofluorescence demonstrated the presence of equatorin at the equatorial segment in capacitated and acrosome-reacted (perivitelline) sperm. These results suggest involvement of equatorin in sperm-oocyte fusion *(103)*. Addition of a synthetic peptide corresponding to a specific region of the mouse acrosomal transmembrane protein cyritestin lowered IVF rate to 30% of the normal value *(104)*. This report supports the involvement of the disintegrin domain of cyritestin in the ovum-receptor binding site of the acrosome-reacted spermatozoon. Other efforts have implicated mouse sperm fertilin alpha and beta subunits in adhesive functions relevant to sperm-ovum binding *(105,106)*.

Methods for detection of cytoskeletal and nuclear architectural structures in mouse oocytes during fertilization and methods used in exploring their regulation by intracellular calcium ion imaging have been well described by Simerly and Schatten *(107)*. These authors pointed out that methods for mammalian IVF have led to many important basic discoveries including genomic imprinting, gametic recognition involving unique receptors and galactosyl-transferases, atypical maternal inheritance patterns of the centrosome in mice, both paternal and maternal inheritance of mitochondria, and unexpected signal transduction pathways for fertilization and cell-cycle regulation. Unlike most species, the centrosome is derived from maternal sources during fertilization in the mouse (for review, *see* ref. *108*). Ultrastructural studies combined with extension of methods developed through earlier applications in the mouse model have made possible a better understanding of the fate of sperm mitochondria and sperm tail structures *(109)*, and the removal of the sperm perinuclear theca and its association with the oocyte surface during bovine fertilization *(110)*.

Initial success in growing preantral mouse oocytes from secondary follicles coupled with in vitro oocyte maturation (IVM) and IVF to obtain offspring was reported by Eppig and Schroeder in 1989 *(111)*. Subsequently, complete oocyte development was achieved by Eppig and O'Brien *(112)*. Primordial follicles were first allowed to develop in newborn mouse ovarian culture for 8 d to become secondary follicles. Then methods developed earlier were applied, i.e., culture of isolated oocyte-granulosa cell complexes for 14 d followed by IVM and IVF. Development from 2-cell to blastocyst stages was around 2%. Transfer of 198 2-cell stage embryos resulted in 2 offspring. One died shortly after birth and the survivor had impaired health that led to early death (*112*; for review, *see* ref. *113*).

DEVELOPMENT OF IVF IN DOMESTIC ANIMALS

Bovine

Among domestic species, greatest progress in developing IVF and complementing technology has resulted from emphasis on bovine reproduction (for reviews, *see* refs. *114,115*). As with development of IVF procedures in laboratory animals a major challenge involved development of sperm treatments for ovum penetration. Initial success was facilitated by models made available by rabbit in vitro capacitation and through studies of bull sperm interaction with zona-free hamster ova (for review, *see* ref. *116*). In 1977, initial success with IVF and comparison with in vivo fertilization and early cleavage development was documented by ultrastructural observations *(117)*. This involved insemination of in vivo matured ova with high ionic strength-treated ejaculated bull spermatozoa. In the same year, Iritani and Niwa *(118)* reported penetration and activation of around 20% of follicular oocytes following maturation of the oocytes for 20–24 h at 37°C in modified KRB. This oocyte treatment had been found earlier to result in approx 60% development to metaphase II *(119)*.

Sperm penetration, as observed 19–24 h after in vitro insemination, was favored by ova recovered from follicles and/or oviducts near the time of induced ovulation when compared with those recovered from unstimulated 2–5 mm follicles and cultured for 18–25 h before insemination *(120)*. Such observations point to sperm-penetration influencing factors associated with female gametes. Ultrastructural studies revealed loss of cortical granules and presence of sperm remnants in ova and embryos resulting from in vivo and in vitro fertilization *(121)*. Extension of these efforts led to publication in 1982 of a repeatable procedure for bovine IVF, with documentation including the first IVF calf born in June, 1981 *(122)*. In vivo matured ova were retrieved after treatment of donors with prostaglandin $F_2\alpha$ followed by PMSG (eCG). In one experiment, frozen-thawed semen was successfully employed, but usually fresh semen was incubated, high ionic strength-treated, and subsequently incubated in DM prior to insemination of ova. A range of fertilization results was observed according to different bulls that provided semen; spermatozoa from one bull fertilized 22 (62.9%) of 35 tubal ova. In vitro development proceeded to the 8-cell stage. Vigorous progressive sperm motility and acrosome integrity were important features of good sperm samples capable of penetrating zona-free hamster ova and cow oocytes *(122)*.

Initial success evidenced by live calves after transfer of IVF embryos into recipients involved surgical procedures for ovum recovery and transfer *(122,123)*. Improvement in the procedure followed laparoscopic recovery of follicular oocytes from hormonally treated cows just before ovulation without impairment of the donor's fertility *(124–127)*. Sirard and Lambert *(128)* found 68% of the recovered oocytes to be mature and approx one-half of them could be fertilized upon incubation with capacitated spermatozoa from selected bulls.

Variability in obtaining suitable ova following hormonal treatments, difficulties inherent in directly working with the animals, and high costs led scientists to devote serious attention to maturing oocytes easily obtained from small ovarian follicles at slaughter. In vitro matured slaughterhouse oocytes represent valuable experimental material for developing improved treatments for capacitation and the acrosome reaction. Proteoglycans and glycosaminoglycans (GAGs) are among the capacitating agents present at the normal site of fertilization in vivo (for reviews, *see* refs. *129,130*). By 1986, Parrish et al. had described an effective heparin treatment to enable cryopreserved bull spermatozoa to fertilize in vitro *(131)*. The glycosaminoglycan, heparin, has been extensively studied *(132,133)* and is most widely used in bull-sperm treatments to effect in vitro capacitation. Interestingly, relationships are now recognized between the degree of affinity for heparin by heparin-binding proteins (HBPs) in spermatozoa *(134)* and in patterns of binding of seminal vesicle-derived HBPs on the sperm surface *(135)*, with bull fertility in artificial insemination (AI) use. Although heparin/heparan sulfate is the group of GAGs implicated as most likely to be responsible for physiologically effecting capacitation in estrual cows *(136)*, available evidence also implicates other classes of GAGs, bicarbonate, calcium, and complementary roles for many additional factors in the physiological preparation of spermatozoa for fertilization.

Hyaluronic acid (HA) has been suggested as a capacitating agent for bull sperm *(137)*. Swim-up procedures through columns of HA-supplemented media have enabled selection of viable, fertile bull spermatozoa for use in IVF *(138,139)*. By traversing the HA-containing medium, the sperm surface is subjected to high shearing forces that might remove decapacitation factors thereby contributing to the capacitation process. An unrelated positive influence involving supplementation of chemically defined culture media with HA (1 mg/mL) was recently found to significantly enhance bovine embryo development to the blastocyst stage after IVM and IVF *(140)*.

In addition to those mentioned previously, successful approaches employed in preparing bull sperm for IVF include a synergistic combination of heparin and caffeine *(141)*, brief treatment with the calcium ionophore A23187 with or without caffeine in DM *(26)*, Percoll separation followed by incubation with hypotaurine or caffeine *(142,143)*, and calcium-free Tyrodes at pH 7.6 *(144)*.

For frozen-thawed spermatozoa of (at least) some bulls, it is possible to greatly simplify conditions with defined media for in vitro capacitation *(145,146)*. Thus, with completely defined media (i.e., protein-free, with PVA replacing BSA in modified DM) for in vitro capacitation, IVF and embryo culture, caffeine (1.0 mg/mL), and penicillamine (0.5 mg/mL) were adequate to replace the usual addition of heparin in the capacitation treatment for optimal results. Thus, of immature oocytes selected for IVM 76, 69, and 63% reached morula, blastocyst and expanded blastocyst stages, respectively, under these conditions. Resulting embryos appeared morphologically normal with a mean of 91 cells at 216 h post insemination. Further evidence of viability followed challenge of 96 late morulae and early blastocysts (144 h post-insemination) by vitrification. After thawing, 67% had survived as determined at 72 h and 82% of these reached the expanded blastocyst stage by 96 h of culture *(146)*.

In similar chemically defined IVF medium but with elevated bicarbonate, Tajik and Niwa *(147)* subjected cumulus-free ova to spermatozoa of 5 different bulls to study effects of caffeine (5 mM) with and without heparin (10 µg/mL) and interactions with glucose (13.9 mM). Sperm penetration took place only in the presence of caffeine and/or heparin. Regardless of the presence of glucose, similar proportions of ova were penetrated in the heparin-containing medium with (73 and 83%) and without (36 and 41%) caffeine, but with caffeine alone a higher penetration rate was observed in the presence (41%) than in the absence (27%) of glucose. When ova inseminated in medium containing caffeine and heparin with or without glucose were cultured in a chemically defined, protein-free medium, 90 and 72% reached at least the 2-cell stage (by 48 h) and 21 and 9% reached blastocyst stages (by 192 h post-insemination), respectively. In these conditions, glucose was beneficial and caffeine and heparin synergism was not explained by caffeine's reversal of glucose inhibition of heparin-induced capacitation *(147)*.

A part of bull-sperm treatments for IVF involves selection of the most progressively motile sperm cell populations for insemination. This is commonly done by allowing the cells to swim up into media over an interval of 30–60 min after washing the sperm cells by centrifugation. Another useful means for accomplishing this has involved centrifugation of spermatozoa through a gradient of 45 and 90% Percoll. Parrish et al. *(148)* found cleavage rates after IVF to be significantly higher with swim-up selected spermatozoa, than after Percoll separation. Comparable cleavage and blastocyst rates were also reported after IVF with frozen-thawed bull spermatozoa separated with glass wool and by swim-up techniques *(149)*. Another interesting approach, transmigration (TM) advocated by Rosenkranz and Holzmann *(150)*, selects motile spermatozoa in a target chamber after swimming from a test chamber through a unipore membrane (with 8 μm diameter pores) against a stream of capacitating medium (5 mL h^{-1}). Using this system, bull-ejaculated spermatozoa did not need any additives, as heparin, hypotaurine, and epinephrine, to promote capacitation and to increase motility *(151)*. Using a TALP medium *(152)* supplemented with pyruvate, BSA, heparin, hypotaurine, and epinephrine, spermatozoa from TM samples penetrated 39.3% of ova by 5 h post-insemination, whereas with swim-up samples first instances of penetration were observed only 2 h later (4.2%). By this time a normal-looking pronucleus was observed in 16.4% of ova in the TM group. Polyspermy was seen only after 7 h of incubation. This nonstatic method may provide a better means for avoiding sperm penetration of ova that become aged along with accompanying abnormal fertilization that may be more common when swim-up separated spermatozoa are used *(150)*.

Complete functional oocyte maturation—including nuclear, cytoplasmic, and membrane components—is necessary for the ooplasm to promote male pronuclear development and to launch ongoing mitotic development of the new individual after fertilization (*see* Chapter 3). Many experiments during the past two decades have revealed positive influences on ovum quality as judged by improved embryonic development following in vitro insemination. Addition of luteinizing hormone (LH) (100 μg/mL) to serum-containing medium for IVM enabled development in culture to 8- to 16-cell stages without extraneous cells for co-culture, and pregnancies could be initiated with the resulting IVF embryos following transfer *(153)*. Earlier, to avoid subjecting recently cleaved IVF embryos to inadequate culture conditions, laparoscopic oviductal transfer was shown to facilitate term development after IVM and IVF *(154)*. By 1993, undefined conditions incorporating selected serum, hormones, and other active agents, and cellular constituents or their contributions to support in vitro production of bovine embryos enabled achievement of IVF (cleavage) of 85% and blastocyst development of 40% of oocytes selected for IVM (for review, *see* ref. *155*). These efforts along with realization that IVM was best supported by certain cow sera, proestrous *(156)* or estrous *(157,158)*, that contained high LH concentrations led to replacement of serum with purified bovine LH (USDA-bLH-B-5) for supplementation of modified tissue culture medium (TCM)-199 to provide defined conditions for IVM *(159,160)*. Defined conditions for IVM coupled with semidefined conditions (i.e., with purified BSA present) for IVF and cell-free embryo culture enabled IVF of 74% and blastocyst development of 28% of selected immature oocytes *(155)*.

It seems likely that part of the beneficial effect of high concentrations of biological preparations of gonadotropins may reflect presence of biologically active contaminants, e.g., activin A *(161–163)*, and/or growth hormone *(164)*. Epidermal growth factor (EGF) *(165)* and insulin-like growth factor-1 (IGF-1), *(166–168)*, act synergistically with gonadotropins to improve oocyte, and resulting embryo quality. Combination of follicle stimulating hormone (FSH) and platelet-derived growth factor (PDGF) or EGF ± PDGF during IVM also enhanced blastocyst development *(169)*. Transforming growth factor-α (TGF-α), binds to the EGF receptor and similarly enhances bovine IVM *(170)*. Further refinement of conditions for IVM include replacement of biological gonadotropin preparations by human recombinant gonadotropins *(171,172)*. Optimal blastocyst production followed inclusion of 10 ng/mL r-hFSH in the Medium 199-based defined milieu for IVM *(172)*. This enabled 73.9, 41.3, 33.7, and 25.0% development of ova to cleavage, morula, blastocyst, and expanded blastocyst stages, respectively, in completely chemically defined conditions.

Much contemporary research involves improvement of in vitro culture media to support development to blastocyst stages (for reviews, *see* refs. *173,174* and Chapter 8). Interleukin-1 (IL-1) added at 8–10 h after insemination (at 0.1–1 ng/mL) increased development to the blastocyst stage when embryos were cultured at high density (~25–30/drop) but had no effect on development when cultured at low density (~10/drop) suggesting involvement of some other embryo-derived product *(175)*. The effect of IL-1 on embryonic development was maintained in completely denuded embryos, indicating that cumulus cells do not mediate the actions of IL-1. The effective treatment also increased embryo cell number at d 5 post-insemination by increasing the proportions of embryos that reached the 9- to 16-cell stage, but IL-1 had no effect on the proportion of blastocysts when added at d 5 post-insemination *(175)*. Several growth factors, e.g., PDGF, EGF, IGF-1, have been shown to be efficacious in promoting morula to blastocyst stages (for review, *see* ref. *176*). Protection from oxidative damage by maintaining a physiological O_2 tension (i.e., 5–8%) and lowered initial glucose concentration *(177)* and by bolstering intracellular glutathione by inclusion of mercaptoethanol or cysteamine *(178)* have had positive influences on blastocyst development after IVF.

Proportions of blastocysts resulting from bovine IVF procedures reflect not only the composition of media for support of IVM, sperm preparation, IVF (i.e., in vitro insemination), and in vitro culture (IVC) but interactions between treatments for each biological step constituting the entire IVMFC system. Also, embryos develop better in less dilute conditions due to beneficial influences of autocrine/paracrine factors. The optimal volume in culture drops is related to changes in medium *(179)* which, in turn, must be balanced against build-up of ammonium ions or other toxic by-products of embryo metabolism (for review, *see* ref. *173*). Modifications of synthetic oviduct fluid, SOF *(180)* with glutamine or citrate and nonessential amino acids (g-SOF + NEA or c-SOF + NEA) *(181)* and with BSA replaced by PVA have proven effective for support of zygote to blastocyst stages after IVF, with IVMFC in completely defined media *(146,172)*. Culture conditions were improved by use of a more complex TCM-199-based medium with recombinant growth factors for support of morula to blastocyst stages *(168)*. The ability to produce bovine embryos in completely defined conditions should facilitate advances in optimization of proportions of immature oocytes that can become viable, transferrable embryos. Such defined conditions will also be of great importance in control of disease.

Porcine

Cheng et al. *(182)* reported the first successful IVF piglets. Mattioli et al. *(183)* developed an oocyte maturation procedure incorporating the whole wall of everted follicles. Earlier difficulties in obtaining normal male pronuclear development were overcome after insemination with Percoll-separated spermatozoa, and blastocyst formation, pregnancies and birth of live piglets after IVF were reported *(184)*. The presence of cumulus cells is important in stabilizing the distribution of cortical granules to maintain the ability of the oocyte to undergo sperm penetration *(185)*. Mattioli et al. *(186)* found choline uptake, unlike uridine uptake, by LH-treated cumulus-intact oocytes was significantly higher than in FSH-treated or control oocytes. After 44 h of maturation culture, the percentage of oocyte reaching metaphase II was significantly higher in the presence of LH (76%) and FSH (86%) than in the controls (35%). The percentage of oocyte supporting male pronuclear formation was 48.4% in the control and 44.3% in FSH-treated oocyte, whereas 72.7% of LH-treated oocyte supported male pronuclear development. The observation that LH selectively increases the uptake of choline suggested that changes in metabolic coupling during maturation are not only quantitative but also qualitative, probably accounting for the regulatory effect of the cumulus cells. Mattioli et al. *(187)* demonstrated influences of LH on cyclic AMP (cAMP) and the ability of cAMP to maintain meiotic arrest, or for a transient increase in cAMP to facilitate meiosis *(see* Chapter 3). Funahashi et al. *(188)* applied these concepts to increase homogeneity of oocyte nuclear maturation by exposing cumulus oocyte complexes to dibutyryl cAMP for the first 20 h of culture. The incidence of embryos that developed to the blastocyst stage after IVF was higher following exposure to dbcAMP (21.5 vs 9.2% for controls). After transfer of experimental embryos to four recipient gilts, three delivered 19 live piglets *(188)*.

Harrison *(189)* has emphasized the importance of bicarbonate in affecting the architecture and functioning of boar spermatozoa. Recent work on membrane changes provoked by cooling has indicated similarities with capacitational changes and therefore cooling may induce premature capacitation (and destabilization). Initiation of premature capacitation by cryopreservation has been demonstrated for bull spermatozoa *(190)*. Studies of sperm-zona interaction using cryopreserved cumulus-free immature oocytes led to conclusion that the strength of attachment reflected the area of sperm head in contact with the zona rather than any physiologically specific binding, and zona attachment was not a functional or temporal indicator of zona penetration *(191)*.

Wang et al. *(192)* investigated combination of 10% pig follicular fluid and cysteine (0.57 m*M*, 1:1) with NCSU 23 medium, TCM-199, or modified Whitten's medium for IVM and found no differences in nuclear maturation, cortical granule distribution, sperm penetration, male pronuclear formation, polyspermy, and cleavage in oocytes matured in the three media. However, the NCSU 23-based medium gave significantly better results in glutathione content, cortical granule exocytosis, blastocyst development (30%), and number of cells in blastocysts (36.8 ± 17.0), indicating improvement in cytoplasmic maturation of porcine oocytes *(192)*. When follicular shell pieces were included for IVM, significantly higher proportions of blastocysts were obtained than following IVF of ova matured in absence of follicular shell pieces *(193)*. Ova matured with pieces of follicular shells also had higher glutathione concentrations. Resulting embryos were viable as demonstrated by term development *(193)*. In recent work, porcine ova were successfully matured in a protein-free medium with subsequent development to the blastocyst stage

(194). In other efforts glucocorticoids were shown to directly inhibit the meiotic, but not cytoplasmic, maturation of porcine ova in vitro *(195)*.

Investigation of morphological characteristics of in vitro matured vs in vivo matured ova revealed differences with in vitro ova exhibiting greater cytoplasmic density in the cortex, thinner zonae that were less resistant to pronase digestion, and lacking affinity for a lectin specific for beta-D-Gal (1-3)-D-GalNAc *(196)*. Although comparable in ability to release cortical granules on sperm penetration, the polyspermy rate was significantly higher for in vitro matured oocytes (65%) than for ovulated oocytes (28%). The results suggested oviductal alterations in functional blocking of polyspermy in porcine ova *(196)*. Morphological evaluation of embryos produced in vitro vs in vivo revealed abnormalities in 27% of 2-cell, 74% of 3-cell, 51% of 4-cell, and 74% of 5- to 8-cell IVF embryos *(197)*. Abnormalities (not seen in in vivo embryos) included fragmentation and/or binucleation. Staining by rhodamine-phalloidin with confocal microscopic examination revealed fewer or no perinuclear actin filaments in blastomeres of IVF embryos. There were significantly more cells in d 5 (136.5 ± 60.4 nuclei per blastocyst) and d 6 (164.5 ± 51.9 nuclei per blastocyst) in vivo blastocysts than were present in d 6 in vitro-produced blastocysts (37.3 ± 11.7 nuclei per blastocyst). These results implicate abnormal actin filament distribution in abnormal cleavage and resultant small numbers of cells in porcine embryos produced in vitro *(197)*.

Ovine

The first lambs resulting from ovine IVF were reported in 1986 by Cheng et al. *(182)*. Ten offspring were delivered by 7 of 16 recipients after transfers 16 h after in vitro insemination. Crozet et al. *(198)* achieved IVF with ovulated and in vitro matured ova and a lamb was born from one of the ovulated ova. Ultrastructural study of oocytes 20–24 h after insemination indicated that IVF approximated in vivo events. Temporal development of fertilization was identical to in vivo development reported earlier. Sperm incorporation into ooplasm was seen as early as 2 h post-insemination; abstriction of the second polar body, by 3–4 h post-insemination; male and female pronuclear formation, by 5 h post-insemination; and development of the first mitotic spindle was seen at 21 h post-insemination *(199)*. Impairment of cytoskeletal function was likely caused by a high incidence of polyspermy (27% of penetrated ova) as reflected in retarded or absent pronuclear migration *(199)*.

Additional efforts were reported by Fukui et al. *(200,201)*. Marked differences in IVF were recognized according to individual rams providing spermatozoa. Elevation of the calcium concentration in the modified DM fertilization medium was found to stabilize the fertilization rate afforded by various rams *(202)*. These conditions led to fertilization of 82.6% of ovulated ova and 61.7% were monospermic *(203)*. Transfer of oocytes taken 17 h after insemination resulted in pregnancies and offspring.

Recent progress by Wang et al. *(204)* demonstrated significant enhancement of oocyte maturation by FSH and LH as compared to hCG alone. Ova fertilized in vitro with spermatozoa treated with calcium ionophore A23187 and caffeine in DM provided significantly greater embryonic development in vitro than when swim-up separated spermatozoa in synthetic oviduct fluid supplemented with estrus ewe serum was used *(205)*. Their IVF procedure was also documented by birth of lambs. Ovine IVF has also been used recently to examine differences between sheep with and without the Booroola gene *(205)*. Other experiments have shown that induction of the acrosome reaction in spermatozoa before intracytoplasmic sperm injection is unnecessary, whereas a capacitating treatment of spermatozoa is required before IVF *(206)*.

Caprine

In 1985, Hanada *(207)* reported the birth of a kid resulting from IVF of in vivo matured oocytes with A23187-treated spermatozoa. In vitro-capacitated epididymal spermatozoa fertilized goat follicular oocytes in early work of Song and Iritani *(208)*. Modified DM was found to be superior to TALP or modified H-M199 for caprine-sperm capacitation and better results were obtained with IVM, than with oocytes harvested after hormonal treatments of does *(209)*. After IVM with a high concentration of LH, 39.5% of the oocytes were fertilized and three pregnancies were initiated after oviductal transfer of 2- and 4-cell IVF embryos *(209)*. DeSmedt et al. *(210)* obtained IVM to metaphase II of 86% of oocytes from 2–6-mm diameter follicles but only 24% for oocytes from 1–2 mm follicles. Using their capacitation treatment for ram spermatozoa, this group obtained a high fertilization rate but also found polyspermy in almost 20% of inseminated ova. By 41 h after insemination, 58% of the IVM-IVF ova reached 2- and 4-cell stages. Comparable results were also reported by Chauhan and Anand *(211)*.

By 1994, conditions were described for IVM, IVF, and IVC (IVMFC) enabling immature oocyte to develop into morulae *(212)* and to kids after embryo transfer *(213)*. Procedural improvements allowed consistent in vitro development to the blastocyst stage, and successful uterine transfers of morulae after IVF with birth of normal offspring *(214)*. Oocyte cumulus complexes were matured during 27 h in TCM-199 supplemented with 20% fetal bovine serum (FBS), 100 μg LH/mL, 0.5 μg FSH/mL, and 1 μg estradiol 17-β/mL at 38.5°C in a humidified 5% CO_2, 5% O_2, and 90% N_2 atmosphere. Freshly collected spermatozoa were washed and incubated for 5 h in mDM-containing 20% FBS, then treated with 7.35 mM calcium lactate in the presence of ova for 14 h, followed by IVC on a cumulus-cell monolayer in HEPES buffered TCM-199 with 10% FBS under paraffin oil. Thirty microliters of spent medium was replaced by an equal volume of fresh HM-199 every 24 h. These conditions supported development of 31.8% inseminated ova to the blastocyst stage *(214)*.

In further work, the feasibility of using frozen-thawed semen in caprine IVF outside the breeding season was demonstrated *(215)*. The highest proportion of blastocysts (35.7% of oocytes inseminated) resulted from use of spermatozoa diluted in a skim milk extender, heparin capacitation, and insemination in mDM supplemented with lamb serum *(215)*. In this work the defined IVC medium used for bovine zygotes (i.e., c-SOF + NEA) *(181)* proved effective for caprine IVC.

Poulin et al. *(216)* reported that out of the breeding season a higher polyspermic fertilization rate (41% vs 13–15%) occurred when 5 μg heparin/mL vs 0.2 and 1 μg/mL, respectively, was included in the fertilization medium; the latter consisted of modified DM with 20% heat-inactivated estrous sheep serum. Only 18% of cleaved ova developed to the blastocyst stage in the 5 μg/mL heparin group compared to 40% in the other groups. In the breeding season the blastocyst yield from cleaved ova was similar with or without heparin in the IVF medium, but after transfer of 2 blastocysts per recipient 8/9 recipients gave birth to 11 kids (developmental rate of 61%) in the control group and only 5/10 gave birth to 5 kids (developmental rate of 25%) in the heparin group. Poulin et al. *(216)* concluded that limited success in producing live offspring in the goat with IVM-IVF ova could be due to use of heparin as a capacitating agent for buck spermatozoa.

An extension of efforts to produce caprine embryos out of the normal breeding season involved development of a procedure for intracytoplasmic sperm injection (ICSI). A significant improvement in fertilization and blastocyst development over the IVF control was achieved by this approach. Thus, oocytes can be obtained from does out of the normal breeding season, matured in vitro, fertilized by injection of frozen-thawed spermatozoa (after manipulation to break their tails), and cultured to blastocysts (25% of oocytes) in defined medium *(217)*.

Equine

In 1991, Palmer et al. *(218)* reported the first foal derived by IVF, and Bezard et al. *(219)* reported the second the following year. In this work preovulatory oocytes were fertilized by calcium ionophore-A23187-treated stallion spermatozoa. Most IVF efforts in the literature with in vivo or in vitro matured oocytes have resulted in development of pronuclear or early cleavage stages, but conditions for oocyte maturation, sperm capacitation, and embryo culture are not well developed to accommodate in vitro embryo production in this species. Greatest progress has followed implementation of procedures for ICSI. In 1996, Squires et al. *(220)* reported the first pregnancy after equine ICSI. By ICSI, Dell'Aquila et al. *(221)* obtained 2 pronuclei or cleavage of 29.8% (17/57) vs 8.7% (9/103) of slaughterhouse oocytes inseminated in vitro. Similarly, fertilization was reported following ICSI in additional efforts *(222,223)*. Recently pregnancies have also followed injection of frozen-thawed sperm cells into in vivo matured oocytes *(224)* and ICSI involving oocytes obtained from pregnant mares *(225)*. Squires et al. *(226)* pointed out the potential utility of ICSI for assessing the viability of variously treated oocytes and the need for improved culture systems. Only 7% of 204 sperm-injected oocytes developed beyond the 8-cell stage although around 40% cleaved at least once *(227)*.

Canine

Efforts to achieve IVM of canine oocytes collected at random stages of the estrous cycle led to germinal vesicle breakdown of only 24.5% of the oocytes within 72 h *(228)*. Following insemination with dog sperm incubated for 7 h to effect capacitation, oocytes at any stage could be penetrated *(228,229)*. Improved results followed use of preovulatory oocytes recovered from ovaries of beagle bitches after hormonal treatment *(230)*. After culture for 72 h in modified Krebs-Ringer bicarbonate supplemented with 10% FCS approx 32% of oocytes reached metaphase II, and by 8 h following insemination with 4-h preincubated dog spermatozoa male and female pronuclei were seen. Sperm penetration of the zona pellucida began around 1 h post-insemination. Transfer of oocytes at 18–20 h after insemination into Whitten's medium enabled cleavage by 48 h post-insemination. Development of 15 of 45 inseminated oocytes to 2- to 8-cell stages was reported *(230)*. Successful term development following canine IVF has not been reported. Interest in canine IVF technology extends beyond applications for pets to include several endangered species *(231)* including the gray wolf (Canis lupis), the red wolf (Canis rufus), the Simien fox (Canis simensis), the San Joquin kit (Vulpes macrotis mutica), and the northern swift fox (Vulpes velox hebes).

Feline

Initial successful IVF in cats resulted from insemination of oviductal ova with uterine spermatozoa recovered after mating to assure capacitation *(25)*. Additional evidence for IVF followed use of spermatozoa obtained from the epididymis and ductus deferens

(232,233). Goodrowe et al. *(234)* reported the birth of kittens following oviductal transfer of 2- to 4-cell stage IVF embryos. Oocytes were recovered by laparoscopy after PMSG (eCG) and hCG treatments and spermatozoa were collected by electroejaculation. Sperm capacitation included a swim-up procedure. The IVF success rate was highly dependent on the time interval between PMSG and hCG treatments as well as the hCG dose. Overall fertilization (48.1%) and cleavage (45.2%, at 30 h post-insemination) rates were highest following an 80 h PMSG to hCG interval combined with a 100 IU hCG dose. Five of 6 cats receiving 6–18 embryos became pregnant and produced 1–4 kittens/litter. The gona-dotropin-treated queens subjected to follicular aspiration produced normal corpora lutea as judged visually at embryo transfer and by circulating progesterone values similar to control cats *(234)*. This work has provided a useful basis for extension to non-domestic endangered Felidae.

Pope et al. *(235)* classified cumulus oocyte complexes according to their cytoplasmic morphology as type A = good, type B = fair, and type C = poor, and matured them for 24 h in TCM-199 with gonadotropins (eCG, FSH, hCG ,or FSH/hCG). Frequency of cleavage after IVF for type A (54%), B (41%), and C (26%) oocytes was similar to the IVM frequency of the equivalent type. Development of morulae was similar among types (47–58%), but higher percentages of types A and B reached blastocysts, 31 and 29%, respectively, than of type C (15%). Transfer of d 6 (n = 32) morulae and blastocysts to three d 5 recipients resulted in pregnancies and birth of 4 live kittens *(235)*.

Kanda et al. *(236)* compared several media and culture types and achieved their best results when follicular ova were fertilized and cultured in modified Earle's balanced salt solution (MK-1) supplemented with 10% human serum (HS); the fertilization rate was 94.7% and 50% reached the blastocyst stage. When the same medium was used in a sus-pension culture dish (in contrast to a tissue culture dish), 47.2 and 71.7% of IVF-derived embryos developed to blastocysts at 120 and 144 h post-insemination, respectively. When 6 embryos per cat were transferred to the uterine horns of recipients 8 of 10 recip-ients that received early blastocysts (120 h) became pregnant *(236)*.

APPLICATIONS OF IVF

Research

Recently developed IVF technology offers unprecedented opportunities for research to improve mammalian reproductive efficiency and to understand basic mechanisms involved in early development. An important avenue involves comparative studies of gene expression for assessment of normal development. The effects of a semi-defined culture system on temporal mRNA expression patterns of 10 developmentally important genes analyzed in bovine oocytes and embryos produced in vitro were recently reported *(237)*. The transcriptional pattern assessed by reverse transcription-polymerase chain reaction (RT-PCR) of IVF morulae and blastocysts was compared with that of their in vivo counterparts. Compared with in vivo-derived embryos, bovine embryos derived from IVF, in general, appear different by light and electron microscopy, differ in num-ber of cells, size, developmental rate, temperature sensitivity, freezability, viability, and pregnancy rates after transfer *(238)*. Earlier, Wrenzycki et al. *(239)* discovered a qualita-tive difference at transcription. Post-implantation events influenced by culture condi-tions are thought to be involved in the delivery of abnormally large fetuses or offspring after transfer of bovine embryos grown in vitro *(240)*. The most prominent correlation is that the high serum content of the media is a major relevant factor *(241)*. Genes analyzed by Wrenzycki et al. *(237)* were chosen to characterize effects of a widely used bovine IVF system on physiological processes involved in compaction and cavitation, glucose metabolism, RNA processing, stress, and early differentiation. Evidence for expression of gap junction protein connexin 43 (Cx43) was detected in blastocysts derived in vivo but not in those derived in vitro. This was not due to a difference between serum and BSA supplementation of media *(237,238)*. Characterization of influences of improved chemically defined conditions for in vitro embryo production in this way should be valuable in efforts to produce physiologically normal embryos (*see* Chapter 8).

Additional avenues of research are opening with further development of microinjection approaches building on current IVF technology, e.g.. bovine ICSI *(242–245)*. Much can be learned of fertilization, appropriateness of gamete preparation, and of cytological events through further development of these potentially useful research tools.

Animal Breeding

Bovine embryos resulting from IVF have already received much commercial interest *(246–248)*. A major boon to practical applications followed development of transvaginal oocyte retrieval capabilities introduced by Pieterse et al. in 1988 (*249*; for review, *see* ref. *250*). In vitro production (IVP, also used as abbreviation for in vitro produced) of bovine embryos may enable replacement of currently practiced artificial insemination since direct embryo transfer after cryopreservation should prove to be a more efficient means for pregnancy initiation. The latest statistics reported by the International Embryo Transfer Society noted over 30,000 IVP embryos were transferred into recipient cows in 1997 *(251)*. Bousquet et al. *(252)* combined IVP with embryo sexing *(253)* and embryo transfer in a commercial setting. This group demonstrated that IVF procedures can effectively replace conventional in vivo embryo production methods when a predetermined number of pregnancies of known sex are needed within a short interval of time *(252)*. Also, bovine IVF provides a means to decrease the generation interval *(254–256)*; to produce calves via sexed semen *(257)*; to overcome infertility *(252)*; to expand reproductive potential of pregnant animals *(258)*; to extend reproductive life; to assist in propagation of endangered cattle breeds *(259)*; to produce large numbers of half-siblings simultaneously; to extend valuable semen via sperm injection *(242,260)*; to assess gamete performance; to provide pronuclear ova for DNA microinjection *(261)*; and to provide the framework for a variety of gamete manipulations including cytoplasmic transfer, nuclear transfer *(262)*, and cloning by blastomeric recycling *(263)*.

Opportunities for utility of IVF are promised by recent advances in preservation of functionality after cryopreservation of embryos (for review, *see* refs. *264,265*), and of bovine oocytes (*266,267; see* Chapter 10*)*. All of the aforementioned should gain impetus from further optimization of chemical and physical conditions for IVP of embryos. This can be facilitated through use of currently available chemically defined conditions for bovine IVM, IVF, and IVC *(146,171,172,176)*.

Prediction of porcine fertility by homologous in vitro penetration of immature oocytes enabled discrimination between boars used for AI characterized as low (<20%), intermediate (40–60%) and high (>80%) fertility groups *(268)*. Parameters of motility, normal morphology, normal apical ridge, viability with eosin-nigrosin stain, hypo-osmotic swelling test, osmotic resistance test, and functional membrane integrity with carboxyfluorescein diacetate were useful in detecting sperm with poor fertility but not precise enough to discriminate between an ejaculate with higher fertility than the herd median. Only the penetration percentage (10.24 ± 1.45 vs 55.13 ± 3.35 vs 84.72 ± 1.73) and sperm number per oocyte (1.29 ± 0.07 vs 11.29 ± 1.79 vs 25.86 ± 1.43) were parameters with a predictive capacity to discriminate between the three fertility groups *(268)*. Another approach to assessing semen quality involved IVF of in vitro matured oocytes *(269)*. In this test, all measures of sperm fertilizing ability were different among boars (all $p < 0.05$) and use of different semen dilutions for IVF allowed further discrimination of apparent sperm quality among boars. For all semen dilutions, estimated potential embryo production rate accounted for up to 70% of the variation in litter size obtained with 3×10^9 sperm per AI dose, and the number of sperm attached per oocyte was a major factor accounting for variation in litter size obtained with 2×10^9 sperm per AI dose *(269)*. These IVF variables hold promise as indicators of boar sperm quality for use in AI. Successful implementation of IVM-IVF with X- and Y-bearing spermatozoa using USDA sperm-sexing technology included surgical embryo transfers and birth of piglets of predetermined sex *(270)*. Recent development of a nonsurgical approach for embryo transfer in pigs *(271)* can be anticipated to further enhance practical uses of porcine IVF technology.

Many of the practical applications in development for farm animals are already feasible for mice. Thus, IVF offers much to efforts to make procreation possible or more efficient in a variety of research circumstances.

Preservation of Endangered Species

In the past 200 years more than 50 mammalian species have vanished and over 200 species are currently being threatened by extinction. The need for extending IVF to scarce gametes of endangered species is obvious but species differences have imposed major technological barriers (for review, *see* ref. *272*). The potential of IVF for conservation of endangered mammalian species is nonetheless tremendous (for review, *see* ref. *273*). Success has been attained using IVF to produce offspring in the Indian desert cat *(274)* and in the Siberian tiger *(275)* as well as several species of non-human primates. Experimentation with zebra led to IVF of 38% of oocytes and 16% development to morula or blastocyst stages *(276)*. Progress in understanding fertilization mechanisms can be obtained through heterologous IVF, as was recently demonstrated with spermatozoa from endangered African antelope, the scimitar-horned oryx, and domestic cow oocytes *(277)*. Cow oocytes were fertilized by spermatozoa from all oryx males tested, and 34 (61.8%) of 55 2-cell embryos produced developed to at least the 8-cell stage; polyspermy was detected in 7 (29.2%) of 24 uncleaved oocytes *(277)*.

CONCLUSIONS AND FUTURE PROSPECTS

Progress in IVF is evidenced by the ability to achieve gamete union and pregnancies following embryo transfer in common laboratory and domestic animals. Additionally, defined conditions are available for support of oocyte maturation, sperm capacitation, IVF, and embryo culture for several species. These and other advances in complementing technologies provide great impetus for acceleration of additional refinements in IVF to afford better ways to enhance reproductive efficiency and to understand physiological events at the molecular level.

Greater prominence can be anticipated for IVF in research and practical applications. The facility to produce embryos by combining previously cryopreserved gametes (*see* Chapter 10) will be useful in breeding of laboratory, domestic, and zoo animals. Technology developed in the course of animal IVF experimentation should provide a good basis for further advances, especially ICSI (*see* Chapter 7), cloning (*see* Chapters 13–17), and improved means for genetic engineering in animals. Refinements in animal IVF systems promise better ways to test for contraceptive development and models for improving assisted human reproduction.

ACKNOWLEDGMENTS

The author gratefully acknowledges Genex Cooperative, Inc. (Ithaca, NY) and Reproductive Biology Associates, Inc. (Atlanta, GA) for support and Ms. Joanne Foster for secretarial assistance.

REFERENCES

1. Austin CR. Observations on the penetration of sperm into the mammalian egg. Aust J Sci Res 1951;B4: 581–589.
2. Chang MC. Fertilizing capacity of spermatozoa deposited in the fallopian tubes. Nature (Lond) 1951; 168:697–698.
3. Austin CR. The capacitation of the mammalian sperm. Nature (Lond)1952;179:326.
4. Thibault C, Dauzier L, Winterberger S. Etude cytologique de la fecondation in vitro de loeuf de la lapine. Compt Rend Soc Biol 1954;148:789–790.
5. Brackett BG. In vitro fertilization of mammalian ova. In: Raspe G, ed. Advances in the Biosciences 4: Schering Symposium on Mechanisms Involved in Conception, Berlin, 1969. Pergamon, New York, NY, 1970, pp. 73–94.
6. Moricard R, Bossu J. Premieres etudes du passage du spermatozoid autravers de la membrane pellucida d'ovocytes de lapine fecondes in vitro. Bull Acad Nat Med 1949;133:659.
7. Smith AU. Fertilization in vitro of the mammalian egg. Biochem Soc Symp 1951;7:3.
8. Chang MC. Fertilization of rabbit ova in vitro. Nature (Lond) 1959;184:466–467.
9. Thibault C, Dauzier L. Analyse des conditions de la fecondation in vitro de l'ouef de la lapine. Ann Anim Biol Biochem Biophys 1961;1:277.
10. Bedford JM, Chang MC. Fertilization of rabbit ova in vitro. Nature (Lond) 1962;193:898.
11. Brackett BG. Effects of washing the gametes on fertilization in vitro. Fertil Steril 1969;20:127–142.
12. Brackett BG. In vitro fertilization of rabbit ova: time sequence of events. Fertil Steril 1970;21:169–176.
13. Seitz HM Jr, Brackett BG, Mastroianni L Jr. In vitro fertilization of ovulated rabbit ova recovered from the ovary. Biol Reprod 1970;2:262–267.
14. Brackett BG, Mills JA, Jeitles GG. In vitro fertilization of rabbit ova recovered from ovarian follicles. Fertil Steril 1972;23:898–909.
15. Mills JA, Jeitles GG Jr, Brackett BG. Embryo transfer following in vitro and in vivo fertilization of rabbit ova. Fertil Steril 1973;24:602–608.
16. Bishop DW. Oxygen concentration in the rabbit genital tract. Intl Congr Anim Reprod 1956;3:53.
17. Mastroianni L, Jones R. Oxygen tension within the rabbit fallopian tube. J Reprod Fertil 1965;9:99.
18. Brackett BG, Williams WL. Fertilization of rabbit ova in a defined medium. Fertil Steril 1968;19: 144–155.
19. Bishop DW. Metabolic conditions within the oviduct of the rabbit. Intl J Fertil 1957;2:11.
20. Brinster RL. Culture of two-cell rabbit embryos to morulae. J Reprod Fertil 1970;21:17–22.
21. Kane MT. Energy substrates and culture of single-cell rabbit ova to blastocysts. Nature (Lond) 1972; 238:468.
22. Kane MT, Foote RH. Factors affecting blastocyst expansion of rabbit zygotes and young embryos in defined media. Biol Reprod 1971;4:41.
23. Brackett BG. Extracorporeal fertilization of mammalian ova. In: Gold JJ, ed. Gynecologic Endocrinology, 2nd ed. Harper & Row, New York, NY, 1975, pp. 621–644.
24. Brackett BG, Oliphant G. Capacitation of rabbit spermatozoa in vitro. Biol Reprod 1975;12:260–274.
25. Hamner CE, Jennings LL, Sojka NJ. Cat (Felis catus L.) spermatozoa require capacitation. J Reprod Fertil 1970;23:477–480.
26. Hanada A. In vitro fertilization in cattle with particular reference to sperm capacitation by ionophore A23187. Jpn J Anim Reprod 1985;31:56–61.

27. Seitz HM Jr, Rocha G, Brackett BG, Mastroianni L Jr. Influence of the oviduct on sperm capacitation in the rabbit. Fertil Steril 1970;21:325–328.

28. Brackett BG, Server JB. Capacitation of rabbit spermatozoa in the uterus. Fertil Steril 1970;21:687–695.

29. Soupart P. Sperm capacitation: methodology, hormonal control and the search for a mechanism. In: Moghissi KS, Hafez ESE, eds. Biology of Mammalian Fertilization and Implantation. Charles C. Thomas, Springfield, IL, 1972, pp. 54–125.

30. Brackett BG, Mills JA, Oliphant G, Seitz HM, Jeitles GG, Mastroianni L. Preliminary efforts to capacitate rabbit sperm in vitro. Intl J Fertil 1972;17:86–92.

31. Ogawa S, Satoh K, Hamada M, Hashimoto H. In vitro culture of rabbit ova fertilized by epididymal sperms in chemically defined media. Nature (Lond) 1972;238:270–271.

32. Brackett BG, Hall JL, Oh YK. In vitro fertilizing ability of testicular, epididymal, and ejaculated rabbit spermatozoa. Fertil Steril 1978;29:571–582.

33. Oliphant G, Brackett BG. Immunological assessment of surface changes of rabbit sperm undergoing capacitation. Biol Reprod 1973;9:404–414.

34. Reyes A, Oliphant G, Brackett BG. Partial purification and identification of a reversible decapacitation factor from rabbit seminal plasma. Fertil Steril 1975;26:148–157.

35. Ericsson RJ, Buthala DA, Norland JF. Fertilization of rabbit ova in vitro by sperm with adsorbed Sendai virus. Science 1971;173:54.

36. Akruk SR, Humphreys WJ, Williams WL. In vitro capacitation of ejaculated rabbit spermatozoa. Differentiation 1979;13:125–131.

37. Rogers BJ. Mammalian sperm capacitation and fertilization in vitro: a critique of methodology. Gamete Res 1978;1:165–223.

38. Hosoi Y, Niwa K, Hatanaka S, Iritani A. Fertilization in vitro of rabbit eggs by epididymal spermatozoa capacitated in a chemically defined medium. Biol Reprod 1981;24:637–642.

39. Bedford JM. Some caveats of mammalian gamete research. In: Alexander NJ, ed. Animal Models for Research on Contraception and Fertility. Harper and Row, Hagerstown, MD, 1979, pp. 254–268.

40. Oliphant G, Eng LA. Collection of gametes in laboratory animals and preparation of sperm for in vitro fertilization. In: Mastroianni K Jr, Biggers J, eds. Fertilization and Embryonic Development In Vitro. Plenum, New York, NY, 1981, pp. 11–26.

41. Viriyapanich P, Bedford JM. The fertilization performance in vivo of rabbit spermatozoa capacitated in vitro. J Exp Zool 1981;216:169–174.

42. Brackett BG, Bousquet D, Dressel MA. In vitro sperm capacitation and in vitro fertilization with normal development in the rabbit. J Androl 1982;3:402–411.

43. Kane MT. Bicarbonate requirements for culture of one-cell rabbit ova to blastocysts. Biol Reprod 1975;12:552–555.

44. Yanagimachi R, Chang MC. Fertilization of hamster eggs in vitro. Nature 1963;200: 281.

45. Yanagimachi R, Chang MC. In vitro fertilization of hamster ova. J Exp Zool 1964;156:361–376.

46. Yanagimachi R. Time and process of sperm penetration into hamster ova in vivo and in vitro. J Reprod Fert 1966;11:359.

47. Barros C, Austin CR. In vitro acrosomal reaction of golden hamster spermatozoa. Anat Rev 1967;157:348.

48. Barros C, Austin CR. In vitro fertilization of golden hamster ova. Anat Rev 1967;157: 209.

49. Yanagimachi R. In vitro capacitation of hamster spermatozoa by follicular fluid. J Reprod Fertil 1969;18:275.

50. Yanagimachi R. In vitro acrosome reaction and capacitation of golden hamster spermatozoa by bovine follicular fluid and its fractions. J Exp Zool 1969;170:269–280.

51. Lui CW, Cornett LE, Meizel S. Identification of the bovine follicular fluid proteins involved in the in vitro induction of the hamster sperm acrosome reaction. Biol Reprod 1977;17:34–41.

52. Hall JL, Stephenson R, Mathias C, Brackett BG. Hormonal dependence of cyclic patterns in hamster uterine fluid proteins. Biol Reprod 1977;17:738–774.

53. Meizel S, Liu CW, Working PK, Mrsny RJ. Taurine and hypotaurine: their effects on motility, capacitation and acrosome reaction of hamster sperm in vitro and their presence in sperm and reproductive tract fluids of several mammals. Dev Growth Differ 1980;22:483–494.

54. Bavister BD. A consistently successful procedure for in vitro fertilization of golden hamster eggs. Gamete Res 1989;23:139–158.

55. Seshagiri PB, Bavister BD. Phosphate is required for inhibition by glucose of development of hamster 8-cell embryos in vitro. Biol Reprod 1989;40:607–614.

56. McKiernan SH, Bavister BD. Environmental variables influencing in vitro development of hamster 2-cell embryos to the blastocyst stage. Biol Reprod 1990;43:404–413.
57. McKiernan SH Bavister BD, Tasca RJ. Energy substrate requirements for in vitro development of hamster 1- and 2-cell embryos to the blastocyst stage. Hum Reprod 1991;6:64–75.
58. Schini SA, Bavister BD. Two-cell block to development of cultured hamster embryos is caused by phosphate and glucose. Biol Reprod 1988;39:1183–1192.
59. Barnett DK, Bavister BD. Hypotaurine requirement for in vitro development of golden hamster one-cell embryos into morulae and blastocysts, and production of term offspring from in vitro-fertilized ova. Biol Reprod 1992;47:297–304.
60. Whittingham DG. Fertilization of mouse eggs in vitro. Nature 1968;220:592.
61. Whitten WK, Biggers JE. Complete development in vitro of the preimplantation stages of the mouse ova in a simple chemically defined medium. J Reprod Fertil 1968;17:399.
62. Cross PC, Brinster RL. In vitro development of mouse oocytes. Biol Reprod 1970;3:298.
63. Iwamatsu T, Chang MC. Further investigation of capacitation of sperm and fertilization of mouse eggs in vitro. J Exp Zool 1970;175:271.
64. Toyoda Y, Yokoyama M, Hosi T. Studies on the fertilization of mouse eggs in vitro. I. In vitro fertilization of eggs by fresh epididymal sperm. Jpn J Anim Reprod 1971;16:147–152.
65. Toyoda Y, Yokoyama M, Hosi T. Studies on the fertilization of mouse eggs in vitro. II. Effects of in vitro pre-incubation of spermatozoa on time of sperm penetration of mouse eggs in vitro. Jpn J Anim Reprod 1971;16:152–157.
66. Miyamoto H, Chang MC. Development of mouse eggs fertilized in vitro by epididymal spermatozoa. J Reprod Fertil 1972;30:135.
67. Mukherjee AB. Normal progeny from fertilization in vitro of mouse oocytes matured in culture and spermatozoa capacitated in vitro. Nature 1972;237:397.
68. Oliphant G, Brackett BG. Capacitation of mouse spermatozoa in media with elevated ionic strength and reversible decapacitation with epididymal extracts. Fertil Steril 1973;24:849.
69. Hoppe PC, Pitts S. Fertilization in vitro and development of mouse ova. Biol Reprod 1973;8:420–426.
70. Fraser LR, Drury LM. The relationship between sperm concentration and fertilization in vitro of mouse eggs. Biol Reprod 1975;13:513–518.
71. Hogan B, Beddington R, Costantini F, Lacy E. Manipulating the Mouse Embryo: A Laboratory Manual, 2nd ed. Cold Spring Harbor Laboratory Press, Cold Spring Harbor, NY, 1994, p. 497.
72. Miyamoto H, Chang MC. In vitro fertilization of rat eggs. Nature 1973;241:50.
73. Toyoda Y, Chang MC. Capacitation of epididymal spermatozoa in a medium with high K/Na ratio and cyclic AMP for the fertilization of rat eggs in vitro. J Reprod Fertil 1974;36:125.
74. Yanagimachi R. In vitro fertilization of guinea pig ova. Anat Rec 1972;172:430.
75. Biggers JD, Whitten WK, Whittingham DG. The culture of mouse embryos in vitro. In: Daniel JC Jr, ed. Methods of Mammalian Embryology. Freeman, San Francisco, CA, 1971, pp. 86–116.
76. Yanagimachi R. Penetration of guinea pig spermatozoa into hamster eggs in vitro. J Reprod Fertil 1972;28:477.
77. Hanada A, Chang MC. Penetration of zona-free eggs by spermatozoa of different species. Biol Reprod 1972;6:300.
78. Yanagimachi R, Yanagimachi H, Rogers BJ. The use of zona-free animal ova as a test-system for the assessment of the fertilizing capacity of human spermatozoa. Biol Reprod 1976;15:471–476.
79. Barros C, Gonzalez J, Herrera E, Bustos-Obregon E. Fertilizing capacity of human spermatozoa evaluated by actual penetration of foreign eggs. Contraception 1978;17:87.
80. Imai H, Niwa K, Iritani A. Penetration in vitro of zona-free hamster eggs by ejaculated boar spermatozoa. J Reprod Fertil 1977;51:495–497.
81. Slavik T, Kopecny V, Fulka J. Developmental failure of hybrid embryos originated after fertilization of bovine oocytes with ram spermatozoa. Mol Reprod Dev 1997;48:344–349.
82. Chatot CL, Ziomek CA, Bavister BD, Lewis JL, Torres I. An improved culture medium supports development of random-bred 1-cell mouse embryos in vitro. J Reprod Fertil 1989;86:679–688.
83. Lawitts JA, Biggers JD. Optimization of mouse embryo culture media using simplex methods. J Reprod Fertil 1991;91:543–556.
84. Lawitts JA, Biggers JD. Culture of preimplantation embryos. In: Wassarman PM, DePamphilis ML. eds. Guide to Techniques in Mouse Development. Methods in Enzymology, vol 225. Academic, San Diego, CA, 1993, pp. 153–164.

85. Lane M, Gardner DK. Increase in postimplantation development of cultured mouse embryos by amino acids and induction of fetal retardation and exencephaly by ammonium ions. J Reprod Fertil 1994; 102:305–312.

86. Lavitrano M, Camaioni A, Fazio VM, Dolci S, Farace MG, Spadafora C. Sperm cells as vectors for introducing foreign DNA into eggs: genetic transformation of mice. Cell 1989;57:717–723.

87. Zaccagnini G, Maione B, Lorenzini R, Spadafora C. Increased production of mouse embryos in in vitro fertilization by preincubating sperm cells with the nuclease inhibitor aurintricarboxylic acid. Biol Reprod 1998;59:1549–1553.

88. Sasagawa I, Ichiyanagi O, Yazawa H, Nakada T, Saito H, Hiroi M, Yanagimachi R. Round spermatid transfer and embryo development. Arch Androl 1998;41:151–157.

89. Songsasen N, Tong J, Leibo SP. Birth of live mice derived by in vitro fertilization with spermatozoa retrieved up to twenty-four hours after death. J Exp Zool 1998;280:189–196.

90. Nakagata N, Takeshima T. High fertilizing ability of mouse spermatozoa diluted slowly after cryopreservation. Theriogenology 1992;37:1283–1291.

91. Songsasen N, Betteridge KJ, Leibo SP. Birth of live mice resulting from oocytes fertilized in vitro with cryopreserved spermatozoa. Biol Reprod 1997;56:143–152.

92. Songsasen N, Leibo SP. Cryopreservation of mouse spermatozoa. I. Effect of seeding on fertilizing ability of cryopreserved spermatozoa. Cryobiology 1997;35:240–254.

93. Songsasen N, Leibo SP. Cryopreservation of mouse spermatozoa. II. Relationship between survival after cryopreservation and osmotic tolerance of spermatozoa from three strains of mice. Cryobiology 1997;35:255–269.

94. O'Neil L, Paynter SJ, Fuller BJ. Vitrification of mature mouse oocytes: improved results following addition of polyethylene glycol to a dimethyl sulfoxide solution. Cryobiology 1997;34:295–301.

95. Songsasen N, Leibo SP. Live mice from cryopreserved embryos derived in vitro with cryopreserved ejaculated spermatozoa. Lab Anim Sci 1998;48:275–281.

96. Wakayama T, Whittingham DG, Yanagimachi R. Production of normal offspring from mouse oocytes injected with spermatozoa cryopreserved with or without cryoprotection. J Reprod Fertil 1998;112: 11–17.

97. Vergara GJ, Irwin MH, Moffatt RJ, Pinkert CA. In vitro fertilization in mice: strain differences in response to superovulation protocols and effect of cumulus cell removal. Theriogenology 1997;47:1245–1252.

98. Visconti PE, Galantino-Homer H, Ning XP, Moore GD, Valenzuela JP, Jorgez CJ, et al. Cholesterol efflux-mediated signal transduction in mammalian sperm. J Biol Chem 1999;274:3235–3242.

99. Adham IM, Nayernia K, Engel W. Spermatozoa lacking acrosin protein show delayed fertilization. Mol Reprod Dev 1997;46:370–376.

100. Naz RK, Zhu X. Recombinant fertilization antigen-1 causes a contraceptive effect in actively immunized mice. Biol Reprod 1998;59:1095–1100.

101. Burruel VR, Raabe OG, Wiley LM. In vitro fertilization rate of mouse oocytes with spermatozoa from the F1 offspring of males irradiated with 1.0 Gy 137Cs gamma-rays. Mutat Res 1997;381:59–66.

102. Oliveira RG, Tomasi L, Rovasio RA, Giojalas LC. Increased velocity and induction of chemotactic response in mouse spermatozoa by follicular and oviductal fluids. J Reprod Fertil 1999;115:23–27.

103. Toshimori K, Saxena DK, Tanii I, Yoshinaga K. An MN9 antigenic molecule, equatorin, is required for successful sperm-oocyte fusion in mice. Biol Reprod 1998;59:22–29.

104. Linder B, Heilein UA. Decreased in vitro fertilization efficiencies in the presence of specific cyritestin peptides. Dev Growth Differ 1997;39:243–247.

105. Evans JP, Kopf GS, Schultz RM. Characterization of the binding of recombinant mouse sperm fertilin beta subunit to mouse eggs: evidence for adhesive activity via an egg beta1 integrin-mediated interaction. Dev Biol 1997;187:79–93.

106. Evans JP, Schultz RM, Kopf GS. Characterization of the binding of recombinant mouse sperm fertilin alpha subunit to mouse eggs: evidence for function as a cell adhesion molecule in sperm-egg binding. Dev Biol 1997;187:94–106.

107. Simerly C, Shatten G. Techniques for localization of specific molecules in oocytes and embryos. Methods Enzymol 1993;225:516–553.

108. Schatten G. The centrosome and its mode of inheritance: the reduction of the centrosome during gametogenesis and its restoration during fertilization. Develop Biol 1994;165:299–335.

109. Sutovsky P, Navara CS, Schatten G. Fate of the sperm mitochondria, and the incorporation, conversion, and disassembly of the sperm tail structures during bovine fertilization. Biol Reprod 1996;55: 1195–1205.

110. Sutovsky P, Oko R, Hewitson L, Schatten G. The removal of the sperm perinuclear theca and its association with the bovine oocyte surface during fertilization. Develop Biol 1997;188:75–84.

111. Eppig JJ, Schroeder AC. Capacity of mouse oocytes from preantral follicles to undergo embryogenesis and development to live young after growth, maturation and fertilization in vitro. Biol Reprod 1989; 41:268–276.

112. Eppig JJ, O'Brien MJ. Development in vitro of mouse oocytes from primordial follicles. Biol Reprod 1996;54:197–207.

113. Eppig JJ, O'Brien MJ. Comparison of preimplantation developmental competence after mouse oocyte growth and development in vitro and in vivo. Theriogenology 1998;49:415–422.

114. Brackett BG. In vitro fertilization of farm animals. In: Lauria A, Gandolfi F, eds. Embryonic Development and Manipulation in Animal Production: Trends and Applications. Portland Press, Chapel Hill, NC, 1992, pp. 59–76.

115. Brackett BG. 1948–1998: Artificial insemination to current gamete biotechnology. In: Lauria A, Gandolfi F, Enne G, Gianaroli L, eds. Gametes: Development and Function. Serono Symposia, Rome, 1998, pp. 31–68.

116. Brackett BG. In vitro fertilization and embryonic development in cattle. Proceedings Indo-US Workshop on Ovum Implantation. Indian Council of Medical Research, New Delhi, 1984, pp. 81–91.

117. Brackett BG, Oh YK, Evans JF, Donawick WJ. Bovine fertilization and early development in vivo and in vitro. 10th Ann Mtg Soc Study Reprod 1977; Abstr 86, 56–57.

118. Iritani A, Niwa K. Capacitation of bull spermatozoa and fertilization in vitro of cattle follicular oocytes matured in culture. J Reprod Fertil 1977;50:119–121.

119. Satoh E, Iritani A, Nishikawa Y. Factors involved in maturation of pig and cattle follicular oocytes cultured in vitro. Jpn J Anim Reprod 1977;23:12.

120. Brackett BG, Evans JF, Donawick WJ, Boice ML, Cofone MA. In vitro penetration of cow oocytes by bull sperm. Arch Androl 1980;5:69–71.

121. Brackett BG, Oh YK, Evans JF, Donawick WJ. Fertilization and early development of cow ova. Biol Reprod 1980;23:189–205.

122. Brackett BG, Bousquet D, Boice ML, Donawick WJ, Evans JF, Dressel MA. Normal development following in vitro fertilization in the cow. Biol Reprod 1982;27:147–158.

123. Brackett BG, Keefer CL, Troop CG, Donawick WJ, Bennett KA. Bovine twins resulting from *in vitro* fertilization. Theriogenology 1984;21:224.

124. Lambert RD, Bernard C, Rioux JE, Beland R, D'amours D, Montreuil A. Endoscopy in cattle by the paralumbar route: technique for ovarian examination and follicular aspiration. Theriogenology 1983; 20:149–161.

125. Sirard MA, Lambert RD, Menard DP, Bedoya M. Pregnancies following in vitro fertilization of bovine follicular oocytes obtained by laparoscopy. Biol Reprod 1985;32:99.

126. Sirard MA, Lambert RD. Birth of calves after in vitro fertilization using laparoscopy and rabbit oviduct incubation of zygotes. Vet Res 1986;119:167–169.

127. Schellander K, Fayrer-Hosken RA, Keefer CL, Brown LM, Malter H, McBride CE, Brackett BG. In vitro fertilization of bovine follicular oocytes recovered by laparoscopy. Theriogenology 1989;31: 927–934.

128. Sirard MA, Lambert RD. In vitro fertilization of bovine follicular oocytes obtained by laparoscopy. Biol. Reprod. 1985;33:487–494.

129. Miller DJ, Ax RL. Carbohydrates and fertilization in animals. Mol Reprod Dev 1990;26:184–198.

130. Rodriguez-Martinez H, Larsson B, Pertoft H, Kjellen L. GAGs and spermatozoan competence in vivo and in vitro. In: Lauria A, Gandolfi F, Enne G, Gianaroli L, eds. Gametes: Development and Function. Serono Symposia, Rome, 1998, pp. 239–272.

131. Parrish JJ, Susko-Parrish JL, Leibfried-Rutledge ML, Critser ES, Eyestone WH, First NL. Bovine in vitro fertilization with frozen-thawed semen. Theriogenology 1986;25:591–600.

132. Parrish JJ, Susko-Parrish J, Winer MA, First NL. Capacitation of bovine sperm by heparin. Biol Reprod 1988;38:1171–1180.

133. Parrish JJ, Susko-Parish JL, First NL. Capacitation of bovine sperm by heparin: inhibitory effect of glucose and role of intracellular pH. Biol Reprod 1989;41:683–699.

134. Bellin MR, Hawkins HE, Ax RL. Fertility of range beef bulls grouped according to presence or absence of heparin-binding proteins in sperm membranes and seminal fluid. J Anim Sci 1994;72:2441–2448.

135. McCauley TC, Bellin ME, Ax RL. Localization of a heparin-binding protein to distinct regions of bovine sperm. J Anim Sci 1996;74:429–438.

136. First NL, Parrish JJ. Sperm maturation and in vitro fertilization. Proc. 11th Intl Congr Anim Reprod AI 1988;5:160–168.
137. Fukui Y. Effect of follicle cells on the acrosome reaction, fertilization and developmental competence of bovine oocytes matured in vitro. Mol Reprod Dev 1990;26:40–46.
138. Shamsuddin M, Rodriguez-Martinez H, Larsson B. Fertilizing capacity of bovine spermatozoa selected after swim-up in hyaluronic acid-containing medium. Reprod Fertil Dev 1993;5:307–315.
139. Shamsuddin M, Rodriguez-Martinez H. A simple, non-traumatic swim-up method for the selection of spermatozoa for in vitro fertilization in the bovine. Anim Reprod Sci 1994;36:61–75.
140. Furnus CC, deMatos DG, Martinez AG. Effect of hyaluronic acid on development of in vitro produced bovine embryos. Theriogenology 1998;49:1489–1499.
141. Niwa K, Ohgoda O. Synergistic effect of caffeine and heparin on in vitro fertilization of cattle oocytes matured in culture. Theriogenology 1998;30:733–741.
142. Iritani A, Utsumi K, Miyake M, Hosoi Y, Saiki K. In vitro fertilization by a routine method and by micromanipulation. In: Jones HW, and Schrader D, eds. In Vitro Fertilization and Other Assisted Reproduction. Ann NY Acad Sci 1988;541:583–590.
143. Utsumi K, Kato H, Iritani A. Full-term development of bovine follicular oocytes matured in culture and fertilized in vitro. Theriogenology 1991;35:695–703.
144. Ijaz A, Hunter AG. Evaluation of calcium-free Tyrode's sperm capacitation medium for use in bovine in vitro fertilization. J Dairy Sci 1989;72:3280–3285.
145. Brackett BG, and Keskintepe L. Defined sperm treatments and insemination conditions enable improved bovine embryo production in vitro. Theriogenology 1996;45:259.
146. Keskintepe L, Brackett BG. In vitro developmental competence of in vitro-matured bovine oocytes fertilized and cultured in completely defined media. Biol Reprod 1996;55:333–339.
147. Tajik P, Niwa K. Effects of caffeine and/or heparin in a chemically defined medium with or without glucose on in vitro penetration of bovine oocytes and their subsequent development. Theriogenology 1998;49:771–777.
148. Parrish JJ, Krogenaes A, Susko-Parrish JL. Effect of bovine sperm separation by either swim-up or Percoll method on success of in vitro fertilization and early embryonic development. Theriogenology 1995;44:859–869.
149. Stubbings RB, Wosik CP. Glass wool versus swim-up separation of bovine spermatozoa for in vitro fertilization. Theriogenology 1991;35:276.
150. Rosenkranz C, Holzmann A. The effect of sperm preparation on the timing of penetration in bovine in vitro fertilization. Anim Reprod Sci 1997;46:47–53.
151. Rosenkranz C, Holzmann A. Der einflub von samenaufbereitung und kulturmedium auf den IVF-erfolg beim rind. J Vet Med A 1995;42:139–143.
152. Bavister BD, Yanagimachi R. The effects of sperm extracts and energy sources on the motility and acrosome reaction of hamster spermatozoa in vitro. Biol Reprod 1977;16:228–237.
153. Brackett BG, Younis AI, Fayrer-Hosken RA. Enhanced viability after in vitro fertilization of bovine oocytes matured in vitro with high concentrations of luteinizing hormone. Fertil Steril 1989;52:319–324.
154. Fayrer-Hosken RA, Younis AI, Brackett BG, McBride CE, Harper KM, Keefer CL, Cabaniss DC. Laparoscopic oviductal transfer of in vitro matured and in vitro fertilized bovine oocytes resulting in offspring. Theriogenology 1989;32:413–420.
155. Brackett BG, Zuelke KA. Analysis of factors involved in the in vitro production of bovine embryos. Theriogenology 1993;39:43–64.
156. Younis AI, Brackett BG, Fayrer-Hosken RA. Influence of serum and hormones on bovine oocyte maturation and fertilization in vitro. Gamete Res 1989;23:189–201.
157. Sanbuissho A, Threlfall WR. The influence of serum and gonadotropins on bovine oocyte maturation in vitro. Theriogenology 1988;29:301.
158. Schellander K, Fuhrer F, Brackett BG, Korb H, Schleger W. In vitro fertilization and cleavage of bovine oocytes matured in medium supplemented with estrous cow serum. Theriogenology 1990;33:477–486.
159. Zuelke K, Younis AI, Brackett BG. Enhanced maturation of bovine oocytes with and without protein supplementation. Serono Symposium on Fertilization in Mammals, Boston, MA, 1989; Abstr. 1–25, 47.
160. Zuelke KA, Brackett BG. Luteinizing hormone-enhanced in vitro maturation of bovine oocytes with and without protein supplementation. Biol Reprod 1990;43:784–787.
161. Stock AE, Woodruff TK, Smith LC. Effects of inhibin A and activin A during in vitro maturation of bovine oocytes in hormone- and serum-free medium. Biol Reprod 1997;56:1559–1564.

162. Silva CC, Knight PG. Modulatory actions of activin-A and follistatin on the developmental competence of in vitro-matured bovine oocytes. Biol Reprod 1998;58:558–565.
163. Yoshioka K, Suzuki C, Iwamura S. Activin A and follistatin regulate developmental competence of in vitro-produced bovine embryos. Biol Reprod 1998;59:1017–1022.
164. Izadyar F, Hage WJ, Colenbrander B, Bevers MM. The promotory effect of growth hormone on the developmental competence of in vitro matured bovine oocytes is due to improved cytoplasmic maturation. Mol Reprod Dev 1998;49:444–453.
165. Harper KM, Brackett BG. Bovine blastocyst development after in vitro maturation in a defined medium with epidermal growth factor and low concentrations of gonadotropins. Biol Reprod 1993;48: 409–416.
166. Harper KM, Brackett BG. Bovine blastocyst development after IGF-1 treatment for oocyte maturation in vitro. Biol Reprod 1992;46:67.
167. Martins A Jr, Keskintepe L, Brackett BG. In vitro blastocyst development of bovine oocytes matured with IGF-1 and reduced FSH. Biol Reprod 1997;56(Suppl 1): Abstr 329, 165.
168. Martins A Jr, Brackett BG. Development of bovine oocytes matured with low concentrations of gonadotropins and IGF-1 into advanced blastocyst stages after IVF. In: Lauria A, Gandolfi F, Enne G, Gianaroli L, eds. Gametes: Development and Function. Serono Symposia, Rome, 1998, p. 571.
169. Harper KM, Brackett BG. Bovine blastocyst development after follicle-stimulating hormone and platelet-derived growth factor treatment for oocyte maturation in vitro. Zygote 1993;1:27–34.
170. Kobayashi K, Yamashita S, Hoshi H. Influence of EGF and TGF-α on in vitro maturation of cumulus cell-enclosed bovine oocytes in a defined medium. J Reprod Fertil 1994;100:439–446.
171. Martins A, Jr, Keskintepe L, Brackett BG. Use of recombinant gonadotropins for bovine embryo production in vitro. Theriogenology 1998;44:292.
172. Martins A Jr, Brackett BG. Effects of recombinant gonadotropins on bovine embryonic development in chemically defined media. European Embryo Transfer Assn. 14th Scientific Mtg, Venice, 1998 (Abstr 214).
173. Gardner DK. Mammalian embryo culture in the absence of serum or somatic cell support. Cell Biol Intl 1994;18:1163–1179.
174. Bavister BD. Culture of preimplantation embryos: facts and artifacts. Human Reprod Update 1995;1(2): 91–148.
175. Paula-Lopes FF, deMoraes AAS, Edwards JL, Justice JE, Hansen PJ. Regulation of preimplantation development of bovine embryos by interleukin-1. Biol Reprod 1998;59:1406–1412.
176. Brackett BG. Chemically defined media for embryo production (IVMFC). Proceedings of the 16th Annual Convention of the American Embryo Transfer Association, Madison, WI, 1997, pp. 18–35.
177. Iwata H, Akamatsu S, Minami N, Yamada M. Effects of antioxidants on the development of bovine IVM/IVF embryos in various concentrations of glucose. Theriogenology 1998;50:365–375.
178. Takahashi M, Nagai T, Hamano S, Kuwayama M, Okamura N, Okano A. Effect of thiol compounds on in vitro development and intracellular glutathione content of bovine embryos. Biol Reprod 1993;49: 228–232.
179. Martins A Jr, Campos MM, Brackett BG. Improved bovine embryo production by reducing changes of culture medium in defined in vitro conditions. Proceedings of the Brazilian Animal Reproduction Society Mtg., Caxambu, Minas Gerais, Brazil, 1997, pp. 29–31.
180. Tervit HR, Whittingham DG, Rowson LER. Successful culture in vitro of sheep and cattle ova. J Reprod Fertil 1972;30:493–497.
181. Keskintepe K, Burnley CA, Brackett BG. Production of viable bovine blastocysts in defined in vitro conditions. Biol Reprod 1995;52:1410–1417.
182. Cheng WTK, Moor RM, Polge C. In vitro fertilization of pig and sheep oocytes matured in vivo and in vitro. Theriogenology 1986;25:146.
183. Mattioli M, Galeati G, Seren E. Effect of follicle somatic cells during pig oocyte maturation on egg penetrability and male pronucleus formation. Gamete Res 1988;20:173–183.
184. Mattioli M, Bacci ML, Galeati G, Seren E. Developmental competence of pig oocytes matured and fertilized in vitro. Theriogenology 1989;31:1201–1207.
185. Galeati G, Modina S, Lauria A, Mattioli M. Follicle somatic cells influence pig oocyte penetrability and cortical granule distribution. Mol Reprod Dev 1991;29:40–46.
186. Mattioli M, Bacci ML, Galeati G, Seren E. Effects of LH and FSH on the maturation of pig oocytes in vitro. Theriogenology 1991;36:91–105.

187. Mattioli M, Galeati G, Barboni B, Seren E. Concentration of cyclic AMP during the maturation of pig oocytes in vivo and in vitro. J Reprod Fertil 1994;100:403–409.
188. Funahashi H, Cantley TC, Day BN. Synchronization of meiosis in porcine oocytes by exposure to dibutyryl cyclic adenosine monophosphate improves developmental competence following in vitro fertilization. Biol Reprod 1997;57:49–53.
189. Harrison RA. Sperm plasma membrane characteristics and boar semen fertility. J Reprod Fertil 1997;52:195–211.
190. Cormier N, Sirard M-A, Bailey JL. Premature capacitation of bovine spermatozoa is initiated by cryo-preservation. J Androl 1997;18:461–468.
191. Lynham JA, Harrison RA. Use of stored pig eggs to assess boar sperm fertilizing functions in vitro. Biol Reprod 1998;58:539–550.
192. Wang WH, Abeydeera LR, Cantley TC, Day BN. Effects of oocyte maturation media on development of pig embryos produced by in vitro fertilization. J Reprod Fertil 1997;111:101–108.
193. Abeydeera LR, Wang WH, Cantley TC, Rieke A, Day BN. Coculture with follicular shell pieces can enhance the developmental competence of pig oocytes after in vitro fertilization: relevance to intra-cellular glutathione. Biol Reprod 1998;58:213–218.
194. Abeydeera LR, Wang WH, Prather RS, Day BN. Maturation in vitro of pig oocytes in protein-free culture media: fertilization and subsequent embryo development in vitro. Biol Reprod 1998;58:1316–1320.
195. Yang JG, Chen WY, Li PS. Effects of glucocorticoids on maturation of pig oocytes and their subse-quent fertilizing capacity in vitro. Biol Reprod 1999;60:929–936.
196. Wang WH, Abeydeera LR, Prather RS, Day BN. Morphologic comparison of ovulated and in vitro-matured porcine oocytes, with particular reference to polyspermy after in vitro fertilization. Mol Reprod Dev 1998;49:308–316.
197. Wang WH, Abeydeera LR, Han YM, Prather RS, Day BN. Morphologic evaluation and actin filament distribution in porcine embryos produced in vitro and in vivo. Biol Reprod 1999;60:1020–1028.
198. Crozet N, Huneau D, DeSmedt V, Theron MC, Szollosi D, Torres S, Sevellec C. In vitro fertilization with normal development in the sheep. Gamete Res 1987;16:159–170.
199. Crozet N. Fine structure of sheep fertilization in vitro. Gamete Res 1988;19:291–303.
200. Fukui Y, Glew AM, Gandolfi F, Moor RM. In vitro culture of sheep oocytes matured and fertilized in vitro. Theriogenology 1988;29:883–891.
201. Fukui Y, Glew AM, Gandolfi F, Moore RM. Ram specific effects on in vitro fertilization and cleavage of sheep oocytes matured in vitro. J Reprod Fertil 1988;82:337–340.
202. Huneau D, Crozet N. In vitro fertilization in the sheep: effect of elevated calcium concentration at insemination. Gamete Res 1989;23:119–125.
203. Cognie Y, Guerin Y, Guyader C, Poulin N, Crozet N. In vitro fertilization of sheep oocytes matured in vivo. Theriogenology 1991;35:393–400.
204. Wang S, Liu Y, Holyoak GR, Evans RC, Bunch TD. A protocol for in vitro maturation and fertilization of sheep oocytes. Sm Ruminant Res 1998;29:83–88.
205. Cognie Y, Benoit F, Poulin N, Khatir H, Driancourt MA. Effect of follicle size and of the Fec^B Booroola gene on oocyte function in sheep. J Reprod Fertil 1998;112:379–386.
206. Gomez MC, Catt JW, Gillan L, Evans G, Maxwell WM. Effect of culture, incubation and acrosome reaction of fresh and frozen-thawed ram spermatozoa for in vitro fertilization and intracytoplasmic sperm injection. Reprod Fertil Dev 1997;9:665–673.
207. Hanada A. In vitro fertilization in goat. Jpn J Anim Reprod 1985;31:21–26.
208. Song HB, Iritani A. In vitro fertilization of goat follicular oocytes with epididymal spermatozoa capacitated in a chemically defined medium. Proc 3rd AAAP Anim Sci Congr Seoul, Korea 1981;1:463.
209. Younis AI, Zuelke KA, Harper KM, Oliveira MAL, Brackett BG. In vitro fertilization of goat oocytes. Biol Reprod 1991;44:1177–1182.
210. De Smedt V, Crozet N, Ahmed-Ali M, Martino A, Cognie Y. In vitro maturation and fertilization of goat oocytes. Theriogenology 1991;37:1049–1060.
211. Chauhan MS, Anand SR. In vitro maturation and fertilization of goat oocytes. Indian J Exp Biol 1991;29:105–110.
212. Keskintepe L, Darwish GM, Younis AI, Brackett BG. In vitro development of morulae from immature caprine oocytes. Zygote 1994;2:97–102.
213. Keskintepe L, Darwish GM, Kenimer AT, Brackett BG. Term development of caprine embryos derived from immature oocytes in vitro. Theriogenology 1994;42:527–535.

214. Keskintepe L, Luvoni GC, Rzucidlo SJ, Brackett BG. Procedural improvements for in vitro production of viable uterine stage caprine embryos. Sm Ruminant Res 1996;20:247–254.

215. Keskintepe L, Simplicio AA, Brackett BG. Caprine blastocyst development after in vitro fertilization with spermatozoa frozen in different extenders. Theriogenology 1998;49:1265–1274.

216. Poulin N, Guler A, Pignon P, Cognie Y. In vitro production of goat embryos: heparin in IVF medium affects developmental ability. Proc VI Intl Conf on Goats. Beijing, China, Vol. 2, May 6–11, 1996, p. 838.

217. Keskintepe L, Morton PC, Smith SE, Tucker MJ, Simplicio AA, Brackett BG. Caprine blastocyst formation following intracytoplasmic sperm injection and defined culture. Zygote 1997;5:261–265.

218. Palmer E, Bezard J, Magistrini M, Duchamp G. In vitro fertilization in the horse: A retrospective study. J Reprod Fertil 1991;44:375–384.

219. Bezard J. In vitro fertilization in the mare. Proc Intl Sci Conf Biotechnics Horse Reprod Agricultural University of Krakow, Poland, 1992, p. 12.

220. Squires EL, Wilson JM, Kato H, Blaszczyk A. A pregnancy after intracytoplasmic sperm injection into equine oocytes matured in vitro. Theriogenology 1996;45:306.

221. Dell'Aquila ME, Cho YS, Minoia P, Traina V, Fusco S, Lacalandra GM, Maritato F. Intracytoplasmic sperm injection (ICSI) versus conventional IVF on abattoir-derived and in vitro-matured equine oocytes. Theriogenology 1997;47:1139–1156.

222. Dell'Aquila ME, Cho YS, Minoia P, Traina V, Lacalandra GM, Maritato F. Effects of follicular fluid supplementation of in-vitro maturation medium on the fertilization and development of equine oocytes after in-vitro fertilization or intracytoplasmic sperm injection. Human Reprod 1997;12:2766–2772.

223. Grondahl C, Hansen TH, Hossaini A, Heinze I, Greve T, Hyttel P. Intracytoplasmic sperm injection of in vitro-matured equine oocytes. Biol Reprod 1997;57:1495–1501.

224. McKinnon AO, Lacham-Kaplan O, Trounson AO. Pregnancies produced from fertile and infertile stallions by intracytoplasmic sperm injection (ICSI) of single frozen/thawed spermatozoa into in vivo-matured mare oocytes. Proc 7th Intl Symp Equine Reprod 1998;137.

225. Cochran R, Meintjes M, Regio B, Hyland D, Carter J, Pinto C, Paccamonti D, Graff KJ, Godke RA. In vitro development and transfer of in vitro derived embryos produced from sperm injected oocytes harvested from pregnant mares. Proc 7th Intl Symp Equine Reprod 1998;136.

226. Squires EL, McCue PM, Vanderwall D. The current status of equine embryo transfer. Theriogenology 1999;51:91–104.

227. Schmid RL, Kato H, Herickhoff LA, Schenk JL, McCue PM, Chung Y-G, Squires EL. Fertilization with sexed equine spermatozoa using intracytoplasmic sperm injection and oviductal insemination. Proc 7th Intl Symp Equine Reprod 1998;139–140.

228. Mahi CA, Yanagimachi R. Maturation and sperm penetration of canine ovarian oocytes in vitro. J Exp Zool 1976;196:189–196.

229. Mahi CA, Yanagimachi R. Capacitation, acrosome reaction and egg penetration by canine spermatozoa in a simple defined medium. Gamete Res 1978;1:101–109.

230. Yamada S, Shimazu Y, Kawaji H, Nakazawa M, Naito K, Toyoda Y. Maturation, fertilization, and development of dog oocytes in vitro. Biol Reprod 1992;46:853–858.

231. CITES. Convention on International Trade of Endangered Species of Wild Flora and Fauna. 10th Meeting of the Conference of the Parties. Harare, Zimbabwe, 1997.

232. Bowen RA. Fertilization in vitro of feline ova by spermatozoa from the ductus deferens. Biol Reprod 1977;17:144–147.

233. Niwa K, Ohara K, Hosoi Y, Iritani A. Early events of in vitro fertilization of cat eggs by epididymal spermatozoa. J Reprod Fertil 1985;74:657–660.

234. Goodrowe KL, Wall RJ, O'Brien SJ, Schmidt PM, Wildt DE. Developmental competence of domestic cat follicular oocytes after fertilization in vitro. Biol Reprod 1988;39:355–372.

235. Pope CE, McRae MA, Plair BL, Keller GL, Dresser BL. In vitro and in vivo development of embryos produced by in vitro maturation and in vitro fertilization of cat oocytes. J Reprod Fertil 1997;51:69–82.

236. Kanda M, Miyazaki T, Kanda M, Nakao H, Tsutsui T. Development of in vitro fertilized feline embryos in a modified Earle's balanced salt solution: influence of protein supplements and culture dishes on fertilization success and blastocyst formation. J Vet Med Sci 1998;60:423–431.

237. Wrenzycki C, Herrmann D, Carnwath JW, Niemann H. Expression of RNA from developmentally important genes in preimplantation bovine embryos produced in TCM supplemented with BSA. J Reprod Fertil 1998;112:387–398.

238. Greve T, Callesen H, Hyttel P, Avery B. From oocyte to calf: in vivo and in vitro. In: Greppi GF, Enne G, eds. Animal Production and Biotechnology. Elsevier, Paris, 1994, pp. 71–97.

239. Wrenzycki C, Herrmann D, Carnwath JW, Niemann H. Expression of the gap junction gene connexin 43 (Cx43) in preimplantation bovine embryos derived in vitro or in vivo. J Reprod Fertil 1996;108: 17–24.

240. Kruip ThAM, denDaas JHG. In vitro produced and cloned embryos: effects on pregnancy, parturition and offspring. Theriogenology 1997;47:43–52.

241. Thompson JG, Gardner KD, Pugh PA, McMillan WH, Tervit HR. Lamb birth weight is affected by culture system utilized during in vitro pre-elongation development of ovine embryos. Biol Reprod 1995;53:1385–1391.

242. Keefer CL, Younis AI, Brackett BG. Cleavage development of bovine oocytes fertilized by sperm injection. Mol Reprod Develop 1990;25:281–285.

243. Heuwieser W, Yang X, Jiang S, Foote RH. Fertilization of bovine oocytes after microsurgical injection of spermatozoa. Theriogenology 1992;38:1–9.

244. Heuwieser W, Yang X, Jiang S, Foote RH. A comparison between in vitro fertilization and micro-injection of immobilized spermatozoa from bulls producing spermatozoa with defects. Mol Reprod Develop 1992;33:489–491.

245. Rho GJ, Kawarsky S, Johnson WH, Kochhar K, Betteridge KJ. Sperm and oocyte treatments to improve the formation of male and female pronuclei and subsequent development following intracyto-plasmic sperm injection into bovine oocytes. Biol Reprod 1998;59:918–924.

246. Looney CR, Lindsey BR, Gonseth CL, Johnson DL. Commercial aspects of oocyte retrieval and in vitro fertilization (IVF) for embryo production in problem cows. Theriogenology 1994;41:67–72.

247. Hasler JF, Henderson WB, Hurtgen PJ, Jin ZQ, McCauley AD, Mower SA et al. Production, freezing and transfer of bovine IVF embryos and subsequent calving results. Theriogenology 1995;43: 141–152.

248. Van Soom A, de Kruif A. Oocyte maturation, sperm capacitation and pre-implantation development in the bovine: implications for in vitro production of embryos. Reprod Dom Anim 1996;31:687–701.

249. Pieterse MC, Kappen KA, Kruip TAM, Taverna MAM. Aspiration of bovine oocytes during transvaginal ultrasound scanning of the ovaries. Theriogenology 1988;30:751–761.

250. Taneja M, Yang X. Promises and problems of in vitro production of embryos by TVOR-IVF scheme in cows and heifers. Embryo Transfer Newslett 1998;16:10–12.

251. Thibier M. The 1997 embryo transfer statistics from around the world: a data retrieval committee report. Embryo Transfer Newslett 1998;16:17–20.

252. Bousquet D, Twagiramungu H, Morin N, Brisson C, Carboneau G, Durocher J. In vitro embryo production in the cow: an effective alternative to the conventional embryo production approach. Theriogenology 1999;51:59–70.

253. Herr CM, Reed KC. Micromanipulation of bovine embryos for sex determination. Theriogenology 1991;35:45–54.

254. Kajihara Y, Blakewood EG, Meyers MN, Kometani N, Goto K, Godke RA. In vitro maturation and fertilization of follicular oocytes obtained from calves. Theriogenology 1991;35:220.

255. Armstrong DT, Holm P, Irvine B, Petersen BA, Stubbings RB, McLean D, et al. Pregnancies and live birth from in vitro fertilization of calf oocytes collected by laparoscopic follicular aspiration. Theriogenology 1992;38:667–678.

256. Armstrong DT, Kotaras PJ, Earl, CR. Advances in production of embryos in vitro from juvenile and prepubertal oocytes from calf and lamb. Reprod Fertil Dev 1997;9:333–339.

257. Cran DG, Johnson LA, Miller NGA, Cochrane D, Polge C. Production of bovine calves following separation of X- and Y-chromosome bearing sperm and in vitro fertilisation. Vet Rec 1993;132:40–41.

258. Ryan DP, Blakewood EG, Swanson WF, Rodrigues H, Godke RA. The use of follicle stimulating hormone (FSH) to stimulate follicle development for in vitro fertilization during the first trimeter of pregnancy in cattle. Theriogenology 1990;33:315.

259. Solti L, Machaty Z, Barandi Z, Torok M, Vajta G. IVF embryos of known parental origin from the endangered Hungarian grey cattle breed. Theriogenology 1992;37:301.

260. Goto K, Kinoshita A, Takuma Y, Ogawa K. Fertilization of bovine oocytes by the injection of immobilized, killed spermatozoa. Vet Rec 1990;127:517–520.

261. Krimpenfort P, Rademakers A, Eyestone W, van der Schans A, van den Broek S, Kooiman P, et al. Generation of transgenic dairy cattle using "in vitro" embryo production. Bio/Technology 1991;9: 844–847.

262. Stice SL, Robl JM, Ponce de Leon FA, Jerry J, Golueke PG, Cibelli JB, Kane JJ. Cloning: new breakthroughs leading to commercial opportunities. Theriogenology 1998;49:129–138.
263. Trounson A, Gunnl I, Lacham-Kaplan O, Lewis I, McKinnon A, Peura T, Shaw J. Manipulation of development: opportunities for animal breeding. In: Lauria A, Gandolfi F, Enne G, Gianaroli L, eds. Gametes: Development and Function. Serono Symposia, Rome, 1998, pp. 485–499.
264. Bautista JAN, Kanagawa H. Current status of vitrification of embryos and oocytes in domestic animals: Ethylene glycol as an emerging cryoprotectant of choice. Jpn J Vet Res 1998;45:183–191.
265. Vajta G, Booth PJ, Holm P, Greve T, Callesen H. Successful vitrification of early stage bovine in vitro produced embryos with the open pulled straw (OPS) method. Cryo-Letters 1997;18:191–195.
266. Martino A, Songasen N, Leibo SP. Development into blastocysts of bovine oocytes cryopreserved by ultra-rapid cooling. Biol Reprod 1996;54:1059–1069.
267. Mogas T, Keskintepe L, Younis AI, Brackett BG. Effects of EGTA and slow freezing of bovine oocytes on post-thaw development in vitro. Mol Reprod Develop 1999;52:86–98.
268. Gadea J, Matas C, Lucas X. Prediction of porcine semen fertility by homologous in vitro penetration (hIVP) assay. Anim Reprod Sci 1998;56:95–108.
269. Xu X, Pommier S, Arbov T, Hutchings B, Sotto W, Foxcroft GR. In vitro maturation and fertilization techniques for assessment of semen quality and boar fertility. J Anim Sci 1998;76:3079–3089.
270. Abeydeera LR, Johnson LA, Welch GR, Wang WH, Boquest AC, Cantley TC, et al. Birth of piglets preselected for gender following in vitro fertilization of in vitro matured pig oocytes by X and Y chromosome bearing spermatozoa sorted by high speed flow cytometry. Theriogenology 1998;50:981–988.
271. Prather RS, Rieke A, Day BN. Non-surgical embryo transfer in pigs: introduction of new genetics with little risk of disease transmission. Embryo Transfer Newslett 1998;16:14–16.
272. Loskutoff NM, Betteridge KJ. Embryo technology in pets and endangered species. In: Lauria A, Gandolfi F, eds. Embryonic Development and Manipulation in Animal Production. Portland Press, Chapel Hill, NC, 1992, pp. 235–248.
273. Bainbridge DRJ, Jabbour HN. Potential of assisted breeding techniques for the conservation of endangered mammalian species in captivity: a review. Vet Rec 1998;143:159–168.
274. Pope CE, Gelwicks DJ, Wachs KB, Keller G, Maruska EJ, Dresser BL. Successful interspecies transfer of embryos from the Indian desert cat (Felis silvestrus ornata) to the domestic cat (Felis catus) following in vitro fertilization. Biol Reprod 1989;40:61.
275. Donoghue AM, Johnston LA, Seal US, Armstrong DL, Tilson RL, Wolf P, et al. In vitro fertilization and embryo development in vitro and in vivo in the tiger (Panthera tigris). Biol Reprod 1990;43:733–744.
276. Meintjes M, Bezuidenhout C, Bartels P, Visser DS, Meintjes J, Loskutoff NM, et al. In vitro maturation and fertilization of oocytes recovered from free-ranging Burchell's zebra (Equus burchelli) and Hartmann's zebra (Equus zebra hartmannae). J Zoo Wildl Med 1997;28:251–259.
277. Roth TL, Weiss RB, Buff JL, Bush LM, Wildt DE, Bush M. Heterologous in vitro fertilization and sperm capacitation in an endangered African antelope, the scimitar-horned oryx (Oryx dammah). Biol Reprod 1998;58:475–482.

3

Control of Oocyte Nuclear and Cytoplasmic Maturation

Gary D. Smith

CONTENTS

INTRODUCTION
DEFINITIONS
SOMATIC CELL REGULATION
INTRA-OOCYTE SIGNALS REGULATING NUCLEAR MATURATION
REVERSIBLE PHOSPHORYLATION AND NUCLEAR MATURATION
CONTROL OF CYTOOPLASMIC MATURATION
ACKNOWLEDGMENTS
REFERENCES

INTRODUCTION

The ultimate goals of sexual reproduction are propagation of the species and integration of genetic diversity. Central to these goals are growth, development, and chromosomal modifications within the oocyte that yield a gamete capable of fertilization and supporting development of a genetically unique offspring. During early fetal development in mammals, primordial germ cells migrate to the genital ridge and differentiate into oogonia. These oogonia undergo proliferation as a result of numerous mitotic divisions. During late fetal development, mitosis ceases and oocytes enter the first meiotic division. Mammalian oocytes become arrested at prophase I of meiosis during this fetal stage of development and are termed primary oocytes. Meiosis only occurs in male and female germ cells and reduces the number of chromosomes from diploid to haploid. In addition, chromatin crossing-over and homologous recombination occur during early stages of meiosis resulting in the "genetic individuality" of each gamete. At puberty and during adulthood, completion of the first meiotic division occurs only after the oocyte and its surrounding follicle has undergone extensive growth. Following completion of meiosis I, the oocyte will undergo asymmetric cytokinesis yielding a secondary oocyte and a polar body. At this point in development, the oocyte will again enter an arrested meiotic state until the oocyte is penetrated by the spermatozoan. This sperm-induced resumption of

From: *Contemporary Endocrinology: Assisted Fertilization and Nuclear Transfer in Mammals*
Edited by: D. P. Wolf and M. Zelinski-Wooten © Humana Press Inc., Totowa, NJ

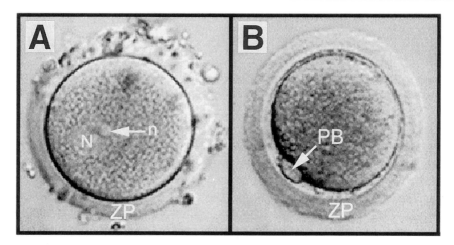

Fig. 1. Photomicrograph of macaque oocytes at different stages of nuclear maturation. (**A**) Fully grown, meiotically-competent, GV-intact oocyte. (**B**) Oocyte that has resumed nuclear maturation, undergone GVB and developed to MII. N, nucleus; n, nucleolus; PB, polar body; ZP, zona pellucida. Note: oocytes are approx110 m in diameter.

meiosis II, also termed oocyte activation, produces a haploid chromosomal complement within the oocyte that is now capable of combining with the sperm's haploid set of chromosomes at syngamy, which results in the diploid zygote. Thus, oocyte maturation is defined as reinitiation of the first meiotic division, progression to metaphase II (MII), and the accompanying cytoplasmic processes occurring within the oocyte that are essential for fertilization and that support early embryo development. From this definition, one can appreciate that both nuclear and cytoplasmic regulations of oocyte maturation are important. In addition, it is becoming increasingly apparent that nuclear and cytoplasmic maturation are not separate entities. There are intricate interactions between these two processes that must occur to support the entire oocyte maturation process. This chapter will address the extrinsic and intracellular regulation of nuclear and cytoplasmic oocyte maturation.

DEFINITIONS

Nuclear Maturation

Oocyte nuclear maturation can be defined as nuclear alterations that take place during the resumption of meiosis producing a haploid chromosomal complement from the previous diploid state. Oocytes arrested at prophase I of meiosis are characterized, at the light microscope level, as having a visible nucleus, also referred to as the germinal vesicle (GV; Fig. 1A). Within the GV is a centrally or peripherally located nucleolus. At meiosis resumption, the most visually recognizable characteristic of the oocyte is the dissolution of the nuclear envelope or breakdown of the GV. Once germinal vesicle breakdown (GVB) is initiated, chromatin within the nucleus condenses into discrete bivalents that align on the meiotic spindle at metaphase I (MI). During anaphase and telophase I, bivalents separate. This separation is complete at MII, which is recognizable at the light microscope level by the presence of the first polar body (Fig. 1B). It is at this point that meiosis again is arrested, awaiting the signal to resume in concert with sperm penetration and the activation of development.

Cytoplasmic Maturation

Whereas nuclear maturation is quite easy to define due to changes in visible characteristics, cytoplasmic maturation is more difficult to understand due to lack of knowledge and absence of definable attributes. Cytoplasmic maturation can be described as processes modifying the oocyte cytoplasm, which are essential for fertilization and developmental competence. Central to the concept of cytoplasmic maturation is the production and presence of specific factors, the relocation of cytoplasmic organelles and the post-transcriptional modification of mRNA's that have accumulated during oogenesis.

Meiotic Competence

In the 1930s Drs. Pincus and Enzmann *(1)* first described the process of spontaneous maturation of mammalian oocytes when they demonstrated that oocytes and/or oocyte-cumulus complexes could be removed from antral follicles and, under appropriate culture conditions, matured to MII. These oocytes are considered to display meiotic competence. However, oocytes from preantral follicles cultured under the same conditions do not mature, and thus exhibit meiotic incompetence. Acquisition of meiotic competence is correlated with oocyte size *(2)*, follicular morphology *(3)*, and species-dependent pre-pubertal chronological age *(2)*. Moreover, oocytes undergo at least two distinct phases of development, a growth phase and a meiotic maturation phase. As oocytes near the completion of their growth phase they become competent to resume meiosis. Acquisition of meiotic competence is also a sequential event *(4–6)*. When fully-grown oocytes first acquire the ability to undergo GVB, they are unable to complete nuclear maturation to MII and become arrested at or around MI. At more advanced developmental states, oocytes are capable of both GVB and progression to MII.

Identification of molecular differences between oocytes of differing meiotic competence is an area of active research in many laboratories; nevertheless, regulators involved in this process have not been clearly defined. GVB-incompetent oocytes display a size-dependent sensitivity to the serine/threonine protein phosphatase inhibitor okadaic acid (OA; for further discussion, *see* section on Reversible Phosphorylation), whereby only larger GVB-incompetent oocytes undergo GVB after OA treatment *(7)*. The use of DNA-binding fluorochromes and immunocytochemistry has relinquished information regarding intracellular morphological differences between GVB-incompetent and -competent oocytes. Chromatin within the nucleus of GVB-incompetent oocytes is diffusely distributed with little heterochromatin foci surrounding the nucleoli, whereas in GVB-competent oocytes, chromatin forms a dense ring adjacent to the nucleoli *(8)*. Microtubular structures also vary with respect to meiotic competence. GVB-incompetent oocytes contain microtubules throughout the cytoplasm with abundant perinuclear arrays. Conversely, GVB-competent oocytes display a reduction in cytoplasmic microtubules accompanied by dense microtubular organizing centers at the nuclear periphery *(9)*. Recently, differences in intracellular trafficking, and thus location of specific molecules, have been investigated in relation to meiotic competence. Both maturation promoting factor (MPF) *(10)* and protein phosphatase-1 (PP1) *(11)* translocate from the cytoplasm to the nucleus in correlation with acquisition of meiotic competence. These observations may help to explain why some larger, more developed GVB-incompetent oocytes display sensitivity to MPF-stimulated *(12)* and PP-inhibited *(13)* resumption of meiosis. The involvement of MPF and PP1 will be discussed in greater detail in the section entitled Reversible Phosphorylation.

SOMATIC CELL REGULATION

Pivotal to understanding control of oocyte maturation is the recognition of mechanisms that control meiotic arrest and those that trigger meiotic resumption. In both situations one cannot consider the oocyte alone; the relationship and interactions between the oocyte and its follicular environment must be appreciated. Ongoing cell-cell communication is critical to the maintenance of meiotic arrest *(14,15)*, whereas disruption of communication is associated with the preovulatory surge of luteinizing hormone (LH) or human chorionic gonadotropin (hCG) administration *(16–19)*. This LH-induced breakdown in communication corresponds with the resumption of meiosis *(14)*. Within the follicle the developing oocyte maintains direct communication with cumulus and mural granulosa cells by way of gap junctions *(20)*, specialized regions in closely opposed membranes of adjacent cells that mediate cell-to-cell communication *(21,22)*. These junctions allow exchange of small nutrients and signal molecules up to 1 kDa in size, and thus coordinate metabolic and electrical coupling between interconnected cells *(23)*. Recently several different gap junctional proteins termed connexins have been identified. Within the ovary, specifically in granulosa and cumulus cells, the primary gap-junction protein is connexin-43 *(24,25)*.

The transition from oocyte meiotic arrest to resumption of meiosis may be due to the blockage of gap junctions between the oocyte and follicular cells *(26)*. Ganot and Dekel *(27)* have demonstrated that LH can modify the gating activity of connexin-43 in ovarian follicles by two mechanisms. The initial response to LH involves phosphorylation of connexin-43 and a reduction in the gating properties. The secondary response is manifested by a reduction in connexin-43 protein levels due to attenuation of its gene expression *(27)*. This information is the premise for a theory by which LH stimulates resumption of oocyte meiosis (Fig. 2). In this scenario, the preovulatory surge of LH, acting through both protein kinase A (PKA) and C (PKC) pathways, causes phosphorylation of connexin-43 resulting in a breakdown in communication between the oocyte and follicle cells, thus blocking delivery to the oocytes of a somatic cell factor that maintains meiotic arrest. Without the meiosis-arresting factor, the oocyte resumes meiosis and progresses to MII, the developmental stage at which the oocyte usually is ovulated.

INTRA-OOCYTE SIGNALS
REGULATING NUCLEAR MATURATION

Determination of the specific somatic cell signal(s) that maintains meiotic arrest has yet to be reported. In addition, there is still the possibility that a positive regulator of meiosis resumption originates from follicular cells and acts upon the oocyte. If such a positive regulator exists, it too remains to be elucidated. However, recent evidence suggests that C_{29} sterols can induce resumption of meiosis and thus may be physiological activators of meiosis *(28)*. Independent of the somatic cell signal, information has accumulated with respect to intra-oocyte signals that maintain meiotic arrest and are altered at meiosis resumption. Several lines of evidence support the hypothesis that elevated levels of intracellular cyclic adenosine monophosphate (cAMP) are involved in maintenance of meiotic arrest in GVB-competent oocytes. The following is a cursory review of research that supports this theory. Treatment of oocytes from antral follicles with membrane-permeable analogs of cAMP will maintain meiotic arrest in these oocytes that

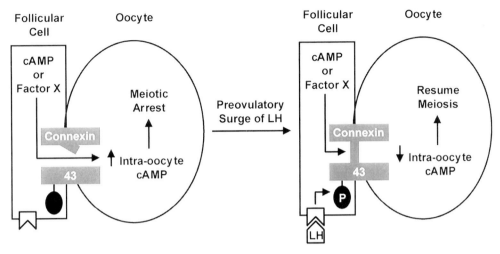

Fig. 2. Schematic diagram representing the theoretical mechanism by which the preovulatory surge of luteinizing hormone (LH) stimulates in vivo resumption of meiosis. When connexin 43, a gap junctional protein, is in a dephosphorylated state, the communication between the follicular cells and the oocytes are open. This allows cAMP and/or some unknown factor (Factor X) to enter the oocyte and maintain elevated (upward arrow) intra-oocyte cAMP, resulting in meiotic arrest. During the midcycle gonadotropin surge LH bind to its receptor in the granulosa cell membrane stimulating the PKA and/or PKC second messenger pathways, ultimately resulting in the phosphorylation of connexin-43. Phosphorylated (P) connexin-43 is believed to undergo a conformational change that closes the gap junction and nullifies the communication between the follicular cells and the oocyte. This results in a decrease (down arrow) in intra-oocyte cAMP that allows the resumption of meiosis.

would otherwise spontaneously resume meiosis *(29,30)*. GVB–competent oocytes can be maintained in meiotic arrest in vitro in the presence of forskolin *(31,32)*, a pharmacological agent that directly stimulates adenylate cyclase, which in turn converts ATP to cAMP. Thus, forskolin catalyzes the production of cAMP, thereby elevating intracellular levels within isolated oocytes, and maintains meiotic arrest in culture for a short period of time. Preventing the reduction of intracellular cAMP that normally accompanies in vitro spontaneous resumption of meiosis, by blocking cAMP phosphodiesterases, also prevents GVB *(33)*. 3-Isobutyl-1-methylxanthine (IBMX) is a phosphodiesterase inhibitor commonly used in such experiments. Lastly, microinjection of oocytes with the catalytic subunit of PKA also inhibits spontaneous GVB *(34)*, and microinjection of an inhibitor of the PKA catalytic subunit induces GVB in oocytes maintained in meiotic arrest in vitro in the presence of IBMX *(34)*. Collectively, these findings suggest that phosphorylation of proteins by the PKA cascade mediates the action of cAMP in the maintenance of meiotic arrest.

Although the aforementioned results strongly support the role of intra-oocyte cAMP in the regulation of nuclear maturation, the focus has been on in vitro maturation and the use of pharmacological agents. These results may not represent the physiologic mechanisms regulating in vivo meiotic arrest and resumption of meiosis. To address this issue, Eppig and colleagues conducted experiments using a follicular culture system in which oocytes were maintained in meiotic arrest by the endogenous physiological pathways of surrounding follicular cells *(35)*. A membrane-permeable antagonist of cAMP, Rp-adenosine-3'5'-cyclic phosphorothioate, was administered to antral follicles in culture, inducing oocyte GVB and leading to the conclusion that a cAMP-dependent pathway participates in the endogenous physiological mechanism maintaining meiotic arrest.

Although evidence for the importance of cAMP pathways in maintenance of meiotic arrest is compelling, the possible role of additional mechanisms cannot be ignored including the PKC system (36), inositol 1,4,5-triphosphate and calcium (for review, see ref. 37), cyclic guanosine monophosphate (38), and purines (for review, see ref. 39). It is quite possible that multiple pathways assist in the maintenance of meiotic arrest, with one pathway being predominant, and others functioning as backup systems. In addition, the relative importance of a particular pathway may be species-dependent.

The next question that arises concerns the origin of intra-oocyte cAMP: is this cAMP produced by the oocyte and/or is it derived from surrounding follicular cells? Oocytes of several species possess adenylate cyclase and produce cAMP in response to forskolin stimulation (40,41). However, whether the oocyte is capable of producing sufficient amounts of cAMP to maintain meiotic arrest is unknown. Evidence exists to suggest that oocyte cAMP also could originate from surrounding follicle cells and be imported through intact gap junctions (17,42,43). The importance of each of these two pathways in maintaining elevated intra-oocyte cAMP, and thus blocking GVB, has not been resolved.

REVERSIBLE PHOSPHORYLATION AND NUCLEAR MATURATION

Regardless of the somatic cell signal, or lack thereof, that initiates GVB, nuclear maturation appears to require reversible protein phosphorylation, a process that is recognized as a major intracellular mechanism in a wide range of eukaryotic cellular events (44). Monumental advances in the understanding of cell signaling have resulted from research characterizing protein kinases and phosphatases and their influences on cellular processes. In this review, we will first consider the kinases, then the phosphatases, and end with a discussion focused on their interactions and specific phosphorylation events implicated in the regulation of meiosis.

MPF was first identified in amphibian oocytes (45,46) and since has been discovered in oocytes of many species and eukaryotic somatic cells undergoing mitosis (47,48). MPF is a complex of two major proteins of 34 and 45 kDa, which correspond to $p34^{cdc2}$ and cyclin B, respectively (49,50). Mammalian oocyte MPF activity has been measured by its ability to induce GVB in starfish oocytes (51) or to cause phosphorylation of histone H1 (52). The $p34^{cdc2}$ component is a serine/threonine kinase that requires dephosphorylation for activity (53), whereas cyclin B requires phosphorylation for activity (54). Protease control of cyclin B turnover has also been implicated in MPF regulation (55). Although the exact regulators of MPF activity remain obscure, it has been speculated that continual phosphorylation of cyclin B is necessary for stability and activity of MPF, and that dephosphorylation results in degradation of MPF (for review, see ref. 39). MPF activity fluctuates during oocyte meiotic progression. For example, MPF activity is undetectable in GV-intact oocytes, is detectable at GVB, peaks in MI oocytes, decreases dramatically during anaphase I and telophase I to low levels at first polar body extrusion, and peaks again at MII (51,52).

Mitogen-activated or microtubule-associated protein (MAP) kinase, also termed extracellular regulated kinase (ERK), is a serine/threonine kinase that has also been implicated in the regulation of oocyte meiosis. Mammalian oocytes possess at least two forms of MAP kinase, p42-ERK 2 and p44-ERK 1 *(56)*, which are regulated by phosphorylation at specific threonine and tyrosine residues *(57,58)*. In mouse oocytes, MAP kinase activity rises following GVB and, as opposed to MPF, remains high throughout maturation (between MI and MII) *(59)*. It has been suggested that MAP kinase plays a critical role in microtubule assembly and chromatin organization *(13,59,60)*. Specifically, MAP kinase activity correlates with bipolar spindle formation following GVB, is involved with maintaining microtubule M-phase configuration between MI and MII, and is related inversely to interphasic morphological organization of microtubules *(59,60)*.

Serine/threonine PP, which remove phosphate groups from phosphoproteins and thus antagonize protein kinases, also have been implicated in regulating oocyte nuclear maturation *(7,61–64)*. Classification of serine/threonine PPs is based on substrate specificity and response to a defined set of inhibitors and activators (for review, *see* ref. 65). Type 1 PP (PP1) is sensitive to heat- and acid-stable endogenous inhibitors, whereas type 2 PPs (PP2s) lack this sensitivity *(66)*. Type 2 PPs can be subclassified into PP2A, PP2B, and PP2C based on cation requirements for activity. An important discovery in phosphatase research was the identification of cell-permeable, PP-specific pharmacological inhibitors, such as OA and calyculin-a (CL-A) *(67)*. Both PP1 and PP2A are sensitive to OA and CL-A inhibition, whereas PP2B and PP2C are essentially insensitive to OA and CL-A *(67,68)*.

OA stimulates GVB in starfish *(69)*, Xenopus *(70,71)*, mouse (7,62,72,73), bovine *(74)*, and macaque *(64)* oocytes. This indicates that the PP involved in regulating oocyte nuclear maturation is PP1 and/or PP2A. Recently, monkey and mouse GVB-competent oocytes were reported to contain both PP1 and PP2A with intracellular localization predominantly nuclear and cytoplasmic, respectively *(11,64)*. Because Rimes and Ozon *(73)* found that OA stimulated GVB in oocytes arrested in the presence of dibutyl-cAMP, it has been speculated that the role of PPs in controlling nuclear maturation occurs between PKA and MPF stimulation. However, this does not preclude the possibility that PP acts downstream to MPF activation at specific phospho-acceptor sites within the oocyte.

Processes that occur in the oocyte during the transition from GV-intact to MII can be divided into at least four specific events, all of which are regulated by either MPF or MAP kinase phosphorylation, and probably by PP1 and/or PP2A dephosphorylation *(13, 75–77)*. These events are represented schematically in Fig. 3. First, GVB is initiated by phosphorylation of nuclear lamins, the major protein located under the nuclear envelope that is important for nuclear membrane integrity *(78)*. Concomitant with GVB, dissolution of the nucleolus occurs. Although this process has not been investigated during meiosis, studies during mitosis suggest that phosphorylation of nucleolar proteins is involved *(75)*. The third event is condensation of chromosomes stimulated by phosphorylation of chromosomal proteins including histones *(79)*. The fourth event involves microtubule nucleation, originating from the centrosomes or microtubule organizing centers, and leading to formation of the spindle apparatus.

The question arises as to the specific phosphorylation signal that triggers these events. In the oocyte and in other cell systems, it is becoming increasingly appreciated that one cannot consider just phosphorylation or dephosphorylation in intracellular phospho-regulated events. In some instances, the important issue is the degree of phosphorylation, which in turn is related to the state of equilibrium between kinase and phosphatase activity. The recent report of MPF in the nucleus of GVB-competent oocytes *(10)*, in conjunction with the presence of PP1 in the nucleus *(11,64)*, forms a basis for the following

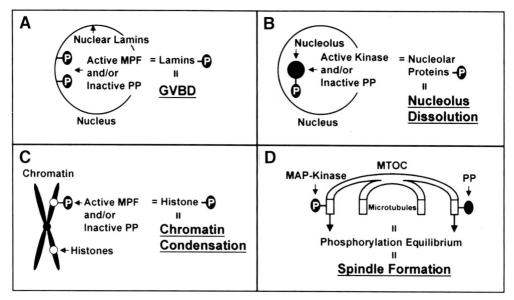

Fig. 3.   Schematic representation of intra-oocyte alterations that are believed to be regulated by reversible phosphorylation (P) during the resumption of meiosis. (**A**) Theoretical mechanism where protein kinase (MPF) and phosphatase (PP) interact resulting in the phosphorylation of nuclear lamins and stimulate GVB. (**B**) Kinase (unknown) and PP interaction that regulates phosphorylation of nucleolar proteins resulting in nucleolar dissolution. (**C**) Interaction between protein kinase (MPF) and PP inducing the phosphorylation of histones that ultimately results in chromatin condensation. (**D**) Relationship between protein kinase (microtubule-associated protein kinase; MAP-kinase) and PP in regulating phosphorylation of microtubule-associated proteins stimulating microtubule nucleation from the microtubule organizing centers (MTOC) and spindle formation. It appears that a state of phosphorylation equilibrium of microtubule-associated proteins is permissive for normal microtubule nucleation, whereas states of hyper-phosphorylation and hypo-phosphorylation are inhibitory.

scenario. As previously mentioned, during GVB a net phosphorylation of nuclear lamins occurs followed by disassembly of the nuclear envelope matrix *(78)*. If we assume that nuclear MPF is active in GVB-competent oocytes, we must ask what maintains the overall dephosphorylated state of nuclear lamins, and thus nuclear membrane integrity, prior to GVB. One explanation could involve nuclear MPF and PP1 acting in an antagonistic manner in the regulation of specific phospho-acceptor sites on nuclear lamins. Therefore, the phosphorylated state of nuclear lamins would depend on relative activities of MPF and PP1. The recent report that OA treatment bypasses the threshold level requirement of p34^{cdc2} kinase activity necessary for spontaneous meiotic resumption would support such a hypothesis *(12)*. This scenario of counteracting nuclear MPF and PP1 regulation of nuclear protein net phosphorylation could explain OA's stimulatory influence on GVB in GVB-competent *(7,60)* and -incompetent oocytes *(12,13)* and merits future investigation.

CONTROL OF CYTOPLASMIC MATURATION

As mentioned earlier, a clear understanding of cytoplasmic maturation is yet to be elucidated. In this section, the processes that comprise cytoplasmic maturation will be discussed in a sequential manner. Early investigators believed that cytoplasmic matura-tion was compromised during in vitro maturation (IVM) as manifested by low rates of fertilization and reduced embryonic developmental competence *(80)*. However, more recent reports have demonstrated that rodents and domestic animal species are capable of quite high fertilization rates and good embryonic development following spontane-ous maturation in culture *(81–83)*. Whether this is also the case in primates has yet to be resolved (*see* Chapters 4 and 16). The ability of oocytes to undergo sperm-induced activation and thus release intracellular stores of calcium is an example of cytoplasmic maturation. Experimentally this calcium release, in response to inositol triphosphate microinjection, is relatively low during early stages of maturation yet increases near the end of nuclear maturation *(84)*. The migration of cortical granules toward the periphery of the oocyte is a process that occurs during oocyte development *(85)* and is important for the release of their enzymatic contents upon sperm penetration. A cortical reaction is critical for the block to polyspermia and to ensure normal fertilization. Thus, intrac-ellular trafficking of cortical granules may be considered a component of cytoplasmic maturation. Once the sperm gains entry to the ooplasm, the sperm nucleus must decon-dense to support normal processing of the male pronucleus. This process involves reduc-tion of disulfide bonds between sperm chromatin–associated proteins. Glutathione has been implicated as the regulatory molecule for this process *(86)*. Formation of the male pronucleus is minimal in GV-intact compared to mature oocytes *(87)* and is caused by reduced levels of glutathione in immature oocytes *(88)*. This is just one specific example of a protein in the oocyte that changes in relation to oocyte function and progression through cytoplasmic maturation. Overall, qualitative and quantitative changes in protein synthesis have also been documented during oocyte maturation *(2,89)*. There are most likely several specific proteins that fluctuate during nuclear maturation that are critical for supporting cytoplasmic maturation. In addition to the production and accumulation of specific proteins during oogenesis, oocytes also acquire surplus mRNAs that are not necessarily translated, but are important during initial stages of embryogenesis, prior to the switch from maternal to embryonic control of development *(90)*. Thus, it is becoming increasingly apparent that essential components of cytoplasmic maturation during oogen-esis and nuclear maturation include transcription, mechanisms that regulate mRNA stability (post-transcriptional regulation), translation, and post-translational processing of specific factors that support early embryogenesis. These are areas that require further investigation to elucidate shortcomings of starting materials and/or culture systems used for IVM of oocytes.

In the past half-century, significant advancements have been made in understanding the endocrine, paracrine, and intracellular regulation of oocyte meiosis, specifically nuclear maturation. Cytoplasmic maturation, the area in which our knowledge is most lacking, may hold the keys to bridging the gap between oocyte meiosis basic science research and the clinical implementation of IVM as a human-assisted reproductive tech-nology. As will be discussed in the following chapter (*see* Chapter 4), IVM holds great promise as a human-assisted reproductive technology. However, currently the ultimate goal of live births following IVM/IVF does not occur at an acceptable rate in comparison to ovarian stimulation/IVF. Without complete knowledge of in vivo processes that regu-late oocyte nuclear and cytoplasmic maturation and embryonic developmental compe-tence, it will be quite difficult to identify, understand, and remedy the shortcomings within the human IVM systems. For this reason, it is imperative that basic science research on oocyte meiosis and IVM continue. The ultimate goal of this research should focus on acquisition of knowledge and implementation of this knowledge into clinical protocols that promote high live birth rates from IVM/IVF.

ACKNOWLEDGMENTS

I am very thankful for the critical reading of this manuscript by Dr. Carrie Cosola-Smith. Research on oocyte maturation in my laboratory is supported by grants HD35125 and HD38134 from the National Institute of Child Health and Human Development of the National Institutes of Health.

REFERENCES

1. Pincus G, Enzmann EV. The comparative behavior of mammalian eggs in vivo and in vitro. I. The activation of ovarian eggs. J Exp Med 1935;62:655–675.
2. Schultz RM, Wassarman PM. Biochemical studies of mammalian oogenesis: protein synthesis during oocyte growth and meiotic maturation in the mouse. J Cell Sci 1977;24:167–194.
3. Erickson GF Sorenson AC. In vitro maturation of mouse oocytes isolated from late, middle, and pre-antral Graafian follicles. J Exp Zool 1974;190:123–127.
4. Iwamatsu T, Yanagimachi R. Maturation in vitro of ovarian oocytes of prepubertal and adult hamsters. J Reprod Fert 1975;45:83–90.
5. Sorenson RA, Wassarman PM. Relationship between growth and meiotic maturation of the mouse oocyte. Dev Biol 1976;50:531–536.
6. Szybek K. In vitro maturation of oocytes from sexually immature mice. J Endocrinol 1972;54:527–528.
7. Gavin AC, Tsukitani Y, Schorderet-Slatkine S. Induction of M-phase entry of prophase-blocked mouse oocytes through microinjection of okadaic acid, a specific phosphatase inhibitor. Exp Cell Res 1991; 192:75–81.
8. Wickramasinghe D, Ebert KM, Albertini DF. Meiotic competence acquisition is associated with the appearance of M-phase characteristics in growing mouse oocytes. Dev Biol 1991;143:162–172.
9. Mattson BA, Albertini DF. Oogenesis: chromatin and microtubule dynamics during meiotic prophase. Mol Reprod Dev 1990;25:374–383.
10. Mitra J, Schultz RM. Regulation of the acquisition of meiotic competence in the mouse: changes in the subcellular localization of cdc2, cyclin B1, cdc 25 and wee1, and in the concentration of these proteins and their transcripts. J Cell Sci 1996;109:2407–2415.
11. Smith GD, Sadhu A, Mathies S, Wolf DP. Characterization of protein phosphatases in mouse oocytes. Dev Biol 1998;204:537–549.
12. de Vantery C, Gavin AC, Vassalli JD, Schorderet-Slatkine S. An accumulation of p34cdc2 at the end of mouse oocyte growth correlates with the acquisition of meiotic competence. Dev Biol 1996;174: 335–344.
13. Chesnel F, Eppig JJ. Induction of precocious germinal vesicle breakdown (GVB) by GVB-incompetent mouse oocytes: possible role of mitogen-activated protein kinases rather than p34^{cdc2} kinase. Biol Reprod 1995;52:895–902.
14. Sherizly I, Galiani D, Dekel N. Regulation of oocyte maturation: communication in the rat cumulus-oocyte complex. Human Reprod 1988;3:761–766
15. Racowsky C, Baldwin KV. In vitro and in vivo studies reveal that hamster oocyte meiotic arrest is maintained only transiently by follicular fluid, but persistently by membrane/cumulus granulosa cell contact. Dev Biol 1989;134:297–306.
16. Gilula NB, Epstein MC, Beers WH. Cell-to-cell communication and ovulation. A study of the cumulus-oocyte complex. J Cell Biol 1978;78:58–75.
17. Moor RM, Smith MW, Dawson RMC. Measurement of intracellular coupling between oocytes and cumulus cells using intracellular markers. Exp Cell Res 1980;126:15–29.
18. Eppig JJ. The relationship between cumulus-oocyte coupling, oocyte meiotic maturation, and cumulus expansion. Dev Biol 1982;89:268–272.
19. Larsen WJ, Wert SE, Brunner GD. Differential modulation of rat follicle cell gap junction populations at ovulation. Dev Biol 1987;122:61–71.

20. Dekel N. Interaction between the oocyte and the granulosa cells in the preovulatory follicle. In: Armstrong D, Freisen HG, Leung PCK, Moger W, Ruf KB, ed. Endocrinology and Physiology of Reproduction. Plenum, New York, NY, 1987, pp.197–209.
21. Gilula NB, Reeves OR, Steinbach A. Metabolic coupling, ionic coupling and cell contacts. Nature 1972; 235:262–265.
22. Loewenstein WR. Junctional intercellular communication: the cell-to-cell membrane channel. Physiol Rev 1981;61:829–913.
23. Pitts JD, Simms JW. Permeability of junctions between animal cells. Intercellular transfer of nucleotides but not of macromolecules. Exp Cell Res 1977;104:153–163.
24. Risek B, Guthrie S, Kumar N, Gilula NB. Modulation of gap junction transcript and protein expression during pregnancy. J Cell Biol 1990;110:269–282.
25. Wirsen JF, Midgley AR Jr. Changes in expression of connexin 43 gap junction messenger ribonucleic acid and protein during ovarian follicular growth. Endocrinology 1993;133:741–746.
26. Piontkewitz Y, Dekel N. Heptanol, an alkanol that blocks gap junctions, induces oocyte maturation. Endocrine J 1993;1:365–372.
27. Granot I, Dekel N. Phosphorylation and expression of connexin-43 ovarian gap junction protein are regulated by luteinizing hormone. J Biol Chem 1994;269:30502–30509.
28. Byskov AG, Andersen CY, Nordholm L, Thogersen H, Guoliang X, Wassmann O, et al. Chemical structure of sterols that activate oocyte meiosis. Nature 1995;374:559–562.
29. Cho WK, Stern S, Biggers JD. Inhibitory effect of dibutyryl cAMP on mouse oocyte maturation in vitro. J Exp Zool 1974;187:383–386.
30. Dekel N, Beers WH. Rat oocyte maturation in vitro: relief of cyclic AMP inhibition with gonadotropins. Proc Natl Acad Sci USA 1978;75:4369–4373.
31. Ekholm C, Hillensjo T, Magnusson C, Rosberg S. Stimulation and inhibition of rat oocyte meiosis by forskolin. Biol Reprod 1984;30:537–543.
32. Dekel N, Aberdam E, Sherizly I. Spontaneous maturation in vitro of cumulus-enclosed rat oocytes by forskolin. Biol Reprod 1984;31:244–250.
33. Schultz RM, Montgomery R, Belanoff J. Regulation of mouse oocyte maturation: implication of a decrease in oocyte cAMP and protein dephosphorylation in commitment to resume meiosis. Dev Biol 1983;97:264–273.
34. Bornslaeger EA, Mattei P, Schultz RM. Involvement of cAMP-dependent protein kinase and protein phosphorylation in regulation of mouse oocyte maturation. Dev Biol 1986;14:453–462.
35. Eppig JJ. Maintenance of meiotic arrest and the induction of oocyte maturation in mouse oocyte-granulosa cell complexes developed in vitro from preantral follicles. Biol Reprod 1991;45:824–830.
36. Urner F, Schoroderet-Slatkine S. Inhibition of denuded mouse oocyte meiotic maturation by tumor-promoting phorbol esters and its reversal by retinoids. Exp Cell Res 1984;154:600–605.
37. Homa S. Calcium and meiotic maturation of the mammalian oocyte. Mol Reprod Dev 1995;40:122–134.
38. Tornell J, Billig H, Hillensjo T. Resumption of rat oocyte meiosis is paralleled by a decrease in guanosine 3',5'-cyclic monophosphate (cGMP) and is inhibited by microinjection of cGMP. Acta Physiol Scan 1990;139:511–517.
39. Eppig JJ. Regulation of mammalian oocyte maturation. In: Adashi EY, Leung PCK, ed. The Ovary. Raven, New York, NY, 1993, pp.185–208.
40. Racowsky C. Effect of forskolin on the spontaneous maturation and cyclic AMP content of hamster oocyte-cumulus complexes. J Exp Zool 1985;234:87–96.
41. Kuyt JRM, Kruip TAM, DeJong-Brink M. Cytochemical localization of adenylate cyclase in bovine cumulus-oocyte complexes. Exp Cell Res 1988;174:139–145.
42. Albertini DF, Anderson E. The appearance and structure of the intercellular connections during the ontogeny of the rabbit ovarian follicle with special reference to gap junctions. J Cell Biol 1974;63:234–250.
43. Downs SM, Coleman DL, Eppig JJ. Maintenance of murine meiotic arrest: uptake and metabolism of hypoxanthine and adenosine by cumulus cell-enclosed and denuded oocytes. Dev Biol 1986;117:174–183.
44. Mumby MC, Walter G. Protein serine/threonine phosphatases: structure, regulation and functions in cell growth. Physiol Rev 1993;73:673–699.
45. Masui Y, Markert CL. Cytoplasmic control of nuclear behavior during meiotic maturation of frog oocytes. J Exp Zool 1971;177:129–146.
46. Ecker RE, Smith LD. The nature and fate of rana pipiens proteins synthesized during maturation and early cleavage. Dev Biol 1971;24:559–576.

47. Sunkara PS, Wright DA, Rao PN. Mitotic factors from mammalian cells induce germinal vesicle break-down and chromosome condensation in amphibian oocytes. Proc Natl Acad Sci USA 1979;76:2799–2802.
48. Kishimoto T, Kuriyama R, Kondo H, Kanatani H. Generality of the action of various maturation-promoting factors. Exp Cell Res 1982;137:121–126.
49. Gautier J, Norbury C, Lohka M, Nurse P, Maller J. Purified maturation-promoting factor contains the product of a Xenopus homolog of the fission yeast cell cycle control gene cdc2. Cell 1988;54:433–439.
50. Langan TA, Gautier J, Lohka M, Hollingsworth R, Moreno S, Nurse P, et al. Mammalian growth-associated H1 histone kinase: a homolog of cdc2+/CDC28 protein kinases controlling mitotic entry in yeast and frog cells. Mol Cell Biol 1989;9:3860–3868.
51. Hashimoto H, Kishimoto T. Regulation of meiotic metaphase by a cytoplasmic maturation-promoting factor during mouse oocyte maturation. Dev Biol 1988;126:242–252.
52. Naito K, Toyoda Y. Fluctuation of histone H1 kinase activity during meiotic maturation in porcine oocytes. J Reprod Fertil 1991;93:467–473.
53. Gautier J, Solomon MJ, Booher RN, Bazan JF, Kirschner MW. cdc25 is a specific tyrosine phosphatase that directly activates p34^{cdc2}. Cell 1991;67:197–211.
54. Roy LM, Singh B, Gautier J, Arlinghaus RB, Nordeen SK, Maller JL. The cyclin B2 component of MPF is a substrate of the c-mos proto-oncogene product. Cell 1990;61:825–831.
55. Sherwood SW, Kung AL, Roitelman J, Simoni RD, Schimke RT. In vivo inhibition of cyclin B degradation and induction of the cell-cycle arrest in mammalian cells by the neutral cysteine protease inhibitor N-acetylleucylnorleucinal. Proc Natl Acad Sci USA 1993;90:3353–3357.
56. Verlhac MH, de Pennart H, Maro B, Cobb MH, Clark HJ. MAP kinase becomes stably activated at metaphase and is associated with microtubule-organizing centers during meiotic maturation of mouse oocytes. Dev Biol 1993;158:330–340.
57. Payne D, Rossomando AJ, Martino P, Erickson AK, Her JH, Shabanowitz J, Hunt DF Weber MJ, Sturgill TW. Identification of the regulatory phosphorylation site in pp42/mitogen-activated protein kinase (MAP kinase). EMBO J 1991;10:885–892.
58. Seger R, Ahn NG, Boulton TG, Yancopoulos GD, Panayotatos N, Radziejewska E, et al. Microtubule-associated protein-2 kinase, ERK1 and ERK2, undergo autophosphorylation on both tyrosine and threonine residues: implications for their mechanism of activation. Proc Natl Acad Sci USA 1991;88:6142–6146.
59. Verlhac MH, Kubiac JZ, Clarke HJ, Maro B. Microtubule and chromatin behavior follow MAP kinase activity but not MPF activity during meiosis in mouse oocytes. Development 1994;120:1017–1025.
60. Verlhac MH, Kubiak JZ, Weber M, Geraud G, Colledge WH, Evans MJ, Maro B. Mos is required for MAP kinase activation and is involved in microtubule organization during meiotic maturation in the mouse. Dev Biol 1996;122:815–822.
61. Rime H, Ozon R. Protein phosphatases are involved in the in vivo activation of histone H1 kinase in mouse oocyte. Dev Biol 1990;141:115–122.
62. Schwartz DA, Schultz RM. Stimulatory effect of okadaic acid, an inhibitor of protein phosphatases, on nuclear envelope breakdown and protein phosphorylation in mouse oocytes and one-cell embryos. Dev Biol 1991;145:119–127.
63. Hampl A, Eppig, JJ. Translational regulation of the gradual increase in histone H1 kinase activity in maturing mouse oocytes. Mol Reprod Dev 1995;40:9–15.
64. Smith GD. Sadhu A, Wolf DP. Transient exposure of rhesus macaque oocytes to calyculin-a and okadaic acid stimulates germinal vesicle breakdown permitting subsequent development and fertilization. Biol Reprod 1998;58:880–886.
65. Cohen P. The structure and regulation of protein phosphatases. Annu Rev Biochem 1989;58:453–509.
66. Ingebritsen TS, Stewart AA, Cohen P. The protein phosphatases involved in cellular regulation. 6. Measurement of type-1 and type-2 protein phosphatases in extracts of mammalian tissues; an assessment of their physiological roles. Eur J Biochem 1983;132:297–307.
67. Ishihara H. Calyculin A and okadaic acid: inhibitors of protein phosphatase activity. Biochem Biophys Res Comm 1989;159:871–877.
68. Cohen P, Schelling DL, Stark MJR. Remarkable similarities between yeast and mammalian protein phosphatases. FEBS Lett 1989;250:601–606.
69. Pondaven P, Cohen P. Identification of protein phosphatases-1 and 2A and inhibitor-2 in oocytes of the starfish Asterias rubens and Marthasterias glacialis. Eur J Biochem 1987;167:135–140.

70. Goris J, Hermann J, Hendrix, Ozon R, Merlevede W. Okadaic acid, a specific protein phosphatase inhibitor, induces maturation and MPF formation in Xenopus laevis oocytes. FEBS 1989;245:91–94.

71. Rime H, Huchon D, Jessus C, Goris J, Merlevede W, Ozon R. Characterization of MPF activation by okadaic acid in xenopus oocyte. Cell Diff Dev 1990;29:47–58.

72. Alexandre H, Van Cauwenberge A, Tsukitani Y, Mulnard J. Pleiotropic effect of okadaic acid on maturing mouse oocytes. Development 1991;112:971–980.

73. Rime H, Ozon R. Protein phosphatases are involved in the in vivo activation of histone H1 kinase in mouse oocyte. Dev Biol 1990;141:115–122.

74. Levesque JT, Sirard MA. Effects of different kinases and phosphatases on nuclear and cytoplasmic maturation of bovine oocytes. Mol Reprod Develop 1995;42:114–121.

75. Peter M, Nakagawa J, Doree M, Labbe JC, Nigg EA. Identification of major nucleolar proteins as candidate mitotic substrates of cdc2 kinase. Cell 1990;60:791–801.

76. Adlakha RC, Rao PN. Molecular mechanisms of the chromosomal condensation and decondensation cycle in mammalian cells. BioEssays 1986;5:100–105.

77. Bailly E, Pines J, Hunter T, Bornens M. Cytoplasmic accumulation of cyclin-B1 in human cells: association with a detergent-resistant compartment and with the centrosome. J Cell Sci 1992;101:529–545.

78. Nigg EA. The nuclear envelope. Curr Opin Cell Biol 1989;1:435–440.

79. Bradbury EM, Inglis RJ, Matthews HR. Molecular basis of control of mitotic cell division in eukaryotes. Nature 1974;249:553–556.

80. Thibault C. Are follicular maturation and oocyte maturation independent processes? J Reprod Fert 1977; 51:1–15.

81. Schroeder AC, Eppig JJ. The developmental capacity of mouse oocyte matured spontaneously in vitro is normal. Dev Biol 1984;102:493–497

82. Vanderhyden BC, Armstrong DT. Role of cumulus cells and serum on the in vitro maturation, fertilization and subsequent development of rat oocytes. Biol Reprod 1989;40:720–728.

83. Sirard MA, Parrish JJ, Ware CB, Leibfried-Rutledge ML, First NL. The culture of bovine oocytes to obtain developmentally competent embryos. Biol Reprod 1988;39:546–552.

84. Fujiwara T, Nakada K, Shirakawa H, Miyazaki S. Development of inositol trisphosphate-induced calcium release mechanism during maturation of hamster oocytes. Dev Biol 1993;156:69–79.

85. Ducibella T, Rangarajan S, Anderson E. The development of mouse oocyte cortical reaction competence is accompanied by major changes in cortical vesicles and not cortical granule depth. Dev Biol 1988; 130:189–192.

86. Perreault SD, Wolff RA, Zirkin BR. The role of disulfide bond reduction during mammalian sperm nuclear decondensation in vivo. Dev Biol 1984;101:160–167.

87. Perreault SD. Regulation of sperm nuclear reactivation during fertilization. In: Bavister BD, Cummins J, Roldan ERS, ed. Fertilization in Mammals. Serono Symposia, Norwell, MA, 1990, pp. 285–296.

88. Perreault SD, Barbee RR, Slott VL. Importance of glutathione in the acquisition and maintenance of sperm nuclear decondensation activity in maturing hamster oocytes. Dev Biol 1988;125:181–186.

89. Kastrop PMM, Bevers MM, Desree OHJ, Kruip TAM. Changes in protein synthesis and phosphorylation patterns during bovine oocyte maturation in vitro. J Reprod Fert 1990;90:305–310.

90. Bachvarova R, De Leon V, Johnson A, Kaplan G, Paynton BV. Changes in total RNA, polyadenylated RNA, and actin mRNA during meiotic maturation of mouse oocytes. Dev Biol 1985;08:325–331.

4

In Vitro Oocyte Maturation
Human Aspects

Jeffrey B. Russell, MD, FACOG

CONTENTS

INTRODUCTION

The successful birth of Louise Brown in 1978 after in vitro fertilization (IVF) was the culmination of the very exciting and innovative work of Robert Edwards, Barry Bavister, and Patrick Steptoe *(1–3)*. Presently, human IVF and embryo transfer (ET) is a widely accepted clinical procedure offered throughout the world to assist couples with infertility. Early research with human IVF involved maturing human oocytes in vitro, but the focus was on fertilization to yield a supply of embryos to study early embryonic development. The team from the University of Cambridge and Oldham General Hospital initiated their studies by collecting oocytes from graafian follicles in Hank's solution containing heparin and tissue culture medium (TCM 199) supplemented with fetal calf serum (FCS).

From: *Contemporary Endocrinology: Assisted Fertilization and Nuclear Transfer in Mammals*
Edited by: D. P. Wolf and M. Zelinski-Wooten © Humana Press Inc., Totowa, NJ

The oocytes were transported from Oldham Hospital to the University of Cambridge and after 38 h in culture many of the "immature" oocytes extruded their first polar body and reached metaphase of the second meiotic division. In vitro insemination was performed at different time intervals to identify the optimal time for fertilization. A key factor in the maturation of these oocytes was that they were matured in a milieu of follicular fluid. These early experiments laid the ground work for future work with IVF using immature oocytes. Therefore, although the first IVF/ET baby was conceived from an in vivo- matured oocyte, its true origination began with the in vitro maturation (IVM) of immature oocytes.

STANDARD ART CYCLE

An IVF/ET cycle as we know it today has evolved in several areas over the past 20 years. The focus of IVF or Assisted Reproductive Technology (ART) has been on recruiting the maximum number of mature oocytes prior to their removal from the ovary *(4)*. The use of human menopausal gonadotropins allows optimal recruitment as well as in vivo oocyte maturation prior to retrieval *(5)*. The challenging laboratory aspect of the process is to provide a compatible environment for fertilization and early embryo development *(6)*.

The retrieval of oocytes began with laparoscopic removal with the assistance of general anesthetics and has evolved from a procedure that required the patient to remain hospitalized for 24 h to ultrasound-guided, transvaginal aspiration on an outpatient basis. Ovulation induction protocols have changed from either a natural *(7)* or clomiphene citrate *(8)* cycle with four times a day urinary luteinizing hormone (LH) measurements, to closely monitored, synchronized stimulations with downregulation of the hypothalamic-pituitary axis *(9)*.

The evolution of ART has been marked with major milestones. One of the most significant advancements over the past 20 years has been the almost complete elimination of male infertility *(10)*. Single-sperm penetration into the ooplasm by manual injection to achieve fertilization has provided many couples, who could not have previously conceived, with children *(see* Chapter 7). In addition, ETs can now be performed after 5 d in culture at the blastocyst stage to reduce the risk of multiple births and increase the rate of implantation *(11)* *(see* Chapter 8). Simple directed techniques and clinical advances continue to improve the technology and clinical success of IVF/ET.

The standard IVF/ET cycle begins after an initial workup of both partners has been completed, including a psychological evaluation *(see* Chapter 9). The cycle is initiated with hypothalamic-pituitary downregulation using a gonadotropin releasing hormone (GnRH) agonist during the luteal phase of the preceding cycle. Downregulation is achieved after a burst of gonadotropins are released from the pituitary gland. Menses usually begins 7–14 d later. The ovaries are evaluated for any residual follicles by ultrasound and a low estradiol level confirms pituitary suppression. A programmed gonadotropin stimulation is initiated with either urinary or recombinant gonadotropins to enhance follicular recruitment. When more than two follicles are greater than 1.8 cm in diameter, human chorionic gonadotropin (hCG) is administered and the patient is then prepared for an in-office, outpatient, oocyte retrieval. Ultrasound-guided transvaginal oocyte retrieval is performed with minimal risk and complications to the patient in usually less than 30 min *(13)*.

The aspirated follicular fluid is scanned under a dissecting microscope until all the oocytes are identified, graded, and placed in culture medium, such as that based on the composition of human tubal fluid (HTF). A sperm sample obtained by ejaculation, fine-needle aspiration from the epididymis, or from testicular tissue is then utilized for fertilization depending upon the male's clinical history. Usually 50–100,000 sperm are added to each individual egg, 4–6 h after oocyte retrieval, in a 5% CO_2, closed, controlled system. Patients with male factor infertility or a poor fertilization history have the opportunity to achieve fertilization with the assistance of intracytoplasmic sperm injection (ICSI; *see* Chapter 7). A single sperm is picked up tail first and injected into the ooplasm. ICSI has been associated with fertilization success (70%) similar to that achieved by conventional insemination techniques *(14)*. Approximately 18 h post-insemination, oocytes are checked for the extrusion of a second polar body and the presence of two pronuclei (2PN). Culture is then maintained over the next 48–96 h before the embryo transfer takes place. At the present time, blastocyst transfer appears to provide pregnancy success rates approaching 60% per ET *(11,12)* (*see* Chapter 8). Supplementation during the luteal phase with human chorionic gonadotropin, progesterone, and estrogen is sometimes employed post-ET.

DISADVANTAGES OF THE ART CYCLE

The disadvantages of an ART cycle involve the expense of the gonadotropins, which can be $2–3,000/month, along with the risk of ovarian hyperstimulation syndrome *(15)* and the time commitment required for alternate or daily monitoring to predict the exact timing of the hCG administration. Also, there are theoretical long-term risks of gonadotropin exposure that are still being investigated *(16,17)*. Moreover, insurance coverage for infertility patients is limited in many geographical areas. These disadvantages provided the stimuli to search for alternative methods to complete the IVF/ET cycle in a safer, as well as more economical and time-efficient manner, with similar success.

Patients that are particularly prone to the complications of IVF/ET such as ovarian hyperstimulation are those with polycystic ovarian syndrome (PCOS) *(15)*. These patients have chronic anovulation or oligoovulation and, because of their large ovaries and multiple small follicles, are potential candidates for an immature oocyte retrieval with in vitro oocyte maturation.

IMMATURE OOCYTE RETRIEVAL

In 1991, Cha et al. *(18)* reported immature oocyte retrieval using surgically removed ovarian specimens to obtain immature follicles. The ovary was then dissected for the identification of antral follicles in the laboratory prior to oocyte recovery, maturation, and fertilization. A successful pregnancy was produced, but the oocytes came from excised ovarian tissue vs the aspiration of immature oocytes by ultrasound guidance as described later.

Based on these clinical observations, Trounson et al. *(19)* retrieved immature oocytes transvaginally in PCOS patients. They were able to retrieve immature oocytes from the ovary under ultrasound guidance; a significant achievement, because it allowed immature oocyte retrieval to become clinically available for all ART patients. The birth of a healthy girl in October of 1996 culminated their work.

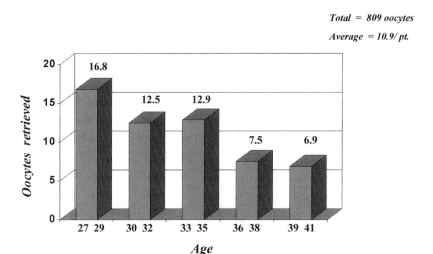

Fig. 1. The number of immature oocytes retrieved when compared to the patient's age.

PATIENT SELECTION

Patients with different diagnoses are now eligible candidates for an immature oocyte cycle. Patients with diagnoses such as PCOS, tubal disease, endometriosis, male factor, or unexplained infertility should be evaluated to rule out all other etiologies and possible therapies prior to their initiation into any ART program.

An immature oocyte cycle begins with a baseline (cycle day [CD] 2 or 3) follicle-stimulating hormone (FSH), estradiol, and progesterone level along with a baseline ultrasound (U/S) to quantify early follicular development and to rule out any residual ovarian or adnexal pathology. A baseline U/S can be predictive of follicular recruitment and provide an estimate of the number of retrievable oocytes *(20)* (*see* Chapter 6). A repeat U/S is performed on CD 6–8 to rule out early selection of the dominant follicle and to assess the thickness of the endometrial lining. The oocytes are retrieved between CD 9 and 11.

RETRIEVAL

The retrieval of immature oocytes is very similar to the retrieval of mature oocytes from stimulated follicles, by transvaginal U/S guidance. First, the vaginal vault is cleansed with antibacterial soap and sterile water. A paracervical block is placed in the lateral fornixes of the vagina with 1% (5 mL) Lidocaine. The vaginal vault is then flushed with culture medium. A sterile biopsy guide is placed on a 5 or 7.5 mHz vaginal probe and inserted into the vagina. All follicles identified between 8 and 12 mm are punctured using 80–100 mm/Hg of pressure. The follicular contents are evacuated and the cells are gently curetted from the sidewalls of the follicle. The fluid is collected with a 17-gauge, 30-cm, short-beveled needle (Cook OB/GYN, Spencer, IN) without flushing the follicle, into a conical tube with 3 mL of culture medium maintained at 37°C. The total number of oocytes retrieved is based on the patient's diagnosis, as well as the patient's age, and averages between 8–12 oocytes/patient. Figure 1 examines the relationship between maternal age and the number of immature oocytes retrieved (*see* Chapter 5). As expected, a decrease in the number of oocytes recovered was associated with increasing patient age.

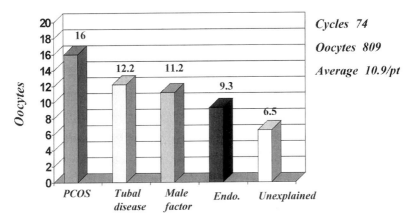

Fig. 2. The number of immature oocytes retrieved based on the patient's diagnosis.

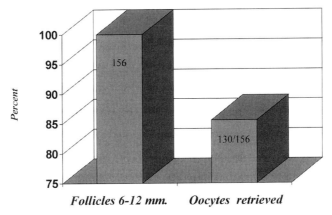

Fig. 3. The number of follicles measured by U/S between CD 6–8 compared with the number of oocytes retrieved.

Figure 2 reviews the number of oocytes retrieved as a function of the patient's diagnosis. Russell et al. *(21)* reviewed retrieval efficiency. The number of follicles as measured on CD 6 or 8 was compared with the number of oocytes retrieved (Fig. 3). A high correlation between the number of follicles identified on CD 6–8 and the number of oocytes retrieved was observed.

RETRIEVAL AND STAGE OF THE MENSTRUAL CYCLE

Cha et al. *(18)* collected oocytes at different phases of the menstrual cycle. A similar number of immature oocytes were retrieved per ovary from the proliferative (12.1/ovary) as compared to the secretory (12.5/ovary) phase of the menstrual cycle. A similar rate of degeneration or atresia was also identified, unrelated to the phase of the menstrual cycle from which these oocytes were isolated. A ratio of 75 to 25% of healthy vs degenerative ova, respectively, was observed regardless of the stage of the menstrual cycle during which the oocytes were retrieved.

Hwang et al. *(22)* showed that immature oocytes can be retrieved from the ovary at the time of delivery. In a case report, they aspirated visible follicles during a cesarean section

from a woman who had consented to be an oocyte donor. The recipient was placed on
conjugated estrogens for 7 d prior to oocyte retrieval. The oocytes retrieved with a 22-
gage needle connected to a syringe, were placed in maturation medium consisting of
TCM 199 with 20% bovine serum albumin (BSA) and 10 IU/mL of pregnant mare serum
gonaotropin (PMSG) and hCG. Seven immature oocytes were recovered; two matured
within 48 h of culture. Both oocytes were fertilized by ICSI and transferred to the patient
after she received progesterone supplementation. The embryos were co-cultured on Vero
cells for 24 h before being transferred at the two-cell stage and a successful pregnancy
occurred.

The possibility of isolating follicles and inducing their growth in vitro has been
described (23). This approach could provide a system for recovering cumulus-enclosed
oocytes for IVM. Preantral and early antral follicles were isolated from women undergoing a laparotomy with an oophorectomy in an attempt to assess maturational requirements. The follicles were measured and only those that were ≥120 µm were isolated.
Once the dissected follicles, often containing immature oocytes, were identified, they
were cultured in 1 mL of minimal essential medium with 5% serum along with antibiotic,
antimycotic solution and highly purified LH with or without the addition of FSH. The
dosages of FSH utilized were either 1.5 IU/mL or 0.1 IU/mL. The addition of 1.5 IU/mL
of FSH induced antral growth of follicles with or without the addition of LH. A critical
size was important in determining which follicles and, hence, immature oocytes, continue maturation.

LABORATORY ASPECTS

Once the follicular contents are collected in 3 mL of heparinized, modified HTF with
HEPES in a 37°C warming block, the fluid is filtered to separate red blood cells from
immature oocytes. Filters (EMCON embryo filter unit 75µ Veterinary Concepts Spring
Valley, WI) must be primed with at least 10 mL of heparinized modified HTF prior to
the addition of aspirates. The cells accumulated on top of the filter are transferred to an
embryo culture dish and immature oocytes are identified under the dissecting microscope, graded, and transferred to Eagle's minimal essential medium (EMEM) or TCM
199 (Sigma Chemical, St. Louis, MO) supplemented with 1µl of 17β- estradiol, 0.075 IU/
mL of urinary FSH, and 0.05 IU/mL of hCG with 3% SSS (Synthetic serum supplement;
Irvine Scientific, Santa Ana, CA). Immature oocytes are observed every 12 h for progression of their maturation.

MORPHOLOGY

Morphology of immature oocytes is categorized into three types based on the cumulus
and corona cells covering the oocyte. The categories are Compact, Bald or Denuded, and
Atretic. Compact oocytes possess one to two and occasionally four to five layers of
corona cells completely covering the oocyte. Bald oocytes have very few coronal cells
covering the zona pellucida and are void of any continuity between cells. The typical
immature oocyte retrieval results in the recovery of all three oocyte types (Fig. 4). As
the patient's age increases, the proportion of atretic oocytes also increases. The trend
towards retrieval in the earlier part of the follicular phase of the cycle is associated with
an increase in Bald oocytes, where the more Compact cells are identified in the mid-to
late follicular phase of the cycle.

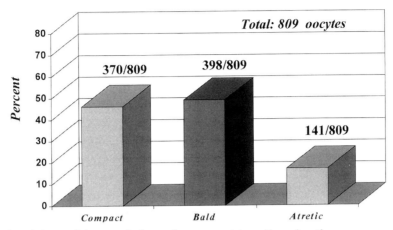

Fig. 4. The breakdown of the morphology of oocytes retrieved based on the presence or absence of coronal cells.

MATURATION

The maturation process, which occurs spontaneously under in vitro conditions, is a critical step in the successful completion of an immature oocyte cycle. Different follicular fluid preparations have been tried, as well as simple salt solutions and co-culture (24,25). The original work of Edwards and coworkers (2) utilized simple salt solutions. Cha et al. (18) utilized follicular fluid from follicles containing mature oocytes from other patients who were undergoing IVF/ET cycles. The follicular fluid was prepared by centrifuging the aspirates to remove blood and granulosa cells. The supernatant was deactivated at 57°C for 30 min followed by double filtration with 0.22-μm filters (Millipore Corporation, Bedford, MA). Trounson and colleagues (19), on the other hand, used EMEM and a mature granulosa cell co-culture with or without hCG supplementation. The granulosa cell co-culture was from a collection of mature oocytes from individually superovulated IVF patients. In addition, TCM 199 containing 10% FCS, 0.075 IU/mL of hMG, and 1 mg of estradiol was used. No differences in maturation rate were observed between media with or without mature follicular fluid, or protein supplement. Oocytes cultured in EMEM with FCS, gonadotropins, and estradiol had the highest maturation rate.

ENDOMETRIAL PRIMING

Endometrial priming and synchronization is an essential part of the IVM cycle. Once oocytes have matured and fertilized, they must be transferred as embryos to a synchronized endometrial cavity. An important strategy is to first retrieve as many immature oocytes as possible during the mid-to-late follicular phase of the cycle, prior to selection of the dominant follicle and without exogenous gonadotropins. Then, embryos must be transferred back to the endometrium in a patient with a shortened follicular phase. The standard IVF/ET cycle involves hCG administration to complete the oocyte maturation process in vivo, oocyte retrieval from the ovary 36 h later, and, in some cases, endometrial priming with supraphysiological levels of progesterone. The day of ovulation arbitrarily dates the endometrium as d 14 (also the day of retrieval) and over the next 7 d, the endometrium must be advanced to provide a window, CD 19–21, for implantation. An

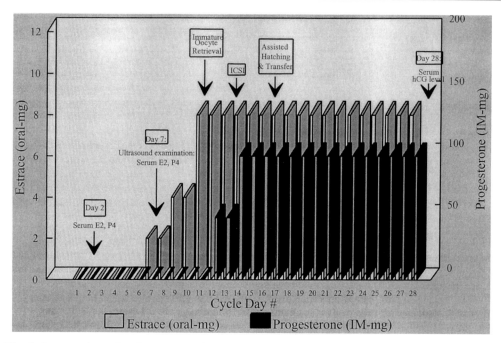

Fig. 5. An overview of patient preparation for endometrial priming with exogenous estrogen and progesterone prior to embryo transfer including blood tests, ultrasound exams, day of retrieval, fertilization, and embryo transfer.

in vitro oocyte maturation cycle does not benefit from the normal interval of exposure to rising estradiol levels, which prepare the endometrium for implantation. In addition, there is loss of hormonal support for the secretory phase of the endometrial cycle from the nonexistent corpus luteum.

To assess endometrial priming, Russell et al. *(26)* initiated early vs midfollicular priming of the endometrium with exogenous estrogens in combination with an immature oocyte retrieval and maturation cycle. Early follicular priming consisted of 2 mg of 17β-estradiol, twice a day, starting on CD 2 or 3 until the oocyte retrieval was performed. The midfollicular endometrial priming consisted of initiating 2 mg of 17β-estradiol on CD 6 and increasing by 1–2 mg/d based on endometrial thickness (Fig. 5). Patients with an endometrial thickness ≤6 mm on CD 6 were increased by 2 mg/d until oocyte retrieval. The patients with an endometrial thickness ≥6 mm were increased by 1 mg/d until retrieval. Both groups were continued on 8 mg/d from the day of retrieval. After retrieval, patients were started on 50 mg IM of progesterone (the first day after the retrieval) followed by 100 mg the second day, until the pregnancy test. Estrogen and progesterone were continued, if the pregnancy test was positive, until 70 d gestation. A significant decrease in the maturation rate and an increase in cleavage arrest was identified with immature oocytes exposed to early exogenous estrogens.

DOMINANT FOLLICLE

During the final selection of the dominant follicle, there appears to be a critical point where existing follicles containing immature oocytes begin to undergo atresia.

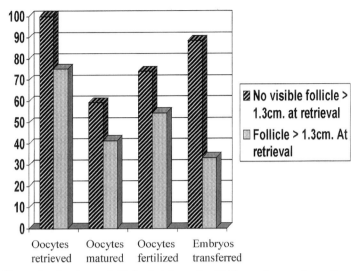

Fig. 6. The effect of a dominant follicle (≥1.3 cm by U/S) on the number of oocytes retrieved, matured, fertilized, and embryos transferred.

Our early experience has shown a dramatic decrease in the rates of maturation, fertilization, and transfer of embryos among patients in which immature oocytes were retrieved when a dominant follicle (≥1.4 cm) was present at the time of retrieval. The key to timing the retrieval is to allow endogenous gonadotropins to enhance an early recruitment of follicles and to initiate early cytoplasmic competence for germinal vesicle breakdown (GVB), which can be completed in vitro, before the selection of the dominant follicle. Figure 6 reveals the reduction in the number of oocytes retrieved, matured, fertilized, and embryos transferred when a dominant follicle was visualized.

THE EFFECT OF ANESTHESIA

One of the most common anesthetic agents used during the oocyte retrieval process is propofol (Propofol [2–6 diisopropylphenol]), a short-acting anesthetic agent. The typical time for immature oocyte retrieval averages around 45 min, which is twice the average retrieval time for a conventional oocyte retrieval. A study was performed by Alsalili et al. *(27)* examining the effects of propofol on IVM of mouse oocytes that were previously exposed to pregnant mare serum gonadotropin (PMSG). They examined and graded the oocytes as either cumulus-free (n = 551) or cumulus-enclosed (n = 222). The oocytes were incubated for 30 minutes in medium containing 0, 100, 1,000, or 10,000 ng/ mL of propofol prior to initiating IVM. Maturation, fertilization, and cleavage rates were compared. A significant difference in the IVM rate was only observed when the cumulus-free and the cumulus-enclosed oocytes were exposed to the highest levels (10,000 ng/ mL) of propofol. Fertilization and embryo cleavage rates were not significantly different. Propofol had previously been found in follicular fluid and, at higher concentrations, has been suspected of causing deleterious effects on the outcome of IVF. A study by Janssens-willen et al. *(28)* showed a significant decrease in blastocyst formation when propofol was added to the medium. Further studies are needed to assess whether the increased duration for retrieving immature oocytes using propofol as the anesthetic may have an adverse effect on the clinical outcome.

CRYOPRESERVATION OF IMMATURE OOCYTES

Oocyte cryopreservation is in the early stages of development, but has shown tremendous promise from a research and clinical aspect (*see* Chapter 10). Successful pregnancies have been observed after cryopreservation of metaphase II oocytes, although inconsistently *(29)*. Possible detrimental effects involve spindle formation, zona pellucida integrity, or cytoplasm changes. Park et al. *(30)* investigated the effects of cryoprotectants as well as low-temperature exposure on the chromosomal and microtubule configurations of human immature oocytes. They selected cumulus-oocyte complexes retrieved from patients undergoing gynecological surgery (oophorectomies) from unstimulated cycles, and randomly divided them into three groups. The first group included 91 cumulus-enclosed oocytes, which were selected as the controls. The second group were cumulus-enclosed oocytes, which were exposed to 1.5 *M* propanediol for 10 min at room temperature followed by 1.5 *M* propanediol containing 0.1 *M* sucrose in phosphate-buffered saline (PBS) for 5 minutes at room temperature. Group III included cumulus-enclosed oocytes that were cryopreserved using a rapid freezing method. Chromosomal abnormalities were ascertained by florescence *in situ* hybridization while spindle integrity was evaluated after immunostaining for tubulin. Their conclusion was that human oocytes, matured in vitro after cryopreservation at the germinal vesicle stage, showed an increased incidence of chromosomal and spindle abnormalities. These abnormalities may impair the capacity for further development of the embryos derived from frozen, thawed immature oocytes.

IN VITRO OOCYTE MATURATION
OF OOCYTES EXPOSED TO GONADOTROPINS

Oocytes retrieved during a stimulated IVF cycle are typically metaphase II with a small number of metaphase I. About 10–15% are GV-intact oocytes that have not responded to the hCG administered in vivo to initiate maturation. A small percentage of these oocytes retrieved at the germinal vesicle (GV) stage mature spontaneously, but the majority do not. Farhi et al. *(31)* looked at the effect of sperm addition to the culture media on the rate of GV oocyte maturation in vitro for oocytes retrieved from a stimulated cycle. The studied oocytes were separated into four groups. The first group included GV-intact oocytes with the cumulus attached. The second group consisted of GV-intact oocytes with sperm cells in the culture media. Group III were "stripped" GV oocytes, i.e., devoid of cumulus cells, and Group IV were stripped GV oocytes with sperm. Oocytes reaching the metaphase II stage of development underwent ICSI and fertilization rates were assessed. A significant difference was found in the oocyte maturation rate. Group I and Group II had 5% and 40% embryos developed. Groups III and IV had 30% and 80%, respectively, of their oocytes reaching the metaphase II stage at 24 and 48 h, 25 and 70%, respectively, embryos developed. GV oocytes in Group IV that were stripped of their cumulus cells and exposed to sperm had the highest rate of embryo production. Although these oocytes were exposed to prior gonadotropin stimulation, they were GV oocytes at the time of retrieval. The mechanism for the effect of the sperm exposure to produce a higher rate of mature oocytes is unknown.

Liu et al. *(32)* reported a unique case where successful IVM was performed on human oocytes not exposed to hCG during the ovulation induction process. The patient inadvertently injected herself with the hCG diluent (saline) instead of the hCG medication. At the time of the retrieval, no oocytes were found until a thorough search through the ovarian tissue in the collection media was undertaken. Once the ovarian tissue was dissected, 5 oocytes were found in tightly packed cumulus-corona cells, which prevented classification of the oocytes. IVM was then initiated in B2 medium supplemented with 50 IU/mL of FSH and 50 IU/mL of hCG. The immature oocytes were incubated at 37°C in 5% CO_2. At 24 h after in-vitro culture, the corona cells loosened from the zona pellucida, making identification possible. After 48 h, polar body extrusion was identified as evidence the oocytes had matured. Fertilization was performed by ICSI with three out of the five oocytes displaying 2 pronuclei. One embryo developed to the four-cell stage and was frozen for subsequent transfer in synchrony with the recipient endometrium. A frozen-thawed cycle was carried out with estrogen and progesterone supplementation to time the window of implantation. The patient conceived and delivered a normal healthy baby. The timetable for these oocytes to mature, fertilize, and develop was very typical for those recovered from nonstimulated cycles.

FUTURE

The future of in vitro oocyte maturation as a therapy for couples attempting to conceive by means of assisted conception is enormous. It could alleviate the medications required to recruit that month's cohort of follicles, reduce the risks of hyperstimulation, and minimize the long-term theoretical implications of exogenous hormonal administration to ovarian cancer. The economic impact could be profound; besides the medication, there would be a reduction in the number of laboratory and U/S analyses required for monitoring. It would also be beneficial in relation to the patients' time required to participate in these analyses. In addition, the initial screening procedure using diagnostic laparoscopy that occurs during the infertility work-up would permit the retrieval of immature eggs for diagnostic purposes and for an assessment of oocyte quality. Oocyte maturation rate may be predictive of clinical outcomes during a stimulated IVF procedure *(33)*. The retrieval of immature oocytes combined with IVM for women in an oocyte donation program, would appeal to individuals concerned about the administration of gonadotropins and the potential short- and long-term side effects.

Our initial research to prime the endometrium with exogenous estrogens combined with IVM revealed a significant decrease in rates of oocyte maturation and embryo cleavage secondary to exogenous estrogen exposure prior to retrieval. Further refinements are clearly needed to advance the uterine environment from a CD day 9 or 10 proliferative endometrium to a CD 19 or 20 secretory endometrium within a short timetable. Endometrial priming is a significant aspect of this procedure. The challenge is to retrieve immature oocytes from the ovary in the mid-to-late follicular phase and then return them to the uterine cavity 4–5 d later. Immature oocytes must be competent to undergo meiosis, cytoplasmic maturation, fertilization, and embryo implantation at an acceptable rate. This process must be synchronized if implantation is to occur. The luteal phase must be supported with enough exogenous estrogen and progesterone to maintain a secretory endometrium until the pregnancy test is performed. If a pregnancy is established, exogenous hormonal administration is continued until the placenta functions independently.

In summary, unstimulated immature oocyte retrieval can be performed successfully in patients with different diagnoses who are candidates for ART. The number of oocytes retrieved depends on the age and diagnosis, as with conventional IVF. Oocytes can be retrieved transvaginally with U/S guidance. The oocyte maturation rate and embryo cleavage rate can be affected significantly by early follicular endometrial priming with exogenous estrogen. Further optimization of nuclear and cytoplasmic maturation (*see* Chapter 3) along with exogenous endometrial priming to synchronize the window of implantation with the ET, could allow the immature oocyte collection and maturation procedure to challenge and possibly even replace the standard stimulated IVF cycle in the near future.

REFERENCES

1. Edwards RG. Maturation in vitro of mouse, sheep, cow, pig, rhesus monkey and human ovarian oocytes. Nature 1965;5008:349–351.
2. Edwards RG. Maturation in vitro of human ovarian oocytes. Lancet 1965;2:926–929.
3. Edwards RG, Steptoe PC. Current status of in vitro fertilization and implantation of human embryos. Lancet 1983;2:1265–1270.
4. Laufer N, DeCherney AH, Haseltine FP, Polan ML, Mezer HC, Dlugi AM, et al. The use of high-does human menopausal gonadotropin in an in vitro fertilization program. Fertil Steril 1983;40:734–741.
5. Pellicer A, Ruiz A, Castellvi RM, Calatayud C, Ruiz M, Tarin JJ, et al. Is the retrieval of high numbers of oocytes desirable in patients treated with gonadotropin-releasing hormone analogues (GnRHa) and gonadotropins? Hum Reprod 1989;4:536–540.
6. Wood C, McMaster R, Rennie G, Trounson A, Leeton J. Factors influencing pregnancy rates following in vitro fertilization and embryo transfer. Fertil Steril 1985;43:245–250.
7. Lemay A, Bastide A, Lambert R, Rioux J. Prediction of human ovulation by rapid luteinizing hormone (LH) radioimmunoassay and ovarian ultrasonography. Fertil Steril 1982;38:194–201.
8. Marrs R, Vargyas J, Shangold G, Yee B. The effect of time of initiation of clomiphene citrate on multiple follicle development for human in vitro fertilization and embryo replacement procedures. Fertil Steril 1984;41:682–685.
9. Wikland M, Borg J, Hamberger L, Svalander P. Simplification of IVF: minimal monitoring and the use of subcutaneous highly purified FSH administration for ovulation induction. Hum Reprod 1994;9:1430–1436.
10. Palermo G, Cohen J, Rosenwaks Z. Intracytoplasmic sperm injection: a powerful tool to overcome fertilization failure. Fertil Steril 1996;65:899–908.
11. Leme Alves da Motta E, Alegretti J, Baracat, E, Olive D, Serafini P. High implantation and pregnancy rates with transfer of human blastocysts developed in preimplantation stage one and blastocyst media. Fertil Steril 1998;70:659–663.
12. Gardner DK, Phil D, Vella P, Lane M, Wagley L, Schlenker T, Schoolcraft WB. Culture and transfer of human blastocysts increases implantation rates and reduces the need for multiple embryo transfers. Fertil Steril 1998;69:84–88.
13. Russell JB, DeCherney AH, Hobbins JC. A new transvaginal probe and biopsy guide for oocyte retrieval. Fertil Steril 1986;47:350–352.
14. Aytoz A, Camus M, Tournaye H, Bonduelle M, Van Steirteghem A, Devroey P. Outcome of pregnancies after intracytoplasmic sperm injection and the effect of sperm origin and quality on this outcome. Fertil Steril 1998;70:500–505.
15. Bergh PA, Navot D. Ovarian hyperstimulation syndrome; a review of pathophysiology. J Assist Reprod Genet 1992;9:429–438.
16. Whittemore AS, Harris R, Itnyre J, the Collaborative Ovarian Cancer Group. Characteristics relating to ovarian cancer risk: collaborative analysis of 12 US case-control studies. II. Invasive epithelial ovarian cancers in white women. Am J Epidemiol 1992;136:1184–1203.
17. Bristow RE, Karlan BY. Ovulation induction, infertility, and ovarian cancer risk. Fertil Steril 1996;66: 499–507.
18. Cha KY, Koo JJ, Ko JJ, Choi DH, Han SY, Yoon TK. Pregnancy after in vitro fertilization of human follicular oocytes collected from nonstimulated cycles, their culture in vitro and their transfer in a donor oocyte program. Fertil Steril 1991;55:109–113.
19. Trounson A. Wood C, Kausche A. In vitro maturation and the fertilization and developmental competence of oocytes recovered from untreated polycystic ovarian patients. Fertil Steril 1994;62:353–362.

20. Chang MY, Chiang CH, Chiu TH, Hsieh T'Sang-T'Ang, Soong YK. The antral follicle count predicts the outcome of pregnancy in a controlled ovarian hyperstimulation/intrauterine insemination program. J Assist Reprod Genet 1998;15:12–17.
21. Russell JB. Immature oocyte retrieval combined with in-vitro oocyte maturation. Hum Reprod 1998; 13:63–70.
22. Hwang JL, Lin YH, Tsai YL. Pregnancy after immature oocyte donation and intracytoplasmic sperm injection. Fertil Steril 1997;68:1139–1140.
23. Abir R, Franks S, Mobberley MA, Moore PA, Margara RA, Winston RML. Mechanical isolation and in vitro growth of preantral and small antral human follicles. Fertil Steril 1997;68:682–688.
24. Barnes FL, Crombie A, Gardner DK, Kausche A, Lacham-Kaplan O, Suikkari AM, et al. Blastocyst development and birth after in-vitro maturation of human primary oocytes, intracytoplasmic sperm injection and assisted hatching. Hum Reprod 1995;10:3243–3246.
25. Krisher RL, Gibbons JR, Gwazdauskas FC. Effectiveness of Menuzo's B2 medium with buffalo rat liver cells for development of in vitro matured/in vitro fertilized bovine oocytes. J Asst Reprod Genet 1998; 15:50–53.
26. Russell, JB, Knezevich, KM, Fabian KF, Dickson JA. Unstimulated immature oocyte retrieval: early versus midfollicular endometrial priming. Fertil Steril 1997;67:616–620.
27. Alsalili M, Thornton S, Fleming S. The effect of anaesthetic, Propofol, on in-vitro oocyte maturation, fertilization and cleavage in mice. Hum Reprod 1997;12:1271–1274.
28. Janssenwillen C, Christiaens F, Camu F. The effect of propofol on parthenogenetic activation, in vitro-fertilization and early embryo development of mouse oocytes. (Abstr. no. 38) J Br Fertil Soc 1,11B.
29. Porcu E, Fabbri, R, Seracchioli R, Ciotti PA, Magrini O, Flamigni C. Birth of a healthy female after intracytoplasmic sperm injection of cryopreserved human oocytes. Fertil Steril 1997;68:724–726.
30. Park SE, Son WY, Lee SH, Lee KA, K JJ, Cha KY. Chromosome and spindle configurations of human oocytes matured in vitro after cryopreservation at the germinal vesicle stage. Fertil Steril 1997;68:920–926.
31. Farhi J, Nahum H, Zakut H, Levran D. Incubation with sperm enhances in vitro maturation of the oocyte from the germinal vesicle to the M2 stage. Fertil Steril 1997;68:318–322.
32. Liu J, Katz E, Garcia JE, Compton G, Baramki TA. Successful in vitro maturation of human oocytes not exposed to human chorionic gonadotropin during ovulation induction, resulting in pregnancy. Fertil Steril 1997;67:566–568.
33. Russell, JB, Rodriguez JA, Sawyers TL, Nichols PA, Trott, EA. Immature oocyte retrieval (IOR) combined with in vitro maturation (IVM) as a diagnostic tool to assess oocyte quality. Poster presentation, ASRM 54th Annual Meeting, 1998, San Francisco, CA.

5

Measurement of Reproductive Potential in the Human Female

Phillip E. Patton, MD

INTRODUCTION

Oocyte depletion is a natural physiologic process, beginning in utero. Approximately 7 million primordial germ cells are formed during mid-gestation, but only 300,000 oocytes remain at menarche. Morphometric studies have been used to examine the process of follicular depletion. The classic model predicts that follicular loss is linear up until age 38, at which time the rate of depletion increases markedly *(1,2)*. Thus, follicular depletion is a biphasic process with an abrupt change in the rate of loss occuring at advanced reproductive ages. The biphasic model of follicular loss fits nicely with other observations of reproductive physiology, including the changing rates of fecundity, and fetal loss noted in older women (Figs. 1 and 2). However, recent studies challenge the classic biphasic model of follicular depletion *(3)*. Based on a reanalysis of oocyte-depletion data, an abrupt increase in the rate of follicular depletion is not apparent. In fact, the rate of follicle loss may actually decrease in the years before menopause. Regardless, it is clear that with the decline in oocyte number, fertility potential is markedly reduced.

Oocyte depletion is not the singular cause of decreasing reproductive potential. Recent work indicates that age-related changes in the physiologic properties of the mature follicle are also important. Follicular fluid aspirates contain higher estrogen and progesterone,

From: *Contemporary Endocrinology: Assisted Fertilization and Nuclear Transfer in Mammals*
Edited by: D. P. Wolf and M. Zelinski-Wooten © Humana Press Inc., Totowa, NJ

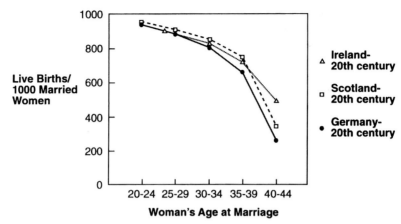

Fig. 1. Live birth rate as a function of age in 20th century European populations. Adapted with permission from ref. *(8)*.

but lower testosterone and insulin-like growth factor (IGF)-1 levels in older compared to younger women *(4)*. As well, granulosa cell cultures obtained from women with decreased ovarian reserve demonstrate decreased inhibin production and an increased rate of apoptosis *(5,6)*. The observed alterations in granulosa cell function may reflect important physiologic changes within follicular cells that are associated with decreasing fertility. Cytoplasmic and nuclear abnormalities are also noted from oocytes of older women. During meiosis, chromosomal segregation requires the complex interplay between cytoplasmic and nuclear elements. As determined by confocal microscopy, both the microtubule matrix and chromosomal alignment are frequently abnormal in older women *(7)*. The increased rates of meiotic spindle abnormalities observed in older women may be responsible for the increased aneuploidy observed from embryos of older women. Taken together, experimental studies indicate that reproductive aging results in not only decreased oocyte numbers, but a diminished oocyte quality.

Longitudinal population studies assessing human fecundity confirm these observations *(8)*. Fecundity rates are relatively stable until age 30, after which a gradual decline is observed that rapidly accelerates after age 40 (Fig. 1). Increased contraception and rates of endometriosis, pelvic inflammatory disease, miscarriage, and decreased coital frequency are all contributing factors, but the process of increased follicular depletion and/or decreased oocyte quality are the predominant explanations for the observed age-related decrease in fecundity. This concept is supported by the results from assisted reproductive programs showing that pregnancy rates, controlled for the effects of confounding factors, decrease with increasing age *(9)*.

Pregnancy potential can be estimated at a given age using fecundity rates. The latter are generally derived from large population studies reflecting a diversity of infertility problems and treatment options. Although such data provide important demographic information, the usefulness of fecundity rates may be limited in the clinical setting. This is because the onset and cessation of ovarian function, and therefore reproductive potential, are unique variables for each woman. The clinical observation of differences in pregnancy potential in women of the same age underscores the argument that age alone is not an accurate index or diagnostic indicator of reproductive potential. Based on these considerations, diagnostic testing that would predict individual reproductive potential would

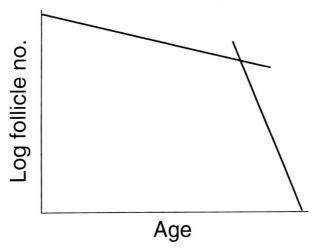

Fig. 2.   The biphasic model of follicular loss that demonstrates a linear loss of follicles with age followed by an accelerated loss of follicles. Adapted with permission from ref. *(3)*.

be enormously helpful. Several new testing paradigms hold promise in accomplishing this goal. The purpose of this chapter is to review the current tests and their role in the clinical setting.

FOLLICLE STIMULATING HORMONE (FSH) TESTING

Predicting pregnancy potential through evaluation of serum FSH levels during the early follicular phase is based on a sound physiological premise. That premise, in the human, is that as FSH levels rise with increasing age *(10)*, there is an associated diminished pool of FSH-responsive follicles and, therefore, reproductive potential. Ultimately, a gradual shortening of the follicular phase occurs reflecting an accelerated process of dominant follicle selection associated with a subtle rise in FSH during the luteal-follicular phase transition.

The rise in FSH precedes any significant derangement in ovarian hormone secretion. In a study of older women (age 40–45), pituitary gonadotropin and ovarian steroid production were compared to a younger cohort (age 20–25) *(11)*. Whereas serum estradiol, progesterone, and luteinizing hormone (LH) levels were indistinguishable between the two groups, 24-h mean FSH levels were significantly higher in the older group. Although a shortened follicular phase occurs in many women with aging, not all women demonstrate menstrual abnormalities in association with rising FSH levels. Regular, predictable, and ovulatory cycles, although the exception, occur up to the time of menopause *(12)*. Therefore, FSH testing is a more sensitive indicator of decreased ovarian reserve than the occurrence of menstrual disturbances.

The use of FSH levels to assess reproductive potential has been evaluated by several groups *(13–16)*. In a large retrospective study, a link between FSH levels and pregnancy outcome was observed *(13)*. Pregnancy levels were highest in women who had low FSH levels (<10 IU/L), and fell dramatically when FSH levels were >25 IU/L (<5%). Based on the observations that women who had the poorest pregnancy rates also had significantly fewer follicles developed, fewer oocytes retrieved, and fewer embryos transferred, the authors concluded that FSH levels were correlated with diminished ovarian reserve.

Table 1
Pregnancy Outcome and Cycle Cancellation as a Function of Basal (D 3) FSH Levels

Reference	FSH (IU/L)	Pregnancy rate (%)	Cancellation rate (%)
Scott *(13)* (n = 755)	<15	24	Not reported
	15–25	13.6	—
	≥25	3.6	—
Toner *(14)* (n = 1478)	<15	~18	6
	15–25	~15	8
	>25	0	30

To address the issue of whether FSH levels represent a better marker of diminished ovarian reserve than age, Toner and coauthors performed a retrospective study of 1,487 in vitro fertilization (IVF) cycles *(14)*. As expected, both FSH values and age were significantly correlated with IVF outcome. As a single marker of ovarian reserve, basal FSH values were better at predicting cancellation rates, peak estradiol levels, egg numbers, and pregnancy rates when compared to age alone (*see* Table 1). In a corollary study, early follicular phase FSH levels were also found to be an independent and more powerful marker of ovarian response than age *(16)*. Numerous studies now confirm the concept that basal FSH levels are strong and meaningful predictors of future reproductive performance, not only for IVF patients but also for women undergoing ovulation induction *(17)*.

During the follicular phase, FSH secretion is regulated by both steroidogenic and peptidergic substances secreted by both ovaries. Therefore, the efficacy of FSH testing in predicting reproductive outcome in women with a single ovary is an important clinical issue. In a retrospective study, 162 women with a single ovary were compared to a control group of 1,066 women with 2 ovaries undergoing IVF. Women with one ovary demonstrated higher basal FSH levels, poorer response to gonadotropin stimulation, and lower pregnancy rates *(18)*. However, when the data were analyzed as a function of basal FSH levels, pregnancy rates between the two groups were comparable. Therefore, based on these results, FSH screening is appropriate in the setting of a single ovary.

To determine the clinical significance of intercycle FSH variability, basal levels in 81 women undergoing IVF were analyzed *(19)*. In those with low mean FSH values (<15 mIU/mL), there was little variability among the cycles compared. In contrast, women who had higher mean basal FSH levels showed significant month-to-month variability. Ovarian responsiveness was assessed in a total of 28 women who had at least one elevated basal FSH value, and who underwent repeated cycles of gonadotropin stimulation. Gonadotropin responsiveness, number of oocytes collected, and fertilization rates were similar among stimulation cycles whether the FSH level was low or high at the time of the initiated cycle.

LIMITATIONS IN FSH TESTING

During the transition from normal ovulatory function to menopause, FSH levels fluctuate from cycle-to-cycle. Because of the variability in FSH levels, there has been concern that the analysis of a single value may not accurately reflect reproductive potential. Consequently, screening of d 3 FSH levels prior to a cycle of gonadotropin stimulation has been advocated *(20)*. In this approach, the results of the pre-stimulation FSH value

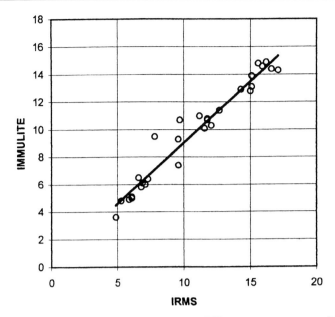

Fig. 3. Correlation of FSH levels between two different assay systems (R = 0.975).

would determine whether or not the cycle is initiated or canceled. Although the rationale for precycle IVF FSH testing is reasonable, there is little confirmatory data that it is clinically efficacious. Martin and coauthors also examined pregnancy outcome as a function of basal FSH level variability *(20)*. A total of 53 cycles were completed in women who evidenced repeatedly high FSH (>20 IU/L) values and no pregnancies occurred. An additional 54 cycles were reviewed where only a single pretreatment FSH value exceeded 20 mIU/mL. Despite a normal FSH value during the treatment cycle, the pregnancy rate was only 5.6%. Based on these results, a single elevated FSH obtained at any time during reproductive life appears to predict diminished ovarian reserve and a low pregnancy potential.

Although FSH testing is available in nearly all clinical laboratories, significant assay variability exists. Consequently, threshold values obtained in one laboratory may be distinctly different from another. Differences in immunoassay standards, antibodies, and testing methodologies emphasize the difficulties in direct comparisons. As a general rule, threshold values should be validated in the clinical setting, or by correlative data from reference institutions. Figure 3 illustrates subtle but important differences in FSH values determined at our institution compared to a large reference laboratory. Although serum sample values correlate between the assay systems, our FSH levels average approx 10% higher. Therefore, the threshold value of FSH used in predicting pregnancy performance would require adjustment for the observed differences between the two assay systems.

FSH thresholds should be used as general guidelines in predicting successful fertility treatment. A very high FSH threshold will accurately predict a poor pregnancy rate. For example, no live births were obtained in women undergoing IVF who had FSH values above 25 IU/L *(14)*. A lower FSH level is less sensitive in the prediction of treatment outcome. Basal FSH values between 15–25 IU/L were associated with a significant decrease in pregnancy rates compared to women who had lower values. Nevertheless, approx 10%

of women with elevated FSH values in this range conceived *(21)*. Furthermore, a normal FSH value does not necessarily predict ovarian responsiveness or outcome. In 12 women with normal FSH values (5.4 ± 2.7 IU/L), Fahri and coauthors reported a persistently poor response to gonadotropin stimulation *(22)*. Within 1 yr, all women had FSH values in the menopausal range. Although an elevated FSH level may be a sensitive marker of limited pregnancy potential, a normal FSH value in itself is not a specific marker of achieving pregnancy.

FSH AND ESTROGEN TESTING

The combination of FSH and estradiol testing during the early follicular phase has been used to assess ovarian reserve because there are situations where measurements of FSH alone are inadequate. The pituitary secretion of FSH and ovarian production of estradiol are interdependent. During the follicular phase of the menstrual cycle, FSH secretion is modulated, in part, by ovarian steroids in a classic negative feedback pathway. The observation of supraphysiologic elevations of FSH during the early follicular phase reflects an unresponsive ovary, decreased estradiol secretion, and a decreased ovarian reserve. However, perimenopausal women with a decreased reproductive potential can exhibit a normal cycle d 3 FSH level secondary to the process of accelerated follicular development. In this situation, supraphysiolosic levels of estradiol occur secondary to rapid follicle development induced by elevated FSH levels during the luteal-follicular phase transition. These elevated estrogen levels suppress FSH levels into the normal range during the early follicular phase.

The prognostic value of both d 3 FSH and estradiol measurements in 225 women representing a total of 292 IVF cycles was recently evaluated *(23)*. Cancellation rates were significantly higher and pregnancy rates lower in women with basal estradiol values >80 pg/mL. Even when cycles with FSH levels >15 mIU/mL were excluded from analysis, an elevated basal estradiol was associated with a significantly reduced IVF outcome. When estradiol levels exceeded 100 pg/mL, no pregnancies occurred, even in women who had a normal d 3 FSH level.

In a corollary study, both d 3 FSH and estradiol levels were evaluated in 394 completed IVF cycles *(24)*. Pregnancy rates were significantly decreased in women with an estradiol value >60 pg/mL and no pregnancies occurred when estradiol values exceeded 70 pg/mL. When both estradiol (>45 pg/mL) and FSH (>17 IU/L) values were elevated, no pregnancies occurred in 31 cycles. Unfortunately, neither FSH nor estradiol testing considered alone was particularly accurate in predicting a poor outcome (Table 2).

The prognostic value of early (cycle days [CD] 2–5) follicular phase FSH, LH and estradiol responses to gonadotropin releasing hormone agonist (GnRH-a) stimulation has also been used to predict ovarian response and pregnancy potential *(25)*. The administration of GnRH-a is used as a dynamic test of ovarian reserve. GnRH-a treatment induces an initial surge of FSH, LH, and estradiol. A poor estradiol response or an abnormal pattern of estradiol secretion is regarded as evidence of a decreased or poor-quality cohort of antral follicles. The pattern of estradiol response was a better predictor of IVF outcome than was baseline or stimulated serum FSH or LH levels. Patterns of estradiol secretion exhibiting either a prompt and persistent rise (C-pattern) or no response (D-pattern) were associated with the poorest pregnancy rates. In contrast, a falling estradiol response (A- and B-patterns) was predictive of a superior pregnancy rate. In a similar

Table 2
Pregnancy Outcome Analyzed as a Function of Basal Estradiol and FSH Levels

Reference	n	Estradiol (pg/mL)	FSH (IU/L)	Pregnancy rate (%)
Liccardi (24)	224	≤45	<17	22.8
	149	>45	<17	17.4
	48	≤45	>17	16.7
	31	>45	>17	0

Reference	n	Estradiol (pg/mL)	Cancellation rate	Pregnancy rate (%)
Smotrich (23)	265	<80	0.4	37
	27	>80	18.5	14.8

study, the response of LH, FSH, and estradiol following GnRH-a administration was evaluated (26). After baseline measurements on cycle d 2 were obtained, 100 μg of buserline nasal spray was administered in a total of 6 doses daily. Serum sampling was repeated on CD 3 and 4 after GnRH-a treatment. Both basal levels of FSH and estradiol to GnRH-a treatment were predictive of the response to ovarian stimulation. Although the change in estradiol response (<180 pg/mL rise) was predictive of cycle cancellation, pregnancy outcome was not reported, therefore the predictive value of the test in determining pregnancy is unknown.

The results of both basal and stimulated estradiol testing add important clinical information over FSH testing alone. The combination may be superior to either test alone in predicting decreased ovarian reserve. However, because basal estradiol testing provides the same diagnostic information as dynamic testing, the need for GnRH-a stimulation is questionable.

LIMITATIONS IN ESTRADIOL AND STIMULATED FSH TESTING

Although mild elevations in basal estradiol levels in women correlate with a decreased pregnancy potential, the estradiol threshold that predicts a negligible pregnancy rate has yet to be established. In addition, studies exist that question the validity of basal estradiol testing. Recently, the prognostic value of d 3 estradiol testing was evaluated in women undergoing IVF and controlled ovarian hyperstimulation (27). Using a threshold value of 80 pg/mL, there was a significant increase in cycle cancellation rates associated with elevated levels. Nevertheless, elevated basal estradiol values were not predictive of pregnancy outcome. Given these concerns, basal estradiol testing in addition to d 3 FSH values may add prognostic value only when estradiol levels are highly elevated (e.g., >80 pg/nL) in conjunction with normal basal FSH values. At the present time, estradiol testing adds prognostic value in the prediction of gonadotropin responsiveness and cycle cancellation. Whether estradiol testing is useful in predicting pregnancy potential remains to be determined.

INHIBIN TESTING

Inhibin is a complex glycoprotein hormone secreted by both the granulosa and theca cells of the ovary. Inhibin-A is composed of an α-subunit, linked by a disulfide bond to one of two β-subunits referred to as βA. Inhibin-B is composed of the same α-subunit linked to the βB subunit. In both human and nonhuman primates, differential ovarian secretion of the dimeric proteins inhibin-A and B occurs *(28,29)*. Expression of the βA-subunit mRNA is highest in the dominant follicle and corpus luteum during the menstrual cycle. The observation that circulating inhibin-A levels peak during the luteal phase and fall with luteal regression supports the concept that inhibin-A is a secretory product of the corpus luteum *(30)*. In contrast, inhibin-B secretion is a product of developing follicles. Serum concentrations are maximal in the early and mid-follicular phases of the menstrual cycle, and fall during the late follicular phase with ovulation. After a brief post-ovulatory rise, the levels reach a nadir at mid-luteal phase. The observation that inhibin-B levels rise in correlation with rising FSH levels suggest that this molecule is regulated by FSH during the early follicular phase *(29)*. Whether or not the degree of inhibin-B expression during the early follicular phase reflects the biologic capacity of the developing cohort of FSH-responsive follicles is a current area of investigation.

The regulation of FSH and inhibin secretion during the menstrual cycle is complex. The rise in inhibin-B noted in the early follicular phase correlates with a rise in FSH. The observation that inhibin-B levels can be manipulated by changing the pulse frequency of intravenously administered GnRH-a in GnRH-deficient women, or by the administration of a GnRH antagonist in ovulatory women, adds support to the concept that inhibin-B production is stimulated by FSH *(29,31)*. Both inhibin-A and B may play a role in the negative feedback inhibition of FSH. The evidence for inhibin-A is the most convincing. Inhibin-A production by the corpus luteum is inversely correlated with FSH, suggesting that inhibin-A suppresses FSH secretion *(32)*. The observation that recombinant inhibin-A administered in the early follicular phase in the nonhuman primate results in persistent FSH suppression confirms this concept *(33)*. The role of inhibin-B in FSH secretion is less clear. The finding of reduced inhibin-B levels in women with rising FSH suggests that inhibin-B may be an important regulator of FSH secretion *(28)*. However, subnormal inhibin-B levels are demonstrable in women with completely normal FSH levels *(34)*. Future studies using recombinant inhibin-B, or inhibin-B-neutralizing antibodies, should clarify the role of inhibin-B on FSH secretory patterns.

Initial studies on the role of inhibin during reproductive life in the human were inconclusive. Using a heterologous polyclonal immunoassay (Monash Assay), analysis of the physiologic role of inhibin during the menstrual cycle provided conflicting results. Because this antisera was directed against amino acids (93–108 in the C-terminus) common to both the α-subunit and α-subunit precursor proteins, it was incapable of distinguishing biologically active dimeric inhibin molecules from α-subunits, or α-subunit precursors. Recently, 2-site, enzyme-linked immunoabsorbent assays (ELISA) have become available that measure either inhibin-A or inhibin-B directly with a high degree of specificity.

Inhibin testing has been used as a marker of reproductive aging and ovarian reserve. Klein and coauthors *(28)* found that elevated follicular phase FSH levels in older women (40–45 yr) were associated with lower inhibin-B levels compared to a younger control group. A significant decrease in inhibin-B levels is thought to reflect a smaller cohort of FSH-responsive follicles than normal. Alternatively, lower inhibin production could reflect a diminished capacity to produce inhibin in a quantitatively normal pool of developing follicles. To test whether inhibin-B levels are reflective of reproductive performance, they were examined during the early follicular phase of the menstrual cycle in women undergoing IVF *(34)*. Estradiol response, the number of oocytes collected, and pregnancy rates were poorer in women with low levels of inhibin-B (<45 pg/mL) compared to cycles with normal levels. After controlling for age, d 3 FSH and estradiol levels, the analysis of the data indicated that inhibin-B levels were still predictive of IVF pregnancy rates.

LIMITATIONS IN INHIBIN TESTING

Based on the published data, physiologic changes in inhibin levels may represent an early marker of ovarian aging and decreased ovarian reserve. Nevertheless, the use of discrete inhibin levels in clinical practice decisions is premature. Currently, inhibin thresholds are based on the 95% confidence intervals in highly selected infertility treatment regimens. As such, inhibin thresholds are not necessarily controlled for age or other factors that may affect the predictive value of the threshold level in the general infertility population. Changes in inhibin methodology add further complexity in the clinical application of inhibin thresholds. With further experience, inhibin testing may provide an early and sensitive marker of ovarian reserve.

CLOMIPHENE CITRATE CHALLENGE TEST

The clomiphene citrate challenge test originally described by Navot and coauthors *(35)* consisted of measuring serum FSH levels on CD 3 and CD 10 after the administration of 100 mg of clomiphene citrate from CD 5–9. The rationale for d 3 FSH testing is as described previously. The addition of a d 10 FSH level is based on the premise that a healthy cohort of developing follicles (FSH-responsive) should respond by producing enough gonadal steroids and inhibiting peptides to suppress FSH levels into the normal range.

In a sense, the test is designed to challenge or test the ability of the ovary to respond to rising FSH levels induced by clomiphene. The administration of clomiphene results in a rise of pituitary gonadotropins. In women with a normal response, LH levels rise more than FSH levels. In women with decreased ovarian reserve, however, FSH levels rise more than LH. In the original study of 51 women over age 35, all had normal d 3 FSH values, and 18 demonstrated an elevated d 10 FSH level *(35)*. Only 1 patient (6%) in the study group with an abnormal test conceived, compared to 42% with normal FSH levels on both d 3 and d 10. The addition of the d 10 FSH measurement was useful in the identification of a previously unrecognized population of women with diminished ovarian reserve.

For screening ovarian reserve, the clomiphene citrate challenge test has several advantages. The test is simple, inexpensive, and safe. Unlike other markers of ovarian reserve, the test has been validated in several distinct diagnostic categories, ranging from the general infertility to the assisted reproductive technology populations. No other marker of ovarian reserve can boast such extensive validation.

The clomiphene citrate challenge test has been applied in a variety of clinical situations (Table 3). Tanbo and colleagues *(36)* evaluated the test in women undergoing IVF who were either over 35 years of age, had a previous oophorectomy, or a history of ovarian endometriomas. Using an FSH threshold of 2-SD from the mean, a total 37 of 91 women had an abnormal challenge test. Only 20 of the women would have been identified using a single d 3 FSH test. A high percentage of cycles were canceled in women with an abnormal test (85%), and no pregnancies were reported in this group. The value of the

Table 3
Ovarian Reserve Testing Using Clomiphene Citrate

Reference	Cases	Frequency with with abnormal FSH (%)	Cancellation rate		Pregnancy rate	
			Normal FSH	High FSH	Normal FSH	High FSH
Navot (35)	51	35[a]	—	—	42[b]	6
Tanbo (36)	91	40[c]	31.5	85.2	11[d]	0
Loumaye (37)	114	17.5[e]	1	25	27.6	0
Scott (38)	236	10[f]	—	—	42.7[g]	9.9

Definition of abnormal FSH.
[a] 95% confidence interval of FSH assay.
[b] $p < 0.05$.
[c] 95% confidence interval of FSH assay.
[d] $p < 0.0001$.
[e] Mean FSH d 5 + FSH d 10 + 2SD.
[f] FSH ≥ 10 IU/L, Becton-Dickinson assay.
[g] $p < 0.004$.

clomiphene citrate challenge test has been assessed in additional studies of women undergoing IVF (37). Using an FSH (FSHd-3 + FSHd-10) threshold based on 2-SD from the mean of the women who conceived, 20 patients were identified who had an abnormal test. In women with an abnormal test, the number of follicles, oocytes collected, and embryos obtained were significantly lower. Importantly, no pregnancies occurred in women with an abnormal test. Subsequent publications confirm the value of the clomiphene citrate challenge test in the prediction of successful achievement of pregnancy.

In distinction to previous tests assessing ovarian reserve, the clomiphene citrate challenge test is the only test examined in the general infertility population (38). The frequency of an abnormal test increases with age, ranging from 3% in women <30 yr of age to 26% for women over age 40. Pregnancy rates are lower (9%) in women with an abnormal test compared to women with a normal test (43%). Importantly, when the independent effects of both age and FSH levels on pregnancy rates are analyzed, an abnormal clomiphene citrate challenge test predicts a poor reproductive outcome independent of age.

LIMITATIONS IN THE CLOMIPHENE CITRATE CHALLENGE TEST

The interpretation of the clomiphene citrate challenge test is dependent on the results of FSH testing and as stated previously, significant variability in FSH assay methodology exists. In order to establish accurately threshold values of FSH, each laboratory needs to validate test results by examining reproductive outcome in a representative infertile population. Alternatively, FSH values can be compared to normative data from reference laboratories. Therefore, clinicians need to establish laboratory-specific threshold values to provide accurate counseling.

It is also important to recognize that the clomiphene citrate challenge test is a more accurate predictor of reproductive failure than success. Longitudinal studies indicate that only 5–10% of women with an abnormal test will conceive. In contrast, variable pregnancy rates are reported in women with normal testing and, of course, these rates diminish with advancing age. Therefore, age remains an additional and important prognostic marker of pregnancy potential in women with normal FSH values.

APPLICATION OF OVARIAN RESERVE TESTING

The decline in reproductive potential in women is an unfortunate but inevitable physiologic process. As pointed out previously, fertility rates diminish as a result of both declining oocyte number and quality, and possibly other factors, but not all women demonstrate a decreased ovarian reserve at similar time points. Therefore, the identification of biomarkers that detect changes in ovarian reserve is clinically important. At the present time, basal FSH and estradiol testing, although useful in predicting reproductive potential for a variety of clinical treatment options, suffers from insensitivity. Inhibin-B may also be a useful biomarker in the general population, however, its limited use in reproductive studies of ovarian reserve is a major drawback. Therefore, the clomiphene citrate challenge test is the method of choice for ovarian reserve assessment at this time.

Ovarian reserve testing is helpful in the general infertility investigation. We screen all women 35 years and older based on the rapidly declining fertility rates observed in this age group. Younger women who are gonadotropin unresponsive, fail IVF repeatedly, or who have repeatedly abnormal or poor-quality embryos may also benefit from testing. Basal estradiol monitoring may provide additional information, particularly when levels are highly elevated or when they are associated with an elevated FSH level. In addition, ovarian reserve testing should be used in screening all couples with unexplained infertility as this group demonstrates a significant increase in abnormal test results compared to other diagnostic categories *(38)*.

When the results of FSH testing are abnormal, clinicians face difficult decisions. Older women (>38) with elevated FSH and estradiol levels have a very poor prognosis, and should strongly consider donor egg IVF or adoption. Younger women with abnormal testing may achieve pregnancy, but success rates are low (<10%). In this age group, less costly fertility treatment regimens are reasonable, but the option of IVF should be discouraged. In our opinion, younger women who have FSH levels ≥ 20 IU/L should be offered donor egg IVF directly, because other forms of treatment are largely unsuccessful with these highly elevated FSH levels. In summary, ovarian reserve testing is a useful screening tool for the infertility population. The consideration of test results, age, associated infertility factors, and clinic-specific success rates will all play important roles in selecting the most beneficial method of treatment for each infertile couple.

REFERENCES

1. Richardson SJ, Senikas V, Nelson JF. Follicular depletion during the menopausal transition: Evidence for accelerated loss and ultimate exhaustion. J Clin Endocrinol Metab 1987;65:1231–1236.
2. Faddy MJ, Gosden RG, Gougeon A, Richardson SJ, Nelson JF. Accelerated disappearance of ovarian follicles in mid-life: implications for forecasting menopause. Hum Reprod 1992;7:1342–1346.
3. Leidy LE, Godfrey LR, Sutherland MR. Is follicular atresia biphasic? Fertil Steril 1998;70:851–859.
4. Klein NA, Battaglia DE, Miller PB, Branigan EF, Giudice LC, Soules MR. Ovarian follicular development and the follicular fluid hormones and growth factors in normal women of advanced reproductive age. J Clin Endocrinol Metab 1996;81:1946–1951.
5. Seifer DB, Gardiner AC, Lambert-Messerlian G, Schneyer AL. Differential secretion of dimeric inhibin in cultured luteinized granulosa cells as a function of ovarian reserve. J Clin Endocrinol Metab 1996; 81:736–739.

6. Seifer DB, Gardiner AC, Ferreira KA, Peluso JJ. Apoptosis as a function of ovarian reserve in women undergoing *in vitro* fertilization. Fertil Steril 1996;66:593–598.
7. Battaglia DE, Goodwin P, Klein NA, Soules MR. Influence of maternal age on meiotic spindle assembly in oocytes from naturally cycling women. Hum Reprod 1996;1:2222–2227.
8. Maroulis GB. Effect of aging on fertility and pregnancy. Semin Reprod Endocrinol 1991;9:165–175.
9. Guttmacher AF. Factors affecting normal expectancy of conception. J Am Med Assoc 1956;161:855–860.
10. Lenton EA, Sexton L, Lee S, Cooke ID. Progressive changes in LH and FSH and LH: FSH ratio in women throughout reproductive life. Maturitas 1988;10:35–43.
11. Klein NA, Battaglia DE, Fujimoto VY, Davis GS, Bremner WJ, Soules MR. Reproductive aging: accelerated ovarian follicular development associated with a menotropic follicle-stimulating hormone rise in normal older women. J Clin Endocrinol Metab 1996;81:1038–1045.
12. Metcalf MG, Donald RA, Livesey JH. Pituitary-ovarian function in normal women during the menopausal transition. Clin Endocrinol 1981;14:245–255.
13. Scott RT, Toner JF, Muasher SJ, Oehninger SC, Robinson S, Rosenwaks Z. Follicle stimulating hormone levels on cycle day 3 are predictive of *in vitro* fertilization outcome. Fertil Steril 1989;51:651–654.
14. Toner JP, Philput CB, Jones GS, Nuasher SJ. Basal follicle stimulating hormone level is a better predictor of *in vitro* fertilization performance than age. Fertil Steril 1991;55:784–791.
15. Muasher SJ, Oehninger S, Simonetti S, Matta J, Ellis LM, Liu H-C, Jones GS, Rosenwaks Z. The value of basal and/or stimulated serum gonadotropin levels in prediction of stimulation response and *in vitro* fertilization outcome. Fertil Steril 1988;50:298–307.
16. Cahill DJ, Prosser CJ, Wardie PG, Ford WCL, Hull MGR. Relative influence of serum follicle-stimulating hormone, age and other factors on ovarian response to gonadotrophin stimulation. Br J Obstet Gynaecol 1994;101:999–1002.
17. Pearlstone AC, Foumet N, Gambone JC, Pang SC, Buyalos RP. Ovulation induction in women age 40 and older: the importance of basal follicle-stimulating hormone level and chronological age. Fertil Steril 1992;58:674–679.
18. Khalifa E, Toner JP, Muasher SJ, Acosta AA. Significance of basal follicle-stimulating hormone levels in women with one ovary in a program of *in vitro* fertilization. Fertil Steril 1992;57:835–839.
19. Scott RT, Hofmann GE, Oehninger S, Muasher SJ. Intercycle variability of day 3 follicle-stimulating hormone levels and its effect on stimulation quality in *in vitro* fertilization. Fertil Steril 1990;53:297–302.
20. Martin JSB, Nisker JA, Tummon IS, Daniel SAJ, Auckland JL, Feyles W. Future *in vitro* fertilization pregnancy potential of women with variably elevated day 3 follicle-stimulating hormone levels. Fertil Steril 1996;65:1238–1240.
21. Scott RT, Toner JP, Muasher SJ, Oehninger S, Robinson S, Rosenwaks Z. Follicle- stimulating hormone levels on cycle day 3 are predictive of *in vitro* fertilization outcome. Fertil Steril 1989;51:651–654.
22. Farhi J, Homburg R, Ferber A, Orvieto R, Ben Rafael Z. Non-response to ovarian stimulation in normogonadotrophic, normogonadal women: a clinical sign of impending onset of ovarian failure pre-empting the rise in basal follicle stimulating hormone levels. Hum Reprod 1997;12:241–243.
23. Smotrich DB, Widra EA, Gindoff PR, Levy MJ, Hall JL, Stillman RJ. Prognostic value of day 3 estradiol on *in vitro* fertilization outcome. Fertil Steril 1995;64:1136–1140.
24. Licciardi FL, Liu H-C, Rosenwaks Z. Day 3 estradiol serum concentrations as prognosticators of ovarian stimulation response and pregnancy outcome in patients undergoing *in vitro* fertilization. Fertil Steril 1995;64:991–994.
25. Padilla SL, Bayati J, Garcia JE. Prognostic value of the early serum estradiol response to leuprolide acetate in *in vitro* fertilization. Fertil Steril 1990;53:288–294.
26. Ranieri DM, Quinn F, Makhlouf A, Khadum I, Ghutmi W, McGarrigle H, Davies M, Serhal P. Simultaneous evaluation of basal follicle-stimulating hormone and 17β-estradiol response to gonadotropin-releasing hormone analogue stimulation: an improved predictor of ovarian reserve. Fertil Steril 1998;70:227–253.
27. Scott RT, Sable DB, Drews MR, Robins ED, Sharara FI, Cohen J, Bergh PA. Abstract PP-20-491. Proceedings of the 10th World Congress on In Vitro Fertilization and Assisted Reproduction; 1997 May 22–25, Vancouver, BC, Canada. Vancouver: The Congress, 1997.
28. Groome NP, Illingworth PJ, O'Brien M, Pai R, Rodger FE, Mather JP, McNeilly AS. Measurement of dimeric inhibin-B throughout the human menstrual cycle. J Clin Endocrinol Metab 1996;81:1401–1405.
29. Welt CK, Martin KM, Taylor AE, Lambert-Messerlian GM, Crowley WF Jr, Smith JA, et al. Frequency modulation of follicle-stimulating hormone (FSH) during the luteal-follicular transition: evidence for FSH control of inhibin-B in normal women. J Clin Endocrinol Metab 1997;82:2645–2652.

30. Roberts VJ, Barth S, El-Roeiy A, Yen SSC. Expression of inhibin/activin subunits and follistatin messenger ribonucleic acids and proteins in ovarian follicles and the corpus luteum during the human menstrual cycle. J Clin Endocrinol Metab 1993;77:1402–1410.
31. McLachlan RI, Cohen NL, Vale WW, Rivier JE, Burger HG, Bremner WJ, Soules MR. The importance of luteinizing hormone in the control of inhibin and progesterone secretion by the human corpus luteum. J Clin Endocrinol Metab 1989;68:1078–1085.
32. Danforth DR, Arbogast LK, Mroueh J, Kim MH, Kennard EA, Seifer DB, Friedman CI. Dimeric inhibin: a direct marker of ovarian aging. Fertil Steril 1998;70:119–123.
33. Molskness TA, Woodruff TK, Hess DL, Dahl KD, Stouffer RL. Recombinant human inhibin-A administered early in the menstrual cycle alters concurrent pituitary and follicular, plus subsequent luteal, function in rhesus monkeys. J Clin Endocrinol Metab 1996;81:4002–4006.
34. Seifer DB, Lambert-Messerlian G, Hogan JW, Gardiner AC, Blazar AS, Berk CA. Day 3 serum inhibin-B is predictive of assisted reproductive technologies outcome. Fertil Steril 1997;67:110–114.
35. Navot D, Rosenwaks Z, Margalioth EJ. Prognostic assessment of female fecundity. Lancet 1987;2:645–647.
36. Tanbo T, Dale PO, Ludne O, Norman N, Abyholm T. Prediction of response to controlled ovarian hyperstimulation: a comparison of basal and clomiphene citrate-stimulated follicle stimulating hormone levels. Fertil Steril 1992;57:819–829.
37. Loumaye E, Billion JM, Mine JM, Psalit I, Pensis M, Thomas K. Prediction of individual response to controlled ovarian hyperstimulation by means of a clomiphene citrate challenge test. Fertil Steril 1990;53:295–301.
38. Scott RT, Leonardi MR, Hofmann GE, Illions EH, Neal GS, Navot D. A prospective evaluation of clomiphene citrate challenge test screening in the general infertility population. Obstet Gynecol 1993;82:539–545.

6

Imaging Technology in Assisted Reproduction

Roger A. Pierson, MS, PHD

CONTENTS

INTRODUCTION

Imaging, in the medical sense of the word, describes the processes with which we visualize the anatomic structures that make up the body. For millennia, we have looked at the outside of the body and tried to imagine what was going on inside. The esteem with which we hold the power to reproduce has made the reproductive system the most intensely pondered of body systems. One only has to read the historical writings of Hippocrates or Soranus to realize the deep mysteries that reproduction holds. Direct visualization of the reproductive organs in cadavers sufficed for centuries as the source of our reproductive knowledge. The drawings of Fabricius, Vesalius, Leonardo da Vinci, and deGraaf represented the standard of knowledge. However, even the most detailed studies of static specimens omit the fundamental processes of life and the inner workings of the systems that we wish to understand. Many discoveries have been made and techniques developed to try to understand the workings of the reproductive system, identification of the reproductively active hormones, and their assay in systemic and organ-specific circulations are some of the most profound. However, only recently has the technology existed to make noninvasive pictures of the inner workings of the reproductive system.

The word fantastic comes to mind when we consider the leaps that have been made in our collective knowledge of reproductive processes over the past half century. The first

From: *Contemporary Endocrinology: Assisted Fertilization and Nuclear Transfer in Mammals*
Edited by: D. P. Wolf and M. Zelinski-Wooten © Humana Press Inc., Totowa, NJ

particularly useful imaging technology applied to reproductive systems was hysterosal-pingography. This technique allowed physicians to determine whether or not the oviducts were patent without invasive surgery. The developments in ultrasonography, magnetic resonance imaging (MRI), and computerized interpretation of the images that these fantastic machines generate have progressed to the point where we may now begin to make functional assessments of the physiologic status of follicles within the ovaries of patients in noninvasive ways. This new information may then be used to diagnose problems never before recognized and direct the course of therapy to ameliorate infertility. Noninvasive imaging of the ovaries and testes are transforming the way that we think about reproductive function. We now have the unprecedented opportunity to observe ovarian function in the same women over time, to determine what happens to individual follicles, and to apply new techniques to age-old puzzles. It is always important to remember that changes in the anatomy and physiology of the reproductive organs form the basis for the images that we see, therefore, reminders of the biology underlying the images are placed where marriage of concept and visualization are critical.

Transvaginal high-resolution diagnostic ultrasonography has become the most important development in the understanding of ovarian function since the development of radio-immunoassay techniques for measuring reproductively active hormones. Relatively high frequency (e.g., 5.0 MHz, 7.5 MHz) or broad-band (4–9 MHz) intravaginal transducers and color-flow Doppler imaging techniques have dramatically increased image resolution, allowing detailed examination of the female reproductive organs. Computer enhancements of the images now facilitate physiologic interpretation of the information in the images. The same techniques are beginning to be applied in animal model systems for the study of the male reproductive organs, although the techniques are not as developed in human studies.

There is a great deal of physiologically important information not readily appreciated by the human eye available in the exquisite detail of the images created by the current generation of ultrasonographic, magnetic resonance, and other imaging instruments. These image data may be evaluated in many forms. The physiologic events underlying ovarian follicular growth and development, ovulation, and luteal function may be evaluated in minute detail using computer-enhanced ultrasonography. Similarly, MRI is emerging as a research tool in ovarian imaging. Future developments in equipment may make MRI as "user-friendly" as ultrasonography is now. Combinations of the information available in ultrasonography, MRI, computer-assisted image analysis, and mathematical modeling are predictive of new era in our understanding of the basic biology of the female and male reproductive processes.

The purpose of this chapter is to identify some of the emerging areas in ovarian imaging and to describe the contributions of imaging technology to our understanding of these problems as they pertain to assisted reproduction. The application of imaging technologies to male reproductive processes is much less developed; however, it is easy to speculate on their uses. The application of imaging techniques to the optical images generated by our microscopes has apparently been limited to digital acquisition of images of oocytes and embryos obtained for the assisted reproductive technologies for database storage and record keeping. An attempt to find any information on structural or functional analysis of oocytes or embryos was unsuccessful. Finally, I will speculate on the applications of emerging imaging technologies to our future understanding of reproductive biology.

FEMALE REPRODUCTIVE SYSTEM

Ovaries

ASSESSMENT OF OVARIAN FOLLICULAR DEVELOPMENT

The follicular population within the ovaries may be evaluated at any time during the menstrual cycle. However, the period of greatest interest usually is the late follicular phase when the development of the follicle physiologically selected to ovulate may be identified and monitored. The dominant follicle appears to be identifiable on the basis of size at approximately d 7 post-menstruation and grows at a rate of approx 2 mm/d *(1–5)*. Serial ultrasound examinations may be performed during the follicular phases of one or more menstrual cycles to ascertain that the processes of follicular selection and growth are occurring within clinically normal limits *(4,7)*. If subtle abnormalities in follicular growth are detected, corrective measures may be taken.

The profiles for serum estradiol concentrations and ultrasonographically determined diameters of preovulatory follicles normally run parallel courses *(4,8)*. Therefore, serial ultrasonography and evaluation of systemic estrogen levels have great potential in the isolation and identification of the causes of follicular phase defects. For example, patients may present with estradiol concentrations that appear to be within clinically normal limits for the preovulatory phase of the menstrual cycle; however, ultrasound examination may reveal the presence of 6–20 follicles of 5–10 mm diameter and the absence of a dominant follicle of preovulatory diameter. Alternatively, ultrasound examination during the late follicular phase of a spontaneous menstrual cycle may reveal a follicle of ostensibly preovulatory diameter (e.g., 22 mm), and the patient may exhibit clinically low estradiol concentrations. In our experience, follicles with this particular pattern of growth and regression have an atypical morphology, appear flaccid, fail to ovulate, and regress over the ensuing week *(9)*. Using serial ultrasonography and assessment of circulating hormone levels, it appears possible to identify subtle defects in the processes of follicular recruitment, development, physiologic selection of the pre-ovulatory follicle, final follicular maturation, and ovulation. Seemingly minor disturbances in the continuum of folliculogenesis may be responsible for much infertility previously classified as idiopathic.

PREOVULATORY FOLLICLES

One way in which the selected preovulatory follicle differs physiologically from the other follicles in its cohort is that they have a more extensive and permeable capillary network *(2,10,11)*. The vascularity that exists around the dominant follicle may allow it to accumulate more of the circulating gonadotropins and thus survive while the other members of its cohort become atretic. However, it is not known whether the enhanced vascularity is a cause or reflection of selection. The patterns and changes in blood flow around preovulatory follicles and during ovulation have been demonstrated by color-flow Doppler ultrasonography *(12*; Pierson, unpublished observations). Follicles imaged after the luteinizing hormone (LH) surge and before ovulation showed pronounced changes in their peripheral vascular flow. There was increased flow at the base of the follicles and concomitant flow at the apex of the follicles. These observations were consistent with histologic and ultrasonographic studies of preovulatory follicles *(2,13)*.

A successful ovarian follicle is one that escapes the overwhelming odds of atresia and ovulates, releasing its oocyte into a realm where it may be fertilized. Ultrasonographic

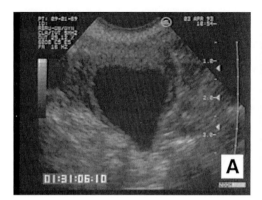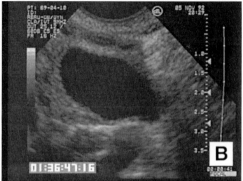

Fig. 1.   Ultrasonographic images of imminently preovulatory follicles recorded within 1 min before the onset of ovulation. The follicular antrum (black) is surrounded by the follicle walls, composed of the stratum granulosum and the theca interna. The follicle wall also is usually discernible from the surrounding ovarian stroma. Note the pronounced stigma projecting from the surface of the ovary in the lower right aspect of the antrum. Stigma formation is observed on most preovulatory follicles. The deep internal walls of preovulatory follicles are typically thicker than the apical portions of the follicle walls.

images of imminently preovulatory follicles are shown (Fig. 1). The follicle destined to ovulate is physiologically selected for preferential development and eventual ovulation, while other follicles in its cohort are condemned to atresia. The processes by which the selection mechanism occurs have not been determined and remain among the great mysteries in reproductive biology. The current concepts regarding physiological selection of the dominant follicle in women and nonhuman primates have been critically evaluated, and it has been determined that the selection process is completed only during the ovarian cycle in which the individual ovulation occurs *(3,6,14)*. In this regard, it has been postulated that selection, final growth, and maturation of the ovulatory follicle may be owing simply to chance development of a follicle within the recruited cohort coincident with luteal regression and increased preovulatory follicle stimulating hormone (FSH) levels. However, the presence of a "carry-over" effect of exogenous gonadotropins administered to superstimulate the ovaries is obvious by the observation that the fertility rates in women who have undergone ovulation induction are substantially higher in the two or three cycles following ovarian stimulation.

ASSESSMENT OF OVARIAN BLOOD FLOW

Transvaginal color-flow Doppler ultrasonographic imaging may be used to identify the ovarian vessels as they enter the ovarian hilus; the intraovarian vascular supply also may be visualized. Resistance to blood flow in the ovarian vasculature has been studied at various times during the ovarian cycle using spectral Doppler techniques; the ovary bearing the preovulatory follicle or corpus luteum exhibits lower resistance to blood flow than the vessels of the contralateral ovary. The lowest impedance to blood flow during the ovarian cycle occurs on the day of the LH peak, whereas highest resistance to blood flow was observed on d 1 of menses *(15)*. However, it was not possible to identify a clear relationship between estradiol, progesterone, and other circulating hormones and the vascular indices of the ovarian and uterine arteries *(16)*.

Color-flow Doppler ultrasonography also has been used to evaluate ovarian blood flow during ovarian stimulation before oocyte retrieval for in vitro fertilization (IVF)

(17–20). In an initial study, peak velocity measurements and resistive indices decreased as the diameter of the follicles increased. This observation was consistent with the idea that the vascularity of the follicles increases as ovulation nears; however, the vascular indices were not useful for predicting the outcome of IVF cycles *(17).* Later studies concluded that there is indeed a physiological relationship between follicular vascular indices and the clinical outcomes of assisted reproduction cycles *(18–20).* A strong correlation was observed between oocyte recovery rates and the level of follicular vascularity, and it was proposed that perifollicular blood flow may be indicative of the appropriate time for human chorionic gonadotropin (hCG) administration for optimal recovery rates *(19).* In addition, it has been proposed that Doppler investigation of individual follicles may provide a direct indication of the health of the follicle and developmental competence of the oocyte *(20).*

Research is just beginning on the assessment of echotextural characteristics and vascular patterns of individual preovulatory follicles to evaluate the probability of ovulation. Studies using transvaginal color-flow mapping to assess blood flow to the follicle and the vascular perfusion of the follicular wall during the dominance phase are ongoing in our laboratory. Although data have not yet been critically evaluated, it appears that there is a very gradual decrease in impedance to blood flow in the vessels immediately surrounding the follicle as the interval to ovulation decreases. Immediately prior to ovulation, the peri-follicular vessels are easily identified and spectral Doppler flow wave forms may be generated. However, it is rare to visualize the peri-follicular vessels in one image plane owing to their tortuous path around the periphery of the follicle *(15;* Pierson, 1999, unpublished observations).

OVULATION

Ovulation occurs on approx d 14 post-menstruation in a classic "textbook" 28-d menstrual cycle and is the culmination of the life of a successful follicle *(1,3,14).* It is a complex series of events that is set into motion with a sudden, brief rise in peripheral LH concentrations, and results in the evacuation of the follicular fluid, collapse of the preovulatory follicle, and expulsion of the oocyte from the follicle *(21–24).* Dissolution of the apex of the follicle, final maturation of the oocyte, and evacuation of the follicular fluid must be closely coordinated for the release of an oocyte capable of being fertilized. Subsequent functional and morphologic changes in the granulosa and luteal cells also must be completed to form the corpus luteum. Direct observation of ovulation (follicular rupture) by laparoscopy or ultrasonography is quite dramatic; however, it must be remembered that the event of ovulation is the result of a long series of biochemical, physiologic, and morphologic changes in the tissues of the follicle (Fig. 2) *(23).*

Transabdominal ultrasound scanning has been used for many years to detect the occurrence of ovulation in women *(25).* However, rupture of the follicle and evacuation of the follicular fluid and cumulus-oocyte complex has only recently been demonstrated by real-time ultrasonography *(26,27)* (Fig. 2). On average, ovulation appeared to take approx 10 min from initiation to complete follicular evacuation. However, the time required for ovulation varied from less than 1 min to more than 20 min. The site of follicular evacuation was immediately detectable. The point of follicular rupture from the surface of the ovary may be recognized for up to a week and the corpus luteum typically remains ultrasonographically detectable until the subsequent ovulatory cycle *(28,29;* Hess and Pierson, 1999, unpublished observations).

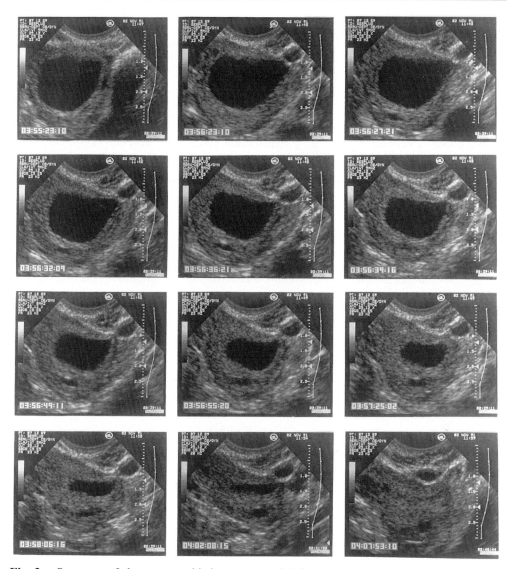

Fig. 2. Sequence of ultrasonographic images recorded during a research study on human ovulation. The ovulation took 10 min and 56 s from onset to complete follicular evacuation. Images are shown at equidistant intervals during ovulation. The first half of the follicular fluid was evacuated in 20 s; the remaining fluid was evacuated over the remaining 10 min and 36 s. Time code values representing hours, minutes, seconds, and video frame are displayed in the lower left corner of each image. Adapted with permission from ref. *(27)*.

Color-flow mapping studies of the follicular vasculature have only recently begun. There is a single report of a single ovulation in the literature *(30)*. Studies regarding vasculature changes during ovulation are ongoing (Pierson 1999, unpublished observations). In our series of color-flow studies, volumetric estimations of the follicular fluid are made from follicular measurements at defined times before and during ovulation. Color-flow maps and spectral Doppler wave forms also are generated at defined times during follicular evacuation. The patterns of blood flow during collapse of the follicle have not yet been critically evaluated. However, variation in resistance to blood flow

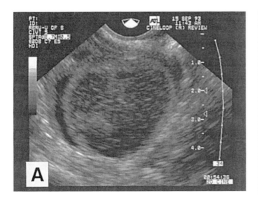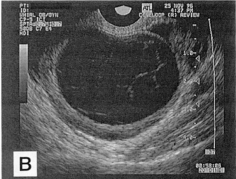

Fig. 3. Ultrasonographic images of anovulatory follicles from women scanned throughout spontaneous menstrual cycles as a part of research into ovulatory failure (**A,B**). The images represent a
luteinized unruptured follicle (LUF) (**A**) and a hemorrhagic anovulatory follicle (HAF) (**B**). The
difference between the two types of ovulatory failure is hypothesized to be primarily the degree of
luteinization of the tissues of the former follicle wall. The LUF (**A**) is surrounded by a visually thicker
wall of apparently luteinized tissue. The internal echoes are consistent with cellular debris and hemorrhage. The internal echoes of the HAF (**B**) are consistent with a semi-organized fibrin network.

appears to be quite dramatically decreased between preovulatory measurements and
those taken following initiation of follicular rupture. Variation in flow characteristics
appear very slight once follicular evacuation has begun. Power-flow Doppler imaging
will have a great deal to add to our knowledge of follicular collapse and luteinization.

OVULATION FAILURE

Evaluation of ovulation and the period of early luteinization in research patients
during spontaneous cycles and patients referred for idiopathic infertility is revealing
previously undescribed flaws in the ovulatory process. Failure of ovulation probably
occurs by one of two mechanisms. The luteinized, unruptured follicle (LUF) syndrome
remains somewhat controversial; however, transvaginal ultrasound has been used to provide detailed descriptions of the process (Fig. 3A) *(31,32)*. The physiologically selected
follicle attains preovulatory diameter and fails to rupture and release the oocyte-cumulus
complex. The oocyte-cumulus complex appears to remain trapped within the lumen of
the follicular structure. The walls of the follicle appear to thicken and acquire echotexture
similar to that of luteinized tissue following normal ovulations. The follicular fluid/
follicle interface acquires hazy, indistinct borders. The LUF remains identifiable for the
duration of the menstrual cycle and apparently regresses following a time-course similar
to that of clinically normal corpora lutea (Pierson 1999, unpublished observations). A
variation of the LUF syndrome is the hemorrhagic anovulatory follicle (HAF), in which
the same series of event occurs, however, there is capillary leakage into the lumen of the
follicle and the same level of peripheral luteinization does not develop (Fig. 3B).

A second proposed mechanism for failure of ovulation appears to involve the growth
of the physiologically selected follicle beyond normal preovulatory diameter without
ovulation. The dysfunctional dominant follicle appears to remain static for one to several
days and then regresses. The rate of follicular regression appears to be highly variable,
although in several instances in our laboratory, the rate of regression has been the same
as the rate of follicular growth. There is no apparent luteinization of the follicular wall,
which appears thin and highly echoic (Fig. 4A). Delamination of the entire granulosa

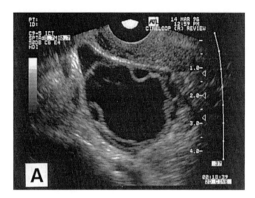 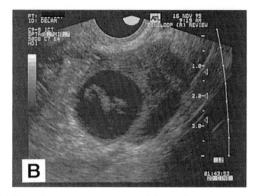

Fig. 4. Ultrasonographic images of anovulatory follicles from women scanned throughout sponta-neous menstrual cycles as a part of research into ovulatory failure (**A,B**). In the first image (**A**) the follicle attained an ostensibly preovulatory diameter of 23 mm, however, it did not ovulate and regressed over the remainder of the cycle. Note the thin, apparently atreic follicle walls surrounding the antrum. The second image (**B**) shows delamination of the stratum granulosum, which is observed floating within the follicular antrum. The follicle wall remaining around the follicle is thin and there is an acute transformation at the fluid-follicle interface.

layer also has been observed; sheets of granulosa cells are observed floating within the follicular antrum (Fig. 4B). The follicular fluid/follicle interfaces appear to remain sharp and distinct.

Corpus Luteum

Following ovulation, the cells of the former follicle must complete the long series of biochemical and morphological steps of luteinization to form the temporary endocrine gland, which produces the progesterone necessary for a successful pregnancy. Ultra-sonographic images of corpora lutea at the beginning, mid-cycle, and end of their tempo-rary lives are shown (Fig. 5). The walls of the follicle are in close apposition immediately following evacuation of the follicular fluid. The cells of the former follicular wall begin the structural and functional transformations of luteogenesis by becoming profoundly vascularized during the 48–72 h following ovulation. There is a slight hemorrhage into the evacuated follicle following ovulation in approx 60% of ovulations (Pierson, 1999, manuscript submitted). The degree of hemorrhage is extremely variable; however, there does not appear to be any relationship between the degree of hemorrhage observed on ultrasound examination and progesterone production during the luteal phase of the men-strual cycle (*29*; Pierson 1999, manuscript submitted).

Because the corpus luteum undergoes profound neoangiogenesis during its develop-ment, is dependent on vascular flow for normal function, and exhibits degradation of the vascular supply during regression, it seems natural to apply sophisticated image analysis regimens to the study of luteal function. The cyclicity in vascularization and the role of the corpus luteum in regulating ovarian function from ovarian cycle to ovarian cycle, in addition to its role in the establishment and maintenance of pregnancy, make the corpus luteum a primary target for research based upon color-flow Doppler ultrasonography.

A pronounced ring of vascularity, which appears to follow the path of the vascular supply surrounding the former preovulatory follicle and which becomes even more appa-rent as the corpus luteum matures, is typically observed upon color-flow Doppler inter-rogation. During active progesterone secretion, resistance to vascular flow is usually

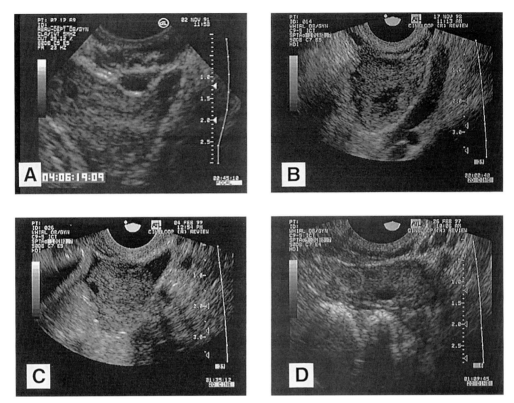

Fig. 5. Ultrasonographic images of the corpus luteum recorded at different times during spontaneous menstrual cycles in research volunteers (**A–D**). Image (**A**) was recorded at complete follicular evacuation immediately after ovulation. The stigma of the former follicle is to the right. A small amount of fluid is observed outside of the ovary just distal to the site of follicular rupture. The thin black line represents the lumen of the former follicle. Images (**B**) and (**C**) represent mid-cycle corpora lutea with (**B**) and without (**C**) a central fluid-filled cavity. The fluid observed in the center of the luteal tissue in image (**B**) is consistent with the echo texture of a blood clot. A corpus albicans is observed in the left aspect of the ovary in image (**D**). The echo texture of the regressed luteal structure is representative of a higher echo signal (brighter) and is well-circumscribed. The corpus albicans is easily discerned from the surrounding ovarian stoma.

low, as would be expected of an active endocrine tissue. As luteal regression ensues, the vascular flow characteristics change profoundly. The color-mapping patterns become much less pronounced and increased resistance to flow is observed within the vessels *(29)*. Definitive studies of the vascular dynamics within the corpus luteum have apparently not yet been performed; however, this is a promising research area with profound ramifications to infertility assessments, the study of maternal recognition of pregnancy and etiology of early embryonic loss. It is highly probable that vascular changes in the corpus luteum may be indicative of impending early embryonic death.

A precise role for color-flow Doppler assessment of luteal vascularity has yet to be defined; it seems probable that there is an important role for this imaging modality in the study of luteal function. Color-flow Doppler imaging combined with high-resolution gray-scale ultrasonography allows evaluation of the functional development of the corpus luteum, as well as other reproductive organs of interest, and provides the ability to locate blood flow in very small vessels that cannot be visualized with conventional gray-scale imaging. In addition, the flow velocity waveforms resulting from spectral Doppler interrogation may be analysed to assess functional integrity. More recently, the addition of power-flow color Doppler provides a technique with which we may study the perfusion of the corpus luteum. Preliminary studies on luteal function have been performed in normal women as well as women with luteal phase defects and LUF syndrome (33–37). High correlations were observed between the levels of circulating progesterone and vascular indices in the luteal phase of the menstrual cycle; although the number of women involved in the study was small, there was no difference in the values recorded in women with normal luteal phases and luteal phase defects (34,36). Follicles which ended their bid for ovulation with a LUF showed reduced blood flow in the follicle walls after the LH surge (37). A new ultrasonographic imaging technique exploiting another aspect of the Doppler effect, power-flow Doppler, may be used to show all the areas of flow within an organ. The technique is currently being actively investigated in several laboratories, however, it remains mostly a clinical curiosity at this point. It has been concluded that color-flow and power-flow Doppler imaging may be used to detect physiologic change in the corpus luteum, however, rigorous studies have not been completed (38).

Transvaginal color-flow ultrasonography evaluation of luteal blood flow in pregnant and nonpregnant women has been demonstrated. Low rates of luteal blood flow were observed in nonpregnant women, whereas the highest rates of blood flow were observed in the corpora lutea glands of women with intrauterine pregnancies (39,40). Color-flow Doppler ultrasonographic mapping is also routinely used to aid in the identification of abnormal adnexal flow patterns associated with the trophoblastic mass in ectopic pregnancies. Women scanned for clinical purposes during early pregnancy may have color-flow Doppler examination to aid clinicians in identification of the corpus luteum (41).

OVARIAN STIMULATION AND OVULATION INDUCTION

In ovarian stimulation, we strive to defeat obligatory atresia and deliver as many competent oocytes as possible into the hands of embryologists wishing to better the odds of natural fertilization. This is currently done by administering exogenous gonadotrophins derived of either biological (human menopausal gonadotropins, hMG) or recombinant sources. Ultrasonographic imaging is essential in determining the numbers and fates of individual follicles induced to grow with gonadotrophins. It is important to understand that the linear relationship between circulating estradiol concentrations and follicular diameter we expect based on the study of unstimulated cycles may not exist during ovulation induction (9,42). Thus, ultrasonography is extremely important in this area. The timing of hCG administration is critical in all ovulation induction protocols. In monitoring the course of an ovulation induction, the responses of individual follicles to the ovulatory dose of hCG may be as important as monitoring the number and rates of growth of the follicles. The number of follicles that ovulate may be discerned and unruptured follicles remaining in the ovaries assessed. If conception does not occur, appropriate actions may be taken for subsequent therapies.

The ovarian response to induction with exogenous gonadotrophins is typically assessed by daily measurement of serum estradiol using standard radioimmunoassay techniques and serial ultrasonographic examinations. Both methods play a complementary role in controlled ovarian hyperstimulation; however, the importance of intensive ultrasonographic monitoring during the stimulation cycle cannot be overemphasized. When the diameter of the largest follicle first attains a predetermined diameter (18–20 mm in our center), 5,000–10,000 IU of hCG is administered to trigger the final phases of follicular maturation leading to ovulation. Oocyte retrieval for the assisted reproductive technologies is typically scheduled for 30–34 h following hCG. Ovulation is expected to occur 34–48 h following the hCG in women who are undergoing intrauterine insemination. In our center, ultrasonographic examinations are continued until all follicles have either ovulated or showed ultrasonographically detectable signs of atresia.

Numerous reports on women studied during spontaneous menstrual cycles have stated that the wide range of values reported for the maximal diameter of preovulatory follicles precludes its use as a single index for the prediction of ovulation (4,25,28). However, follicular diameter was a more accurate predictor of impending ovulation than plasma measurements of FSH, LH, or estradiol (43). Some of the disparity in measurements of preovulatory follicular diameter may, in part, be attributed to different scanning protocols. In most cases, scans were performed daily and measurements were made as much as 24 h prior to ovulation (4,25,28,43), whereas other measurements were taken just prior to ovulation (13,26).

The relationship between follicle size and oocyte maturity has yet to be resolved. In most ovulation induction protocols, hCG is administered when the leading preovulatory follicle attains 18–20 mm. It has been postulated that oocyte maturity may be achieved at a mean follicular diameter of 15–16 mm in hMG-stimulated cycles (44). However, it is possible that follicle diameter does not correlate well with the stage of maturity and quality of the oocyte. The results of one study have been interpreted to demonstrate that there were no differences in the fertilization rate of oocytes aspirated from follicles in the following size categories: 10–14 mm, 15–19 mm, and ≥20 mm, although the lack of differences may also be because of in vitro maturation of the oocytes (45). The characteristics and appropriate sizes of follicles that will produce oocytes in states of maturity appropriate for fertilization remains the subject of much controversy and research. These observations support the necessity of monitoring the development of individual follicles; any follicle attaining a diameter ≥14 mm has the potential to ovulate viable oocytes, which can maximize the benefit of the ovulation induction cycle. Previous reports have suggested that ova from smaller follicles display reduced oocyte quality and fertilization rates (46).

Uterus

The uterus, in addition to its function as the site of embryo implantation in natural conception and of embryo transfer in the assisted reproductive technologies, is comprised of the perimetrium, myometrium, and the endometrium. The endometrial lining is an exquisitely sensitive visual bioassay with which we may infer the relative levels and types of reproductively active hormones in the circulation. Assessment of the changes in patterns of the endometrium during the menstrual cycle were among the first uses of ultrasonography in reproductive medicine (47–50). Ultrasonographic images of the uterus showing each of the important patterns observed during spontaneous menstrual cycles are shown (Fig. 6). Ultrasonographic images of the endometrium during the early part of the cycle change from a thin, simple hyperechoic stripe seen immediately following menstruation to the triple-line pattern indicative of increasing estradiol levels. Then a pronounced triple-line pattern with distinct separation of the stratum basalis and stratum spongiosum is observed with the high estradiol levels associated with the periovulatory period. A heterogenous, fully secretory endometrial pattern indicative of luteinization

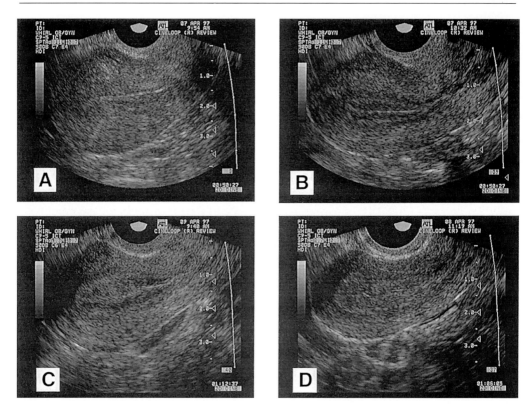

Fig. 6. Ultrasonographic images representing the various stages of endometrial development observed during spontaneous menstrual cycles. Images of the endometrium during the early part of the cycle change from a thin, simple hyperechoic stripe seen immediately following menstruation (**A**) to the triple-line pattern indicative of increasing estradiol levels associated with the early follicular phase of the cycle (**B**). A pronounced triple-line pattern with distinct separation of the stratum basalis and stratum spongiosum is observed with the high estradiol levels associated with the periovulatory period (**C**). A heterogenous, fully secretory endometrial pattern indicative of luteinization and progesterone exposure is seen following ovulation (**D**).

and progesterone exposure is seen following ovulation *(48,51)*. The patterns of endometrial development are well-documented and the endometrial response to circulating estradiol and progesterone are markedly different. However, the responses of individual women are subject to considerable biovariability and the response of the endometrium to precise levels of circulating hormones have not yet been determined.

The use of imaging technology to evaluate the endometrium should not be limited to simple measurements of endometrial thickness. Rather, the full range of endometrial expression and reaction to the reproductively active steroids should be embraced. The patterns displayed by the endometrium undergo predictable, quantifiable changes as estradiol and progesterone are elaborated by the ovaries. Ultrasonography has been used for many years to try to correlate the probability of pregnancy in ovarian stimulation–ovulation induction cycles and IVF programs with varying degrees of success *(49,52,53)*. It appears that implantation may occur as long as the endometrial thickness is greater than 6 mm *(54,55)*. Assessment of the endometrium using traditional ultrasonographic imaging does not appear to have predictive value in estimating the probability of successful implantation; however, it is not known whether or not two- or three-dimensional image mapping may be useful.

Computer-assisted analysis of ultrasonographic images of the uterus remains largely unexplored. However, any of the techniques discussed in other sections of this chapter may be easily applied to images of this important target organ. A preliminary study of changes in the decidual reaction of the endometrium during the first trimester of pregnancy was used to demonstrate that the changes in developing placentation could be documented with this technique (56). However, no further studies using quantitative image analysis appear to have been completed to evaluate the prospects for predicting the probability of pregnancy.

The use of ultrasonographic imaging of the endometrial cavity for embryo replacement in assisted reproduction cycles has been discussed, but it is probably underutilized (57–60). Careful guidance of the embryo transfer catheter using concomitant transabdominal ultrasonography would likely have a real impact upon the rates of successful pregnancy following assisted reproduction cycles (see Chapter 9). Guided transfer would help to avoid the pitfalls associated with difficult anatomical configurations of the cervix and lower uterine segment and would decrease the likelihood of sub-endometrial embryo transfer. In one study, catheter placements done by only tactile placement were ultrasonographically monitored (60). The guiding cannula indented the endometrium in 25% of 121 patients, the transfer catheter was embedded in the endometrium in 33% and sub-endometrial transfers occurred in approx 22% of the patients. In addition, ultrasound guided transfer avoided accidental oviductal transfer in approx 7% of the 121 patients.

There is much work to do with the application of advanced imaging technology to the uterus and endometrium. However, it appears that this is a rich field for exploration.

MALE REPRODUCTIVE SYSTEM

Ultrasonography and image analysis are only beginning to be used in the assessment of male reproductive organs. Transrectal ultrasonography and color-flow Doppler assessment have been used clinically for the evaluation of the distal portions of the vas deferens, seminal vesicles and ejaculatory ducts, and the prostate (61,62). Previously, investigations were limited to operative vasography and computed tomography (CT). Doppler ultrasonography is commonly used for diagnosis and study of varicocele, but this appears to remain a primarily clinical tool. A cause and effect relationship of varicocele and male factor infertility has not been established. Although ultrasonography has made the clinical evaluation of the male organs possible, it appears that little research has been done to explore the possibilities of correlating testicular echotexture with semen quality and characteristics. The primary use of the imaging technology appears to be in the diagnosis of gross anatomic anomalies and some subtle changes such as hypoplasia, seminal vesicle fibrosis, or fibrotic changes in the prostate or ejaculatory ducts (62). Animal models have been used to explore some aspects of image analysis and the male reproductive organs during puberty; however, no human studies appear to have been done (63–65).

Computerized image analysis of sperm motility (CASA) is a common technique in semen analysis, however, its true utility in semen evaluation remains somewhat controversial. Image acquisition and detailed analysis of sperm would make a significant addition to the state of knowledge in automated semen analysis. It seems reasonable that strict morphological evaluation of individual sperm, such as that indicated by the Kruger strict morphology criteria (66,67), could be done as a relatively simple pattern-recognition algorithm. Once the correlations among oocyte capacity for fertilization was established, similar means could be developed for sperm identification. Computer-enhanced images of individual sperm would then provide a rational basis for the selection of individual sperm for ICSI (*see* Chapter 7). This line of inquiry may be especially important for establishing the fertilizing abilities of sperm with specific morphological defects and in the assessment of semen from males requiring enhanced techniques to express their genetic potential.

EMERGING IMAGING TECHNIQUES

Computer-Assisted Ultrasonographic Imaging

Physiologically dominant ovarian follicles are identifiable by ultrasonography at approx d 7 post-menstruation in unstimulated cycles. The attributes of ultrasonographic images of normal preovulatory follicles include thick, low-amplitude walls and a gradual transformation zone at the fluid-follicle interface. We are actively evaluating the acoustic characteristics indicative of viability and atresia of ovarian follicles of different diameters in unstimulated cycles and under ovarian stimulation protocols. The walls of preovulatory follicles are characterized by increased heterogeneity, increased wall breadth, and a more gradual transformation at the fluid-follicle wall interface. Atresia is characterized by thin walls, high numerical pixel value (bright) signals, and highly variable signals from the follicular fluid (68,69).

TIME SERIES IMAGE ANALYSIS

Follicular dynamics in women undergoing ovarian stimulation are extremely variable. Follicle growth profiles are determined and images of the follicles are analyzed using linear time-series techniques. Three-dimensional surface maps of the image are then made to assess the textures of the follicular fluid and the follicle wall using the regional pixel intensity mapping technique at physiologically important time points (e.g., day of hCG administration, day before ovulation). The physiologic status of follicles as small as 10 mm may be determined. Image attributes of physiologically selected small follicles (<6 mm) include higher amplitude walls and smooth echotexture of follicular fluid compared to subordinate follicles of the cohort. Similarly, time-series analyses, combining image attributes of the follicles and their individual growth profiles, show marked differences in the characteristics of ovulatory and atretic follicles (Fig. 7) (68). Follicles that eventually ovulate (Fig. 7A), or provide superior grades of oocytes, exhibit walls that are thicker and of quantitatively lower peak pixel values throughout their development than do the walls of follicles that are destined to atresia (Fig. 7B). In addition, follicles that ovulate typically have smooth, even textures in the areas corresponding to follicular fluid, whereas images of follicles that do not ovulate exhibit rough surfaces in the fluid areas and higher (brighter) walls. The correlations among the computer-assisted analyses, follicular fluid hormonal analyses, and histological appearances appear to be very high (68–70). The implications for timing oocyte retrieval from small follicles for in vitro maturation are profound. If acoustic markers for follicle and/or oocyte competence are determined, oocyte retrieval and in vitro maturation from 4–6 mm follicles may become a routine clinical procedure.

IMAGE ANALYSIS AND OVARIAN STIMULATION

Computer-assisted image analysis and ultrasonographic assessment of ovarian follicular development are natural extensions of the technologic advances in ovulation induction therapy. The overall ovarian response, growth profiles, and ultrasonographically

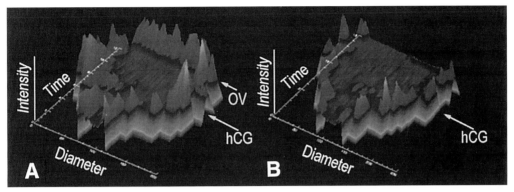

Fig. 7. Time-series images of concatenated numerical pixel values generated from ultrasound image data of two follicles mapped during a research project on follicular development and ovulation during ovarian stimulation (**A,B**). The images were taken from a follicle that ovulated (**A**) and one that did not ovulate (**B**). The x axis represents numerical pixel value, the y axis represents follicular diameter, the z axis represents day of the ovarian stimulation protocol. The point of hCG administration is labeled. Note the thicker, higher amplitude values of the portion of image representing the follicular walls in the ovulatory follicle. The high-amplitude echoes across the distal aspect of the ovulatory follicle are indicative of follicular collapse at ovulation. The follicles followed similar growth curves, yet responded to the ovulation induction agent quite differently. Adapted with permission from ref. *(68)*.

detectable characteristics of individual follicles, doses, and types of stimulatory agents may be interactively evaluated as therapeutic manipulation of the ovaries unfolds. The response of the individual follicles to the ovulation-inducing dose of hCG may be as important as the number and rates of growth of the follicles. Follicles may be as individual as patients in their response to stimulation. Thus, assessment of the development and fates of individual follicles is critical in tailoring ovarian stimulation to individual patients in order to increase the probability of conception.

The corpus luteum may also be evaluated using computer-assisted imaging technology. In an in vitro study, the echotextural characteristics of the bovine corpus luteum were highly correlated with systemic progesterone production and the histologic state of development or regression *(71)*. A similar study done in vivo was equally convincing in demonstrating that the physiologic status of the corpus luteum could be accurately determined using only imaging criteria *(72)*. Human studies to address these same issues are currently ongoing.

SURFACE EVALUATION OF ECHO TEXTURE

Once an ultrasound image has been digitally acquired by the computer, it may be manipulated like any other graphics file. In our laboratory, a series of digital processing steps, which includes, but is not limited to, narrow band-width amplification and pixel-by-pixel numerical value analysis, has enabled us to generate a graphic output that we may interpret to provide an indication of the physiologic status of ovarian follicles, or any other structure in which we may be interested. Currently, we are interested in the status of an individual follicle's viability or atresia. The technique hinges upon overlaying a pixel-by-pixel mesh onto follicular images, then generating a shaded three-dimensional surface based on numerical value of the individual pixels comprising the image. The shading algorithms to evaluate surface contours or height of the peaks are done over wire-frame models developed in this manner and they yield a surface that may be used to infer the physiologic status of the follicles. This technique allows a rapid visual assessment of follicle health (state of viability or atresia) and discriminatory examination of the surfaces (Fig. 8). The addition of color to the algorithms makes subtle differences in the surface contours easier to appreciate. Many projects using the same type of imaging technology to examine ultrasonographic and magnetic resonance images of the parenchyma of the ovaries, uterus, testes and secondary sex glands, and breast are currently underway.

TIME-SERIES ANALYSES OF OVARIAN FOLLICULAR DEVELOPMENT

Images of uniquely identified follicles during natural or ovulation induction cycles are digitized in our laboratory using a direct ethernet connection between the ultrasound instrument in our imaging suite and a high-resolution computer graphics workstation. The time-series analysis is done by drawing a line across the image of the follicle and generating a map of the numerical pixel value along the line. A graph is then created that depicts the numerical value of the echo amplitude along the specified line. If a single line is drawn across the image of each follicle on each day of a period of interest, the resulting pixel maps from each day may be concatenated, or strung together, into a composite image. A shading algorithm is applied to the resulting images, which allows visual analysis of the surface contours of the walls and follicular fluid as the follicle grows from the day it is first identified until the day of ovulation or oocyte retrieval (Fig. 8) *(68)*. The time-series analysis method is particularly valuable in the assessment of follicular development during ovarian stimulation protocols.

In the bovine, the correlations among ultrasonographic appearance, hormonal analyses, and histologic appearances are high *(69,70)*. Studies done in the bovine model system are encouraging as a preliminary step in the sequential analysis of the physiologic status of ovarian follicles in women during natural menstrual cycles and under ovarian stimulation conditions. We are now involved in the development of an interactive interpretive program combining the mathematical modeling approach and this type of graphic analysis with which the progress of follicle growth and development may be monitored throughout ovulation induction. The responses of the ovaries, and of individual follicles, to different doses of stimulatory agents may be assessed and appropriate alterations in clinical management may be made. Although the techniques and the biologic foundations to support their interpretation remain under development, computer-enhanced images reveal potentially valuable information regarding changes in the physiology of the follicles. The application of computer-assisted image analysis and ultrasonographic assessment of follicular development are natural extensions of the technologic advances in ovulation induction therapy. As developments progress, it is clear that the ability to visualize the actions of various hormonal manipulations or reproductive technologies using high-resolution ultrasonography and quantitative image analysis will be an integral component of assisted-reproduction protocols. The goal is reliable stimulation of the ovaries to optimize the quality of oocytes retrieved. If reliable noninvasive techniques are developed, immediate improvement in the clinical management of patients who have defects in follicular development and ovulation will follow. The potential for evaluating ovarian response to hormonal stimulation is tremendous. We suspect that follicles may be as individual as patients in their response to stimulation and that assessment of the progress and fates of individual follicles may become important in tailoring ovarian stimulation to individual women to increase the probability of a successful outcome.

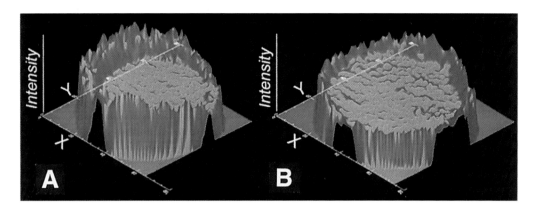

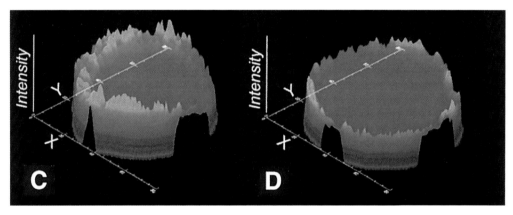

Fig. 8. Surface- (**A,B**) and height- (**C,D**) shaded images of ovulatory (**A,C**) and anovulatory (**B,D**) follicles during a research project on follicular development and ovulation during ovarian stimulation. Both sets of images were created from ultrasonographic image data recorded from 24 h following hCG administration. Color coding is applied to enhance the visual appreciation of the differences between the two types of follicles. Note the higher peak levels and thicker walls of the images from the ovulatory follicle. Images from the anovulatory follicle show a more acute transformation zone at the fluid-follicle interface and comparison of the surface features from the region representing the follicular antrum reveals a rougher texture. Adapted with permission from ref. *(68)*.

Mathematical Modeling of Ovarian Follicular Development

One of the newest methods of investigating ovarian function is mathematical modeling of follicular development. The hypothesis that imaging attributes derived from ultrasonography or MRI may be integrated into a comprehensive model of ovarian folliculogenesis, which includes mathematical description of growth of ovarian follicles in a competitive environment under the influence of estradiol and other hormones such as FSH and LH is under active investigation in our laboratory (Fig. 9) *(73)*. Image attributes from MRI or ultrasonography integrated into the mathematical model appear to allow inference of hormone levels from noninvasive image data and obviate the need for routine hormonal analyses. In the model's simplest form, the growth of every follicle is governed by a first order nonlinear differential equation where the follicle's maturity is measured by the intrafollicular estradiol content, circulating estradiol level, and imaging characteristics determined by ultrasonography and MRI.

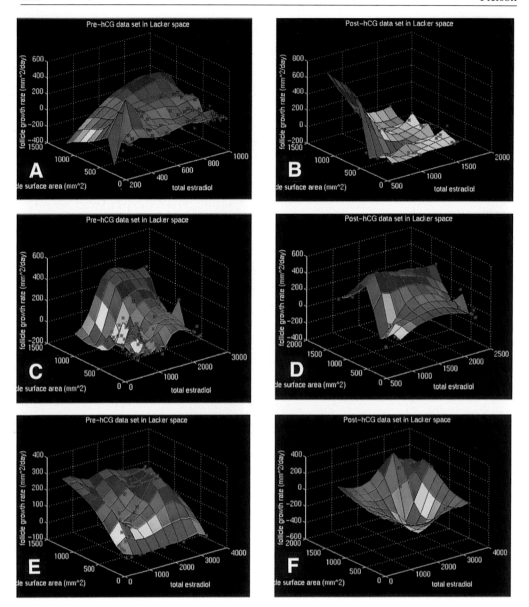

Fig. 9. Mathematical models of follicular development in parametric three-dimensional space (**A–F**). Models are created by a mathematical description of growth of individually identified follicles in a competitive environment under the influence of estradiol, FSH, LH, and ultrasonographic image attributes. In these examples, images (**A**), (**C**), and (**E**) model pre-hCG follicular development in an ovarian stimulation protocol. Images (**B**), (**D**), and (**F**) represent post-hCG responses to the ovulation-inducing agent. Images (**A**) and (**B**) were generated from an ovarian stimulation with a partial ovulation response, which resulted in a conception. Images (**C**) and (**D**) were generated from a stimulation cycle that resulted in good follicular development, but only 1 of 8 follicles ovulated and conception did not occur. Images (**E**) and (**F**) came from a high percentage ovulation cycle (4 of 4 follicles ovulated) and conception occurred. Correlation of the mathematical surfaces with imaging data, follicular growth curves, and estradiol levels is expected to set the stage for interactive software for ovarian-stimulation regimens that will optimize the probability of success, either in the production of oocytes or ovulation, for individual patients based on their individual ovarian response to exogenous gonadotropins.

Although it is too early to tell how applicable this technology will be in wide-spread use, it is providing an unprecedented opportunity to study the relationships among follicles in natural cycles and those stimulated with exogenous gonadotropins. It seems logical to speculate that this type of modeling would be well-suited to predicting the optimal time to collect oocytes for IVF or ICSI, the ovulatory potential for individual follicles, and optimizing the gonadotropin dose for individual patients.

Power Doppler Ultrasonography

Color-flow Doppler has had a great impact on ultrasonographic imaging because the vascular system of the organs being imaged may be directly visualized. Yet, in some ways, the typical method by which color Doppler has been implemented has been arbitrary. Most color Doppler scanners display local blood flow by encoding an estimate of the mean Doppler frequency shifts at a particular position in color. Although this technique has merit, it is not without its difficulties. One problem with employing the mean frequency shift as the characteristic of choice is that the random noise in the ultrasonographic imaging system has a random frequency shift. This is because the noise has random phase, and since frequency is defined as the rate of change of phase, noise can acquire any frequency shift. Therefore, in the mean frequency mode, noise looks like flow in any direction. The more noise there is in an image, the more aberrant flow there appears to be, and consequently, the more the true flow is buried in the background. Mean frequency maps have other problems similar to those of standard Doppler; that is, they alias, which means that they generate some artifactual low-frequency signals when the sampling frequency drops below two times the Doppler signal, and are angle dependent, making it quite difficult to measure flow at normal incidence. These properties can make vessels appear discontinuous and ultimately lead to detection and measurement problems.

A new application of the Doppler technique encodes the power in the Doppler in color. This is fundamentally different from the mean frequency shift. The advantage of using power is in the way the noise appears. Noise always has uniformly low power because of the standard signal-to-noise demands of a color Doppler scanner. Because noise has uniformly low power, when power is written in color the noise appears uniform, not random. Hence, when the sensitivity of the color Doppler unit is raised to image the noise floor, only a uniformly colored background is imaged instead of a random distribution of color. Any true flow having more power in the Doppler signal than the noise appears out of the background. The improvement in flow sensitivity using this technique depends on the machine being used; however, the sensitivity in measuring and displaying vascular flow has been improved dramatically *(74)*.

Power Doppler imaging does not alias and is relatively angle-independent. This is because the total power in the signal is represented by the integral under Doppler power curve, also called the power spectrum. This total power does not change with the mean frequency, and even at perpendicular incidence, there is still some power in the signal *(74)*. The use of power Doppler imaging of the reproductive organs is in its early stages. The technique has, for example, been employed to study neovascularization of the human follicle *(75)* and corpus luteum *(38)*; however, the uterus does not appear to have been studied, with the exception of some pathologic changes of the cervix *(76,77)*.

Three-Dimensional Ultrasonography

The technological sophistication of conventional two-dimensional ultrasonography is now being developed into three-dimensional ultrasonographic imaging, which will allow us to study the anatomy of the female and male reproductive organs quickly and accurately. True, real-time, three-dimensional imaging has been the subject of dreams since the first ultrasound images were generated. Although three-dimensional ultrasonography is not yet a standard imaging technique, the transducers and software for near real-time image reconstruction and display are available in commercial and research settings. The anatomic location of the reproductive organs does produce some physical constraints on the imaging apparatus that other organs do not. The nonpregnant and early-pregnant female organs may be imaged by a transvaginal approach, whereas the male internal organs may only be approached transrectally. The testes may be imaged using standard noncavitary probes. However, the potential applications of being able to see the reproductive organs in accurate spatial configurations are so profound that this area requires exploration even before the best technical apparatus is available.

In conventional two-dimensional imaging, the operator continuously scans over the fetus or other structures of interest in order to build up a mental image of the three-dimensional structures. This limitation has impeded exploitation of its full potential. Three-dimensional imaging presents an opportunity for anyone to visualize the organs and systems of interest with the vision of Leonardo da Vinci at his finest moments of insight.

Although three-dimensional imaging has the potential to make ultrasonography substantially easier to perform and interpret, to be truly useful, three-dimensional imaging must also occur in real-time or near real-time. The technical aspects of three-dimensional ultrasonography pose a difficult problem because of the combined effects of movement and image acquisition speed. Computer speeds are just now at the point where 30 images per second can be acquired and we are still awaiting the computer power to analyze, reconstruct, and display three-dimensional images in near real-time. However, there have been nearly constant improvements in image acquisition techniques, reconstruction algorithms, computer power, and display technology that have made the many previously tedious steps in creating a three-dimensional image nearly invisible to the ultrasonographer. Volume measurements may be made quickly and accurately and surface features are easily evaluated. One of the tremendous advantages of three-dimensional imaging is that, once the images are acquired and reconstructed, the three-dimensional image may be rotated to different viewing planes and evaluated without continued scanning of the patient. Furthermore, the layers of image information may be stripped away, revealing both internal and external features (Fig. 10). The three-dimensional, gray-scale images, displaying either surface-rendered images to evaluate the exterior aspects of an organ, or volume-rendered images to examine interior structures, can then be rotated and examined from many different angles. Views of the organs may be generated that are not possible with standard imaging techniques. Positive space and negative space models can be generated with equal ease, and color may be applied to any set of image data for depth shading, which allows enhanced three-dimensional appreciation of external and internal anatomic detail (Fig. 10). Our research group has developed a functional intravaginal probe for three-dimensional acquisition and the computer software for reconstruction of ultrasonographic images of the ovaries and uterus. Research refining the imaging technique and combining the three-dimensional images with other types of image analysis is well underway.

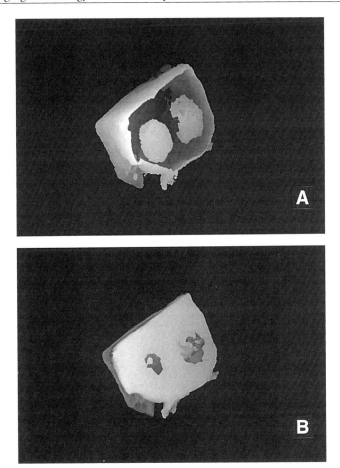

Fig. 10. Three-dimensional ultrasound images of bovine ovaries (**A–D**). Contour data were extracted from the ultrasound images using a multi-resolution texture segmentation algorithm designed for ultrasonographic images. The three-dimensional model was created at a graphics workstation interfaced with the ultrasound instrument. Surface-smoothing and depth-shading algorithms enhance the visual appreciation of the three-dimensional aspects of the images (**A,B**). The images represent positive (**A**) and negative (**B**) space models of the ovary, which contains a dominant preovulatory follicle (left) and a regressing dominant anovulatory follicle (right) from the previous follicular wave. In the positive space model, the surface of the preovulatory follicle is smooth contrasting with the rough texture of the atretic follicle. In the negative space model, the interior surface of the atretic follicle is roughly textured, representing the irregular surfaces in the collapsing follicle. An oocyte-cumulus complex is observed in the antrum of the negative space model.

Magnetic Resonance Imaging (MRI)
of the Ovaries in the Bovine Model

Two-Dimensional MRI

MRI observations from bovine ovaries retrieved from the abattoir, or surgically removed at defined times of the estrous cycle, imaged in vitro have revealed that the nuclear magnetic resonance (NMR) relaxation properties of ovarian follicular fluid appear to depend upon the physiologic status of the follicle *(78,79)*. Typical two-dimensional T1 and T2 MR images of bovine ovaries in vitro are shown (Fig. 11). We have developed the

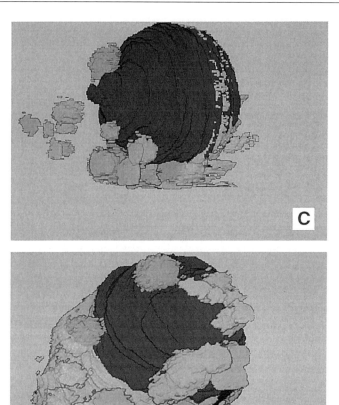

Fig. 10. (Continued). Three-dimensional models may be used to study the growth and development of follicles and corpora lutea (**C,D**). The images were made using a rapid reconstruction algorithm and shows the spatial location of several small (2–4 mm) follicles surrounding a d 6 corpus luteum. The nipple-like projection of the CL is easily seen in image (**C**). Part of the surface of the ovary has been peeled away to reveal the follicles on the front of the CL. Other follicles may be seen embedded in the ovarian stroma on the inferior aspect of the image. Color may be added to the images to enhance visual appreciation. Adapted with permission from ref. *(81)*.

hypothesis that the physiologic status of the follicle will be reflected in the image attributes of T1 and T2 NMR relaxation rates of follicular fluid. Follicles imaged during the early follicular phase (pre-physiologic selection) or during atresia contain fluid that has long T1 and T2 relaxation times at "resting" values of approx 6500 ms and 500 ms respectively. As the time of selection of the dominant follicle approaches in the late follicular phase, both the T1 and T2 times of the fluid decrease as the follicle becomes more endocrinologically active. The T1 time will continue to decrease while the T2 time rapidly recovers to the resting value in dominant follicles just prior to ovulation. If the follicle is committed to atresia, both T1 and T2 times will recover to the resting value, with the T2 recovery time being slower in atretic follicles than the T2 recovery time for the dominant pre-ovulatory follicle. Thus, image attributes from MRI have the potential to discriminate among viable and atretic follicles once selection has occurred.

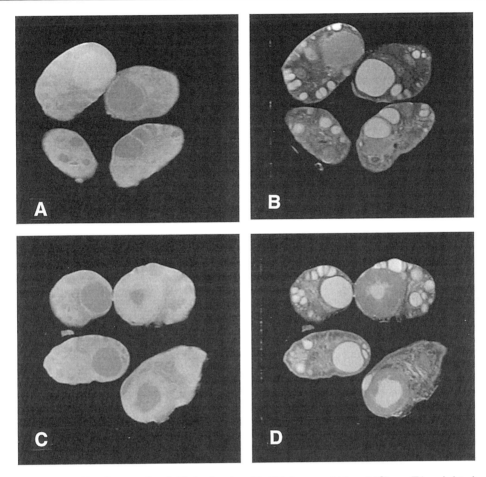

Fig. 11. MRI of bovine ovarian follicles in vitro (**A–D**). Images (**A**) and (**C**) are T1 weighted and images (**B**) and (**C**) are T2 weighted. Note the clarity and spatial resolution of the MRI compared to ultrasonographic images. In T1-weighted images, follicles are dark gray and luteal tissue is lighter. In T2-weighted images, follicles are very light gray and CL are a darker gray. A regressing CL is seen in the upper left set of ovaries and a dominant preovulatory follicle is observed in the upper right ovary in images (**A**) and (**B**). In images (**C**) and (**D**), both sets of ovaries contain mid-cycle CL and dominant anovulatory follicles. The CL have cystic, fluid-filled cavities in their respective antra, which gives a signal similar to that of follicular fluid.

It appears that the T1 value is inversely related to estradiol levels in the follicular fluid, whereas the T2 value reflects an unknown factor associated with the event of dominant follicle selection. Conventional MRI relaxometry may be useful for identifying the physiologic status of ovarian follicles. We expect that improvements in MRI speed and resolution, combined with the use of intravaginal coils, will soon allow relaxometric observations of ovarian follicles in vivo in women.

Three-Dimensional MRI

Three-dimensional MRI coupled with maximum intensity projection display has also been used to study the relationships among bovine follicles in vitro (Fig. 12) *(80)*. The ovary may be studied using fast imaging with steady-state precession imaging sequences

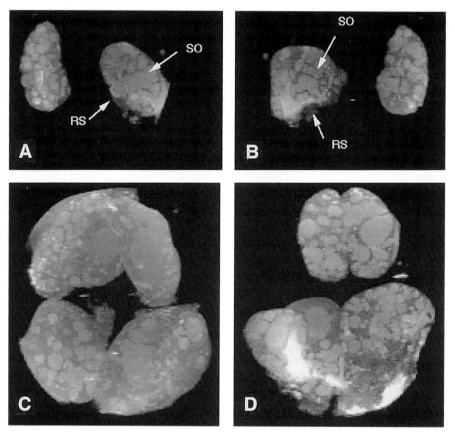

Fig. 12. Three-dimensional MRIs of bovine ovaries in vitro (**A–D**). The three-dimensional data set is rotated in a cine-loop to appreciate the volumetric aspects of the images. Follicles are lighter gray than the surrounding ovarian stroma and CL are detectable within the image matrix. A recent site of ovulation was observed in the upper set of images (**A,B**). The recently collapsed follicle walls (SO) and site of ovarian rupture (RS) are indicated. The lower set of images (**C,D**) represent two pairs of ovaries surgically removed at physiologically important time points. Many small follicles, emerging dominant follicles, and corpora lutea are visible.

using maximum intensity projection, which displays three-dimensional images as a cine-loop of the ovaries rotating in space. Presently, only the in vitro model system is functional, however, recently developed intravaginal probes for MRI are now being used experimentally in humans. Future developments making MRI fast and user-friendly make this a particularly exciting avenue of inquiry for the study of normal and pathologic ovarian function.

CONCLUDING REMARKS

Our understanding of the vital and dynamic processes in reproductive biology has been, and will be, greatly enhanced with the application of advanced imaging technology. Although most of the work to date has focused on reproductive biology in the female, it is only a matter of time before the male factor in reproduction is subjected to similar scrutiny. The door is open for enhanced comprehension of basic ovarian biology, clinical improvement of follicular growth and development, selection of the best gametes for assisted reproduction, suppression of follicular function when desired, control of ovarian cyclicity, determination of the optimal uterine environment for replacement of embryos, and examination of testicular function. If we understand that we can believe what we see, and if we have the vision to wander through this portal and down what may now seem to be a somewhat hazy path, advanced imaging technology will continue to evolve as an indispensable partner in clinical evaluation of the normal and pathophysiologic processes in reproduction.

ACKNOWLEDGMENTS

Original research in Dr. Pierson's laboratory is supported by the Medical Research Council of Canada. The contributions of the members of the Women's Health Imaging Research Laboratory, John Deptuch, Michelle Hanna, Angela Hess, Jennifer Hilton, and Dr. Gord Sarty are gratefully acknowledged.

REFERENCES

1. Hodgen GD. The dominant ovarian follicle. Fertil Steril 1982;38:281–300.
2. Guraya SS. Biology of Ovarian Follicles in Mammals, Springer-Verlag, New York, NY, 1985, p. 320.
3. Baird DT. A model for follicular selection and ovulation: lessons from superovulation. J Steroid Biochem 1987;27:15–23.
4. Bomsel-Helmreich O. Ultrasound and the preovulatory human follicle. Oxford Rev Reprod Biol 1985; 7:1–72.
5. Leerentveld RA, VanGent I, DerStoep M, Wladimiroff JW. Ultrasonographic assessment of Graafian follicle growth under monofollicular and multifollicular conditions in clomiphene citrate stimulated cycles. Fertil Steril 1985;40:461–465.
6. Greenwald GS, Terranova PF. Follicular selection and its control. In: Knobil E, Neill J, eds. The Physiology of Reproduction. Raven, New York, NY, 1988, pp. 387– 446.
7. Renaud RL, Macler J, Dervain I, Ehret MC, Aron C, Plas-Roser S, et al. Echographic study of follicular maturation and ovulation during the normal menstrual cycle. Ferti Steril 1980;33:272–279.
8. Hackelöer BJ, Fleming R, Robinson HP, Adam AH, Coutts JRT. Correlation of ultrasonic and endocrinologic assessment of human follicular development. Am J Obstet Gynecol 1979;135:122–129.
9. Pierson RA, Chizen DR, Olatunbosun OA. Ultrasonographic assessment of ovulation induction. In: Jaffe R, Pierson RA, Abramowicz JS, eds. Imaging in Infertility and Reproductive Endocrinology. Lippincott, Philadelphia, PA, 1994, pp. 155–166.
10. Moor RM, Seamark RF. Cell signalling, permeability, and microvascular changes during follicle development in mammals. J Dairy Sci 1986;69:927–943.
11. Carson R, Findlay J, Mattner P, Brown B. Relative levels of thecal blood flow in atretic and non-atretic ovarian follicles of the conscious sheep. Aust J Exper Biol Med Sci 1986;64:381–387.
12. Brannstrom M, Zackrisson U, Hagstrom HG, Josefsson B, Hellberg P, Granberg S, et al. Preovulatory changes of blood flow in different regions of the human follicle. Fertil Steril 1998;69:435–442.
13. Martinuk SD, Chizen DR, Pierson RA. Ultrasonographic morphology of the human preovulatory follicle wall prior to ovulation. Clin Anat 1992;5:1–14.
14. Gougeon A. Dynamics of follicular growth in the human: a model from preliminary results. Hum Reprod 1986;1:81–87.
15. Collins W, Jurkovic D, Bourne T, Kurjak A, Campbell S. Ovarian morphology, endocrine function and intra-follicular blood flow during the peri-ovulatory period. Hum Reprod 1991;6:319–324.
16. Tinkanen H, Kujansuu E, Laippala P. The association between hormone levels and vascular resistance in uterine and ovarian arteries in spontaneous menstrual cycles: a Doppler ultrasound study. Acta Obstet Gynecol Scand 1995;74:297–301.
17. Balakier H, Stronell RD. Color Doppler assessment of folliculogenesis in in vitro fertilization patients. Fertil Steril 1994:62:1211–1216.
18. Nargund G, Bourne T, Doyle P, Parsons J, Cheng W, Campbell S, Collins W. Associations between ultrasound indices of follicular blood flow, oocyte recovery and preimplantation embryo quality. Hum Reprod 1996;11:109–113.

19. Oyesanya OA, Parsons JH, Collins WP, Campbell S. Prediction of oocyte recovery rate by transvaginal ultrasonography and color Doppler imaging before human chorionic gonadotropin administration in in vitro fertilization cycles. Fertil Steril 1996;65:806–809.

20. Van Blerkom J, Antczak M, Schrader R. The developmental potential of the human oocyte is related to the dissolved oxygen content of follicular fluid: association with vascular endothelial growth factor levels and perifollicular blood flow characteristics. Hum Reprod 1997;12:1047–1055.

21. Balboni GC: Structural changes: ovulation and luteal phase. In: Serra GB, ed. The Ovary: Comprehensive Endocrinology. Raven, New York, NY, 1983, pp. 123–142.

22. Morioka N. Mechanisms of mammalian ovulation. In: Development of Preimplantation Embryos and Their Environment. Alan R. Liss, New York, NY, 1989, pp. 65–85.

23. Espey LL, Lipner H. Ovulation. In: Knobil E, Neill J, eds. The Physiology of Reproduction, 2nd ed. Raven, New York, NY, 1994 pp. 725–780.

24. Tsafriri A, Chun SY. Ovulation. In: Adashi E, Rock JA, Rosenwaks Z, eds. Reproductive Endocrinology, Surgery, and Technology. Lippincott-Raven, Philadelphia PA, 1996, pp. 235–249.

25. Queenan JT, O'Brien GD, Bains LM, Simpson J, Collins WP, Campbell S. Ultrasound scanning of ovaries to detect ovulation in women. Fertil Steril 1980;34:99–105.

26. Pierson RA, Martinuk SD, Chizen DR, Simpson CW. Ultrasonographic visualization of human ovulation. In: Evers JCL, Heineman MJ, eds. From Ovulation to Implantation. Proceedings of the VIIth Reinier de Graaf Symposium, Maastricht, the Netherlands. Excerpta Medica, Amsterdam. 1990, pp. 73–79.

27. Hanna MD, Chizen DR, Pierson RA. Characteristics of follicular evacuation during human ovulation. J Ultrasound Obstet Gynaecol 1994;4:488–493.

28. Lenz S. Ultrasonic study of follicular maturation, ovulation and development of corpus luteum during normal menstrual cycles. Acta Obstet Gynecol Scand 1985;64:15–19.

29. Bächström T, Nakata M, Pierson RA. Ultrasonography of normal and abnormal luteogenesis. In: Jaffe R, Pierson RA, Abramowicz JS, eds. Imaging in Infertility and Reproductive Endocrinology. Lippincott, Philadelphia, PA, 1994, pp. 143–154.

30. Bourne TH, Jurkovic J, Waterstone J, Campbell S, Collins WP. Intrafollicular blood flow during human ovulation. J Ultrasound Obstet Gynecol 1991;1:53–59.

31. Haines CJ. Luteinized unruptured follicle syndrome. Clin Reprod Fertil 1987;5:321–332.

32. Katz E. The luteinized unruptured follicle and other ovulatory dysfunctions. Fertil Steril 1988;50:839–845.

33. Kupesic S, Kurjak A. The assessment of normal and abnormal luteal function by transvaginal color Doppler sonography. Eur J Obstet Gynecol Reprod Biol 1997;72:83–87.

34. Kalogirou D, Antoniou G, Botsis D, Kontoravdis A, Vitoratos N, Giannikos L. Transvaginal Doppler ultrasound with color flow imaging in the diagnosis of luteal phase defect (LPD). Clin Exp Obstet Gynecol 1997;24:95–97.

35. Kupesic S, Kurjak A, Vujisic S, Petrovic Z. Luteal phase defect: comparison between Doppler velocimetry, histological and hormonal markers. Ultrasound Obstet Gynecol 1997;9:105–112.

36. Glock JL, Brumsted JR. Color flow pulsed Doppler ultrasound in diagnosing luteal phase defect. Fertil Steril 1995;500–504.

37. Zaidi J, Jurkovic D, Campbell S, Collins W, McGregor A, Tan SL. Luteinized unruptured follicle: morphology, endocrine function and blood flow changes during the menstrual cycle. Hum Reprod 1995;10:44–49.

38. Miyazaki T, Tanaka M, Miyakoshi K, Kasia K, Yoshimura Y. Power and colour Doppler ultrasonography for the evaluation of the vasculature of the human corpus luteum. Hum Reprod 1998;13:2836–2841.

39. Zalud I, Kurjak A. The assessment of luteal blood flow in pregnant and non-pregnant women by transvaginal color Doppler. J Perinat Med 1990;18:215–221.

40. Glock JL, Blackman JA, Dadger GJ, Brumstead JR. Prognostic significance of morphologic changes of the corpus luteum by transvaginal ultrasound in early pregnancy monitoring. Obstet Gynecol 1995;85:37–41.

41. Durfee SM, Frates MC. Sonographic spectrum of the corpus luteum in early pregnancy: gray scale, color, and pulsed Doppler appearance. J Clin Ultrasound 1999;27:55–59

42. Marrs R, Vargyas D, March C. Correlation of ultrasonic and endocrinologic measurements in human menopausal gonadotropin therapy. Am J Obstet Gynecol 1983;145:4–11.

43. Bryce RL, Shuter B, Sinosich MJ, Stiel JN, Picker RH, Saunders DM. The value of ultrasound, gonadotropin, and estradiol measurements for precise ovulation prediction. Fertil Steril 1982;37:42–45.

44. Silverberg KM, Olive DL, Burns WN, Johnson JV, Groff TR, Schenken RS. Follicular size at the time of human chorionic gonadotropin administration predicts ovulation outcome in human menopausal gonadotropin stimulated cycles. Fertil Steril 1991;56:296–303.

45. Haines CJ, Emes AL. The relationship between follicle diameter, fertilization rate and microscopic embryo quality. Fertil Steril 1991;55:205–207.

46. Veek LL, Wortham JWE, Witmyer J, Sandow BA, Acosta AA, Garcia JE, et al. Maturation and fertilization of morphologically immature human oocytes in a program of in vitro fertilization. Fertil Steril 1983; 39:594–599.

47. Brandt TD, Levy EB, Grant TH Marut E, Leland H. The endometrial echo and its significance in female infertility. Radiology 1985;157:225–229.

48. Fleischer AC, Kalemeris GC, Endman SS. Sonographic depiction of the endometrium during normal cycles. Ultrasound Med Biol 1986;12:271 –277.

49. Fleischer AC, Herbert CM, Sacks GA, Wentz AC, Entman SS, James AE. Sonography of the endometrium during conception and non-conception cycles of in vitro fertilization and embryo transfer. Fertil Steril 1986;46:442–447.

50. Forrest TS, Elyaderani MK, Muilenburg MI, Bewtra C, Kable WE, Sullivan P. Cyclic endometrial changes: US assessment with histologic correlation. Radiology 1988:167:233–237.

51. Lindenberg S. Ultrasonographic assessment of the endometrium during the normal menstrual cycle. In: Jaffe R, Pierson RA, Abramowicz JS, eds. Imaging in Infertility and Reproductive Endocrinology. Lippincott, Philadelphia, PA, 1994, pp. 47–52.

52. Dickey RP, Olar TT, Curole DN, Taylor SN, Rye PH. Endometrial pattern and thickness associated with pregnancy outcome after assisted reproduction technologies. Hum Reprod 1992;7:418–421.

53. Ueno J, Oehninger S, Brzyski RG, Acosta AA, Philput CB, Muasher SJ. Ultrasonographic appearance of the endometrium in natural and stimulated in-vitro fertilization cycles and its correlation with outcome. Hum Reprod 1991;6:901–904.

54. Gonen Y, Casper RF. Prediction of implantation by the sonographic appearance of the endometrium during controlled ovarian stimulation for in vitro fertilization (IVF). J In Vitro Fert Embryo Transf 1990; 7:146–152.

55. Czemiczky G, Wramsby W, Johannisson E, Landgren B.-M. Endometrial evaluation is not predictive for in vitro fertilization treatment. J Assisted Reprod Genet 1999;16:113–116.

56. Richards N, Pierson RA. Transvaginal ultrasonography of the uterine decidual reaction in early human pregnancy. Ultrasound Intl 1996;2:174–180.

57. Strickler RC, Christianson C, Crane JP, Curato A, Knight AB, Yang V. Ultrasound guidance for human embryo transfer. Fertil Steril 1985;43:54–61.

58. Hurley VA, Osborn JC, Leoni MA, Leeton J. Ultrasound-guided embryo transfer: a controlled trial. Fertil Steril 1991;55:559–562.

59. al-Shawaf T, Dave R, Harper J Linehan D, Riley P, Craft I. Transfers of embryos into the uterus: how much do technical factors affect pregnancy rates? J Assist Reprod Genet 1993;10:31–36.

60. Woolcott R, Stranger J. Potentially important variables identified by transvaginal ultrasound-guided embryo transfer. Hum Reprod 1997;12:963–966.

61. Dhabuwala CB, Parulkar BG. Doppler flow analysis and conventional ultrasonography for evaluation of the infertile male. In: Jaffe R, Pierson RA, Abramowicz JS, eds. Imaging in Infertility and Reproductive Endocrinology. Lippincott, Philadelphia, PA, 1994, pp. 207–216.

62. Kuligowska E. Transrectal ultrasonography in diagnosis and management of male infertility. In: Jaffe R, Pierson RA, Abramowicz JS, eds. Imaging in Infertility and Reproductive Endocrinology. Lippincott, Philadelphia, PA, 1994, pp. 217–230.

63. Chandiola RK, Honamarooz A, Omeke BC, Pierson RA, Beard AP, Rawlings NC. Assessment of development of the testes and accessory glands by ultrasonography in bull calves and associated endocrine changes. Theriogenology 1996;48:119–132.

64. Chandiola RK, Bartlewski PM, Omeke BC, Beard A, Rawlings NC, Pierson RA. Ultrasonography of the developing reproductive tract in ram lams: effects of a GnRH agonist. Theriogenology 1997;48:99–117.

65. Evans ACO, Pierson RA, Garcia A, McDougall LM, Hrudka F, Rawlings NC. Changes in circulating hormone concentrations, testes histology and ultrasonography of the testes during sexual maturation in beef bulls. Theriogenology 1996;46:345–357.

66. Menkveld R, Stander F, Kotze T, Kruger T, van Zyl JA. The evaluation of morphological characteristics of human spermatozoa according to stricter criteria. Hum Reprod 1990;5:586–592.

67. Ombelet W, Menkveld R, Kruger TF, Steeno O. Sperm morphology assessment: historical review in relation to fertility. Hum Reprod Update 1995;6:543–557.
68. Pierson RA, Adams GP. Computer-assisted image analysis, diagnostic ultrasonography and ovulation induction: strange bedfellows. Theriogenology 1995;43:105–112.
69. Singh J, Pierson RA, Adams GP. Ultrasound image attributes of bovine ovarian follicles: endocrine and functional correlates. J Reprod Fertil 1998;112:19–29.
70. Tom JW, Pierson RA, Adams GP. Quantitative echotextural analysis of bovine ovarian follicles. Theriogenology 1998;50:339–346.
71. Singh J, Pierson RA, Adams GP. Ultrasound image attributes of the bovine corpus luteum: structural and functional correlates. J Reprod Fertil 1997;109:35–44.
72. Tom JW, Pierson RA, Adams GP. Quantitative echotextural analysis of bovine corpora lutea. Theriogenology 1998;49:1345–1352.
73. Sarty GE, Pierson RA. Analysis of ovarian follicular response to superstimulation in a three dimensional parametric space. Fertil Steril 1998;70(Suppl 3):S183.
74. Zagzebski J. Doppler Instrumentation. In: Essentials of Ultrasound Physics. Mosby-Year Book, Inc., St. Louis, MO, 1996, pp. 87–108.
75. Chui DK, Pugh ND, Walker SM, Gregory L, Shaw RW. Follicular vascularity: the predictive value of transvaginal power Doppler ultrasonography in an in-vitro fertilization programme: a preliminary study. Hum Reprod 1997;12:191–196.
76. Umesaki N, Nakai Y, Honda K, Kamamura N, Kanaoka S, Ishiko O, Ogita S. Power Doppler findings of adenoma malignum of uterine cervix. Gynecol Obstet Invest 1998;45:213–216.
77. Suren A. Osmers R, Kuhn W. 3D Color power angio imaging: a new method to assess intracervical vascularization in benign and pathological conditions. Ultrasound Obstet Gynecol 1998;11:133–137.
78. Sarty GE, Kendall EJ, Pierson RA. Magnetic resonance imaging of bovine ovaries in vitro. Mag Res Mat Physics Biol Med (MAG*MA)1996;4:205–211.
79. Hilton JE, Sarty GE, Adams GP, Pierson RA. Magnetic resonance imaging of bovine ovarian follicles during development and regression: an in vitro model study. Proc 20th Conf Canada West Soc Reprod Biol 1998;Abstracts:24.
80. Sarty GE, Adams GP, Pierson RA. Semi-transparent 3D magnetic resonance imaging for the study of ovarian follicular dynamics. Proc 20th Conf Canada West Soc Reprod Biol 1998;Abstracts:34.
81. Pierson RA, Brown HK, Lees WR, Rubin JM, Yang YH, Mattox JH, Jaffe R. New directions in imaging in infertility and reproductive endocrinology. In: Jaffe R, Pierson RA, Abramowicz JS, eds. Imaging in Infertility and Reproductive Endocrinology. Lippincott, Philadelphia, PA, 1994, pp. 389–398.

7

Intracytoplasmic Sperm Injection or Conventional Fertilization to Maximize the Number of Viable Embryos

Susan E. Lanzendorf, PhD
and Catherine Boyd, BS

CONTENTS

FERTILIZATION OF THE HUMAN OOCYTE WITH INTRACYTOPLASMIC SPERM INJECTION

History of Sperm Injection

The earliest recorded attempt to inject sperm directly into eggs occurred around 1914 when a scientist named G.L. Kite injected star-fish oocytes [1]. Since then, sea urchin and hamster oocytes have been utilized in investigations of oocyte activation and post-fertilization events [2–7]. Studies aimed at assessing fertilization and embryonic development following sperm injection have also been performed in several animal species, including the mouse [8], rabbit [9,10], bovine [11], and nonhuman primate [12] (*see* Chapter 16).

From: *Contemporary Endocrinology: Assisted Fertilization and Nuclear Transfer in Mammals*
Edited by: D. P. Wolf and M. Zelinski-Wooten © Humana Press Inc., Totowa, NJ

To determine the feasibility of sperm injection as a treatment for human male infertility, Lanzendorf and coworkers *(13)* injected amorphous and acrosomeless sperm into hamster oocytes. Following injection, sperm decondensation and pronuclear formation was observed, suggesting that sperm of some infertile men may be capable of participation in early fertilization events, provided they are mechanically placed in the ooplasm. To demonstrate that human oocytes could survive the sperm-injection procedure, 20 in vitro-matured human oocytes were injected with human sperm; following a 13-h incubation prior to fixation, all were intact, with one half containing a decondensed sperm head and the other half showing both a male and a female pronucleus *(14)*. A clinical trial was then performed with 16 patients receiving a transfer of embryos resulting from oocytes fertilized by sperm injection, however, no pregnancies were established (Lucinda Veeck, personal communication).

In 1992, Palermo et al. *(15)* reported the first human pregnancies following sperm injection, performed on patients with severely impaired sperm function. Referred to as intracytoplasmic sperm injection (ICSI), the procedure yielded a fertilization rate of 66% in four patients undergoing 8 treatment cycles. All four patients achieved a pregnancy with one preclinical abortion. These same investigators later reported an additional 150 ICSI treatment cycles, resulting in a fertilization rate of 64.2% and a clinical pregnancy rate of 39.2% *(16)*. Since the time of the first reported ICSI pregnancy, attention has focussed on the best methods for oocyte and sperm preparation, the technical aspects of the procedure, and the effect the procedure has on the resulting offspring. To date, ICSI remains the treatment of choice for patients whose sperm are incapable of fertilizing an oocyte following conventional insemination.

Indications for Male Factor Infertility

Routine indications for ICSI include poor semen parameters and poor or failed fertilization on a previous in vitro fertilization (IVF) attempt. However, we have all been faced with the dilemma of counseling couples with a borderline abnormal semen analysis or who fertilized poorly at another IVF center. Many now pose the question as to whether it would not be safer to perform ICSI on all couples undergoing IVF.

In general, IVF programs set criteria for patients considering the ICSI procedure, most commonly, a total motile sperm count below a specified value. Examples would be a total motile count below one million after preparation for IVF or a cut-off of less than five million total motile sperm in the ejaculate. Some programs also factor in the total number of sperm with normal morphology. Patients with parameters below these thresholds are automatically recommended for the ICSI procedure.

Patients who have demonstrated poor fertilization (20–50%) are often counseled regarding ICSI because application of the technique may increase the number of embryos available for transfer. If a patient presents to a new program with a history of poor fertilization at another center and also appears to have normal semen parameters, evaluation may be difficult. One solution is to offer the ICSI procedure on a certain proportion of oocytes in an attempt to determine if the sperm are truly impaired. The hemizona assay, a test that measures the ability of the sperm to bind tightly to the human zona pellucida, may also be used to determine a patient's need for ICSI *(17)*.

In a study performed by Mercan and coworkers *(18)*, patients with a history of poor fertilization by conventional IVF (<50%) showed significantly lower fertilization rates following ICSI (61%) compared to patients with prior total fertilization failure (68%) or with poor semen quality (<one million motile sperm/mL after separation and/or a poor hemizona binding assay; 65%). It may be that samples exhibiting poor fertilization rates after IVF contain a population of sperm that are incapable of participating in early fertilization events even when some steps (zona and oolema penetration) are bypassed by ICSI. In contrast, sperm from patients with prior failed fertilization or poor semen parameters may be deficient in their ability to bind and penetrate the zona pellucida and/or oolema, a defect that is correctable by ICSI.

Most programs will also perform ICSI when a patient has a history of failed fertilization, either at their own center or at another IVF program. Included in this group are patients with both normal and abnormal semen parameters. An evaluation of ICSI cycles, in couples with a history of failed fertilization following conventional IVF but with normal semen parameters, found that implantation and pregnancy rates were significantly lower compared to patients undergoing ICSI secondary to either obstructive azoospermia or impaired semen quality *(19)*. Fertilization rates were not affected leading to the speculation that the impaired pregnancy rate may be owing to a gamete abnormality.

Effect of ICSI on Embryo Quality

Does ICSI have a negative impact on embryo quality? A study performed by Bar-Hava and associates *(20)* compared IVF and ICSI cycles performed during the same time span and found that fertilization rates, embryo quality, and the number of embryos available for cryopreservation, as well as pregnancy rates, were better in the IVF group. The authors suggested that "paternal or maternal factors" and the lack of natural selection during ICSI, resulting in poorer-quality embryos, may explain these findings. The ICSI procedure results in the production of embryos that otherwise would not exist. Evaluations of matched IVF and ICSI groups at the Jones Institute *(21)* have also found that IVF-derived embryos have better cleavage rates and morphology scores than ICSI-derived embryos, however, the implantation rates were similar between the two groups. One must keep in mind that the underlying male infertility, and not just the ICSI procedure itself, may be imparting some negative influence on embryo quality.

In a study performed to evaluate implantation rates for patients with severe teratozoospermia, undergoing IVF with a high insemination concentration or ICSI, Oehninger and coinvestigators *(22)* found that ICSI produced a significantly higher proportion of morphologically superior embryos with a tendency towards a higher implantation rate. In this instance, the benefit of ICSI to embryo quality may be indirect resulting from not having the eggs exposed to extremely high concentrations of sperm and their waste products.

Could ICSI have a positive impact on embryo quality if male factor infertility was not involved? A study by Yang and coworkers *(23)* randomized the eggs of nine nonmale factor couples into two groups and exposed one half to conventional IVF and the remaining half to ICSI. They report that the fertilization rate was similar in both groups, however, the quality of the embryos was significantly better in the ICSI group. The investigators postulate that the inseminating sperm may damage the embryos in the IVF group because sperm have been shown to produce reactive oxygen species *(24,25)*. Because of these conflicting reports, it may be prudent to perform additional randomized studies to determine whether or not ICSI impacts embryo quality, especially in non-male factor patients.

Effect of ICSI on Embryo Cryopreservation

Concern has existed over the cryopreservation of ICSI-produced embryos, secondary to damage that may be induced by the injection needle or by the rupture in the zona, which may cause premature hatching (*see* Chapter 10). Macas and coworkers *(26)* found that ICSI embryos survived the freezing protocol but showed impaired rates of cleavage, embryo morphology, and implantation, which resulted in an increased rate of embryonic loss. The authors speculate that this may result from the cryopreservation of pronuclear stage, ICSI embryos at a suboptimal time; at a shortened time between insemination (injection) and freezing compared to embryos resulting from conventional IVF. In this study, eggs were cryopreserved 20 h after injection with 10% having already reached syngamy.

Two earlier studies found no detrimental effect of ICSI on the cryopreservation of pronuclear stage eggs. Both Al-Hasani and coworkers *(27)* and Hoover and coinvestigators *(28)* found no significant differences in survival or pregnancy rates between frozen-thawed, pronuclear-stage embryos fertilized by conventional IVF or ICSI. Al-Hasani *(27)* also showed similar abortion rates between the two groups. Kowalik and coworkers *(29)* have also demonstrated that ICSI does not have an adverse impact on the survival and implantation of both cryopreserved and cleavage stage embryos.

At the Jones Institute, we have performed 66 transfer cycles in which cryopreserved pronuclear stage embryos were the result of ICSI. Following the thaw of 371 embryos, 275 survived (74%) and, following their transfer on d 2 or 3, 21 clinical pregnancies were established (32%). Eighteen of those pregnancies are ongoing (27%). Although the cryo-survival of pronuclear-stage embryos resulting from ICSI appears to be lower than that seen following conventional IVF, the clinical, ongoing, and implantation rates between the two groups are not different. Under our current pronuclear-stage cryopreservation protocol, embryos resulting from both conventional IVF and ICSI are cryopreserved around 18 h after insemination or injection but this time may range from 16–19 h. Pronuclear stage embryos are not frozen at syngamy.

Should Everyone Be Fertilized with ICSI?

What would be the advantages or disadvantages of using the ICSI procedure to fertilize the eggs of all patients? ICSI offers no natural selection of the sperm and includes exposure of the oocytes to factors that may be harmful (hyaluronidase, light, fluctuations in temperature, mechanical stresses to the zona pellucida, and oolemma, and so forth). However, recent studies have shown that shortened exposure of the oocyte to large numbers of sperm during conventional IVF may be beneficial to subsequent embryo development *(30)*. Therefore, the stress that the oocyte encounters during sperm injection may be balanced by the fact that it is not exposed to the harsh environment of insemination.

Another concern is that the ICSI procedure may result in embryos with a greater rate of genetic abnormalities. This could result from damage occurring to the chromosomes of the gametes or associated structures, such as the meiotic spindle, during the procedure. There is also fear that sperm with abnormal karyotypes are being injected into eggs, resulting in an increased rate of offspring with aneuploidy *(31)*. However, the association of aneuploidy and ICSI is probably not a consequence of the procedure but owing to the high incidence of male patients with Klinefelter's syndrome or 46XY/47XXY-mosaicism *(32)*.

Despite the report cited above that better embryo quality was seen in ICSI embryos from non-male factor cases, multiple studies have found no benefit to performing the procedure in non-male factor couples with tubal-factor infertility. Aboulghar et al. *(33)* randomized couples with tubal-factor infertility to having all oocytes undergo standard IVF (n = 58) or ICSI (n = 58). They found that the normal fertilization rate was significantly higher in the ICSI group, however, no significant differences were noted in the pregnancy rate between the two groups.

Van Steirteghem and coinvestigators *(34)* obtained similar results, however they randomized sibling oocytes from 50 cycles of couples with tubal infertility and normal semen parameters. Although the fertilization was significantly higher in those undergoing ICSI (68%) as opposed to IVF (57%), pregnancy and implantation rates were not different between couples receiving only ICSI or IVF embryos. However, conventional IVF resulted in failed fertilization in four couples, while only one couple failed following ICSI.

When couples present with borderline semen, ICSI has been associated with increased fertilization (60%) compared to sibling oocytes under going IVF (18%) *(35)*. In addition, the use of ICSI in this study prevented the complete fertilization failure that occurred in 49% of the patients following conventional IVF.

Although few in number, these studies suggest that performing ICSI on patients with seemingly normal or borderline semen parameters may prevent unexpected fertilization failure. Should future controlled, randomized studies show that the ICSI procedure does not impair embryo development, increase the risk of genetic abnormalities in the children, or limit the ability to cryopreserve embryos, programs of the future may adopt the use of ICSI for all patients.

ICSI WITH SPERMATOZOA
AND SPERMATIDS OBTAINED FROM THE EPIDIDYMIS OR TESTIS

Recovery and Use of Spermatozoa from the Epididymis

In patients with obstructive azoospermia, sperm recovery from the epididymis for IVF offers the only hope for pregnancy. Unfortunately, rates of fertilization and pregnancy are often low and depend greatly on the number and quality of the sperm collected *(36)*. In 1994, Tournaye and coinvestigators *(37)* reported pregnancies after combining ICSI with microsurgical epididymal sperm aspiration (MESA). The technique involved dissection of the epididymis followed by the opening of an epididymal tubule with microscissors. A small, glass pipet was then inserted into the tubule and epididymal fluid was aspirated. Additional epididymal incisions were performed until motile sperm were recovered. Variations of this procedure have also been reported, including percutaneous epididymal sperm aspiration (PESA) *(38)* and mini-micro-epididymal sperm aspiration *(39)*. Despite the successful use of epididymal sperm for ICSI, many clinicians use testicular sperm (testicular sperm extraction; TESE) for all azoospermic cases, including obstructive azoospermia, because the recovery protocol for testicular sperm is simpler, requires less training, and has a shorter operative time. The TESE procedure can also be performed under local anesthesia and does not require specialized equipment *(40)*.

Recovery and Use of Sperm from the Testis

The use of testicular sperm with ICSI has become common for the treatment of patients with both obstructive and nonobstructive azoospermia *(41–43)*. The collection procedure involves an incision of the scrotal skin and tunica vaginalis followed by excision of a small piece of the extruding testis. The biopsy is then sent to the IVF lab in buffered medium, where it is minced and examined for the presence of sperm. In some instances, when few or no sperm are found, the physician can be notified, and another biopsy performed at another site while the patient is still prepared. Specimen processing typically involves mincing the tissue with sterile glass slides, scissors, needles, or a combination of these tools followed by aspiration of the effluent and concentration of the sperm by centrifugation (43–45). Several investigators have assessed the fertilization and pregnancy rates following ICSI with testicular sperm. Aboulghar and coinvestigators (45) reviewed their experience with abnormal ejaculated sperm, epididymal sperm, testicular sperm obtained from patients with nonobstructive and obstructive azoospermia, and normal ejaculated sperm. They found that cases of nonobstructive testicular sperm had significantly lower rates of fertilization and pregnancy, whereas ICSI using normal sperm had significantly higher rates of fertilization. The authors concluded that because results obtained with testicular sperm were comparable to those obtained with epididymal sperm, TESE could be used in all cases. In addition, these investigators were able to cryopreserve testicular sperm, with 6 patients obtaining an embryo transfer and two pregnancies achieved. Similar results were reported by Madgaret et al. (46). Obstructive azoospermia cases (epididymal aspiration and TESE reported together) had a fertilization and pregnancy rate of 48.4% and 24.0%, respectively, whereas TESE with nonobstructive azoospermia resulted in a fertilization rate of 41.4% and a pregnancy rate of 14.6%.

The ability to cryopreserve testicular sperm has also expanded treatment options for patients with obstructive and nonobstuctive azoospermia. Freidler and coinvestigators (47) found no significant differences in fertilization, implantation, and clinical pregnancy rates comparing cycles using fresh and frozen testicular sperm recovered from cases of nonobstructive azoospermia. Biopsied tissue was shredded and repeatedly aspirated through a tuberculin syringe with the fluid extracts frozen in a test yolk buffer freezing medium diluted 1 to 1 using a two-step LN_2 vapor freezing protocol. Testicular sperm have also been cryopreserved following needle puncture (48). With this procedure, the seminiferous tubules are frozen within 30 min of the biopsy and, upon thaw, the tubules are squeezed with two 25-gauge needles to release sperm. These investigators reported a 46% fertilization rate, and three pregnancies in six patients undergoing five embryo transfers.

The recovery of viable sperm from shredded testicular tissue can often be technically difficult, particularly in cases of nonobstructive azoospermia. To reduce the presence of erythrocytes in the sample, the testicular sperm pellet can be exposed to erythrocyte lysing buffer (ELB) during a 10-min centrifugation (49). This procedure improved sperm collection from samples in which very few sperm could be found. A comparison between ICSI of sibling oocytes from 5 patients found no difference in fertilization and development rates. Crabbe and coworkers (50) also developed a method to maximize testicular sperm recovery from difficult cases such as Sertoli cell-only syndrome or maturational arrest. In this report, no sperm could be recovered from 27 cases after the samples were minced and exposed to ELB, however, following exposure of the tissue to enzymatic digestion with collagenase type IV at 37°C for 1 h, sperm were recovered in seven cases. Five of the seven couples achieved an embryo transfer with one ongoing pregnancy resulting.

Testicular sperm can also be obtained from azoospermic, nonmosaic Klinefelter patients. Using fine-needle biopsy, Reubinoff et al. (51) obtained mature sperm (4 of 6 cases) and following ICSI, one term pregnancy resulted. This pregnancy was obtained following the application of preimplantation genetic diagnosis, a procedure the authors recommend when the risk of gonosomal aneuploidy exists.

Use of Spermatids for ICSI

In 1993, two studies conducted in rodents demonstrated that round spermatids, obtained from the testis, could participate in early fertilization events following injection or electrofusion into hamster or mouse oocytes *(52,53)*. In the mouse model, normal offspring resulted following the injection of cryopreserved round spermatids *(54)*. Clinically, the first ongoing pregnancy was announced in 1995 *(57)* following the injection of immature testicular sperm, in this case, elongated spermatids. Thereafter, pregnancies were described following the injection of round *(58–60)* or elongated spermatids *(56,59–61)*. In 1997, Antinori and coinvestigators *(62)* reported an ongoing pregnancy following the injection of cryopreserved, round spermatids. By way of explanation, during spermiogenesis, haploid spermatids undergo cytodifferentiation to form mature spermatozoa. The different developmental stages of spermatids have been classified into the following groups: Sa, round; Sb1, round with flagellum; Sb2, elongating; Sc, elongating, nucleus fully elongated; Sd1, elongated, head not separated from mid-piece; Sd2, mature, cytoplasmic sheath in the mid-piece *(55,56)*.

Success rates have been lower with round spermatids (Sa and Sb1 types) compared with more mature spermatids (elongated Sb2). Bernabeu and coworkers *(56)* reported nine cases of ICSI using immature sperm; 8 cases were performed using round spermatids (Sa type) collected from either the ejaculate (6 cases) or the testis (2 cases). No pregnancies resulted from these attempts. However, one normal term pregnancy was obtained using elongated spermatids (Sb2 type) obtained from the testis.

As with TESE, the identification of spermatids within minced tissue preparations is often difficult, particularly with round spermatids; therefore, it is recommend that programs perform preclinical experimental work to obtain sufficient experience in the identification of round spermatids before attempting clinical trials. Round spermatids are often distinguished by their size (similar to erythrocytes) and shape *(60,63)*. They contain a round nucleus surrounded by a regular area of cytoplasm. In some, a developing acrosome can be distinguished adjacent to the nucleus. Elongated spermatids are distinguished by the presence of the developing flagellum. Round spermatids (Sa) have also been identified by their deformation when aspirated into the ICSI pipet, and absence of shrinkage when exposed to 10% polyvinyl pyrrolidone *(56)*.

ICSI OF OOCYTES THAT FAIL
TO FERTILIZE FOLLOWING CONVENTIONAL IVF

Low rates of fertilization or total fertilization failure following conventional IVF can occur in couples in which a sperm and/or oocyte defect was not suspected. Prior to the advent of ICSI, many programs attempted the reinsemination of these oocytes, but fertilization and pregnancy rates were typically low. One year after the first successful ICSI pregnancies, Nagy and coworkers *(64)* reported the use of ICSI for the fertilization of 1-d-old oocytes that had failed to fertilize following conventional IVF. An oocyte survival rate of 92%, a fertilization rate of 38%, and a cleavage rate of 84% was quoted. However, the embryos resulting from this study were not transferred.

In another report, Sjogren and coinvestigators *(65)* found that using a fresh sperm sample, collected and prepared the day of the injection of the "day-old" oocytes, increased the fertilization rate from 36 to 56%. Following the transfer of only ICSI-derived embryos, two pregnancies were established (2/9 transfers, 22%). The authors expanded the data in a later report *(66)*, increasing the population to 29 patients receiving a transfer of only ICSI-derived embryos. Again, two established pregnancies were reported, giving a pregnancy rate per transfer of 6.9%.

In a subsequent case report *(67)*, a patient was transferred one oocyte that fertilized the previous day using the standard insemination protocol and two embryos injected on d 2 after they failed to fertilize. The sperm sample utilized for ICSI was the one prepared the day before. A normal, dizygotic twin pregnancy resulted, leading the investigators to conclude that at least one child was derived from the "second day ICSI" procedure.

It seems clear from these reports that both reinsemination using conventional IVF and ICSI on oocytes that fail to fertilize, result in low rates of fertilization. This may be owing to the aging of the oocytes, resulting in either an impairment of early fertilization events or abnormal oocyte activation. Previous studies *(68–70)* performed on oocytes that fail to fertilize or fertilize late have shown a high incidence of chromosomal abnormalities, possibly explaining the low rates of implantation and pregnancy following their fertilization and transfer. Therefore, programs offering assisted fertilization must weight the benefits of second day ICSI against the possibility of producing offspring with genetic abnormalities owing to oocyte aging.

THE USE OF ICSI FOR PREIMPLANTATION GENETIC DIAGNOSIS

Preimplantation genetic diagnosis (PGD) provides couples at risk of passing a genetic defect to their children a method of screening their embryos prior to the initiation of a pregnancy. In 1996, Verlinsky and the International Working Group on Preimplantation Genetics reported that over 300 at-risk couples had undergone PGD during clinical trials in 14 centers around the world *(71)*. For couples at risk of transmitting X-linked or single-gene disorders, evaluation of the blastomeres removed from the cleavage-stage embryo is routinely performed in conjunction with the polymerase chain reaction (PCR) and the birth of 22 children following embryo diagnosis and gene amplification by PCR has been reported *(72)*. The PCR technique allows for the amplification of a single template of a specific gene from a single blastomere. Because PCR is very sensitive, the risk of amplifying a contaminant is real and care must be taken to avoid misinterpretation or even a false-positive report. Possible contaminants include skin and hair from the individual performing the embryo biopsy or the PCR, carryover from other samples, or from contaminating patient cells *(73)*.

The use of ICSI, prior to embryo biopsy and gene amplification by PCR, offers two advantages. The first is that oocytes are stripped of their corona radiata during the hyaluronidase procedure and the second is that mechanical insertion of the sperm by ICSI produces an embryo with no extraneous sperm. The presence of both sperm and corona cells during the biopsy procedure present the danger of having one of these cells inadvertently enter the biopsy pipet, resulting in a potential misdiagnosis of the embryo. For example, if a sperm with a normal gene contaminates a reaction tube containing a blastomere with a homozygous affected karyotype, the embryo may be diagnosed as heterozygous. If that embryo was then transferred, a pregnancy with an affected fetus could be established.

FERTILIZATION OF FROZEN-THAWED OOCYTES

In the human, investigations into oocyte cryopreservation have focused on the potential benefits for the treatment of infertility and patients about to lose ovarian function owing to medical treatments (i.e., radiation and/or chemotherapy). The cryopreservation of human oocytes may prove to be a clinically feasible technique for the enhancement of IVF outcome and provide an alternative to human embryo freezing (*see* Chapter 10). For patients anticipating loss of gonadal function, oocyte cryopreservation would allow for the thaw, insemination, and transfer of embryos at a more appropriate time.

Although there have been pregnancies established using frozen-thawed human oocytes, the success rates were very low (*74,75*). Recently, however, there has been a renewed interest in oocyte cryopreservation owing to three publications describing oocyte survival following thawing, and pregnancy after fertilization by ICSI and transfer (*76–78*).

During the freezing process, a cryoprotectant is used to remove water from the cell and this exposure can induce a precocious release of cortical granules. This in turn may alter the structure of the zona pellucida, the membrane that surrounds the oocyte, resulting in low rates of fertilization (*79*). In 1995, Kazem and coworkers (*80*) subjected frozen-thawed oocytes (n = 220) to insemination by conventional IVF or ICSI. Although thawing survival was only 34%, significantly more oocytes fertilized by ICSI.

The need to assist the fertilization of cryopreserved eggs by ICSI may be dependent on the stage of maturity at which they are frozen. In a study evaluating the cryopreservation of prophase I oocytes (*81*), no statistical difference in the fertilization rate following conventional IVF was noted between frozen-thawed, in vitro matured oocytes (30/52, 57.7%) and nonfrozen control oocytes (52/92; 56.5%). Cryopreservation at the immature stage, prior to the completion of cortical granule migration to the egg cortex, may allow for standard insemination following thaw and in vitro maturation.

THE USE OF ICSI WITH CYTOPLASMIC TRANSFER

There are several reports suggesting that certain undefined cytoplasmic factors within the oocyte influence or control significant genetic, maturational, and developmental properties (*see* Chapter 3). For instance, in the monkey (*82*), it was found that the developmental potential of oocytes matured in vitro could be increased by injecting them with the cytoplasm of oocytes matured in vivo. Following transfer to recipients for in vivo fertilization, 13% of the injected oocytes resulted in a viable pregnancy. No pregnancies were established with the use of sham-injected or nonsurgical control oocytes.

Recently, Cohen and coworkers (*83*) reported the first human pregnancy following the transfer of cytoplasm from donor into recipient eggs. The goal was to provide healthy cytoplasmic "factors" in patients who had repeatedly produced embryos of poor quality, which may have accounted for the patient's inability to achieve pregnancy. Subsequently, two additional pregnancies (one miscarried, one ongoing) were reported using this procedure (*84*). A term, twin pregnancy has also been established at the Norfolk program following the transfer of cytoplasm from cryopreserved donor eggs into the eggs of a 35-yr-old patient who had previously failed to achieve a pregnancy following 6 IVF attempts with very poor embryo morphology.

Because the cytoplasmic transfer procedure itself may activate the oocyte, the sperm is placed into the recipient oocyte along with the donated cytoplasm. The procedure is performed by first immobilizing and loading a sperm into the ICSI pipet, followed by cytoplasm from the donor egg. The pipet is then moved to the patient egg and the donor cytoplasm, along with the sperm, is injected. The addition of donor cytoplasm to the ICSI procedure does not affect the fertilization outcome for the recipient oocytes. In preliminary studies, 70.2% (26/37) of oocytes from 4 patients underwent normal fertilization following the transfer procedure. The use of cryopreserved donor eggs for cytoplasmic transfer was undertaken by the Jones Institute to avoid the need for synchronization of the oocyte donor and recipient cycles. Because the nature of the transferred cytoplasmic factor(s) is unknown, however, it is not yet clear whether cryopreservation has an adverse effect. The previous work by Flood and coworkers *(54)* suggested that the cytoplasmic factor(s) might be heat-labile, possibly a specialized protein or messenger ribonucleic acid that directs subsequent cell-cycle events. It is also possible that the transfer of donor mitochondria confers a benefit to the recipient oocyte.

CONCLUSIONS

Since the first reported ICSI pregnancies *(15)*, the mechanical procedure of placing a single sperm into the human oocyte has revolutionized the way we treat male factor infertility. In the future, sperm injection may become standard practice for the fertilization of oocytes, regardless of the type of infertility being treated. ICSI is also being used in conjunction with other clinical procedures to enhance fertilization and provide patients with improved treatment outcomes. During embryo biopsy and PGD, the use of ICSI allows clinicians a method for decreasing sample contamination and avoiding possible misdiagnosis. The oocyte's ability to undergo activation and development following the mechanical insertion of a sperm and donor cytoplasm may allow investigators to improve embryo quality in selected patients. In addition to the clinical treatment of human male factor infertility, ICSI has provided the opportunity to study early fertilization events in numerous animal species.

REFERENCES

1. Lillie FR. Studies of fertilization VI. The mechanism of fertilization in Arbacia. J Exp Zool 1914;16: 523–590.
2. Hiramoto Y. Microinjection of the live spermatozoa into sea urchin eggs. Exp Cell Res 1962;27:416–426.
3. Uehara T, Yanagimachi R. Microsurgical injection of spermatozoa into hamster eggs with subsequent transformation of sperm nuclei into male pronuclei. Biol Reprod 1976;15:467–470.
4. Uehara T, Yanagimachi R. Behavior of nuclei of testicular, caput and cauda epididymal spermatozoa injected into hamster eggs. Biol Reprod 1977;16:315–321.
5. Keefer CL, Brackett BG, Perreault SD. Behavior of bull sperm nuclei following microinjection into hamster oocytes. Biol Reprod 1986;34(Suppl 1):54.
6. Perreault SD, Naish SJ, Zirkin BR. The timing of hamster sperm nuclear decondensation and male pronucleus formation is related to sperm nuclear disulfide bond content. Biol Reprod 1987;36:239–244.
7. Perreault SD, Barbee RR, Elstein KH, Zucker RM, Keefer CL. Interspecies differences in the stability of mammalian sperm nuclei assessed in vivo by sperm microinjection and in vitro by flow cytometry. Biol Reprod 1988;39:157–167.
8. Kimura Y, Yanagimachi R. Intracytoplasmic sperm injection in the mouse. Biol Reprod 1995;52:709–720.
9. Keefer CL. Fertilization by sperm injection in the rabbit. Gamete Res 1989;22:59–69.
10. Yanagida K, Bedford JM, Yanagimachi R. Cleavage of rabbit eggs after microsurgical injection of testicular spermatozoa. Hum Reprod 1991;6:277–279.
11. Goto K. Bovine microfertilization and embryo transfer. Mol Reprod Dev 1993;288–290.
12. Hewitson L, Takahashi D, Dominko T, Simerly C, Shatten G. Fertilization and embryo development to blastocysts after intracytoplasmic sperm injection in the rhesus monkey. Hum Reprod 1998;13:3449–3455.
13. Lanzendorf S, Maloney M, Ackerman S, Acosta A, Hodgen G. Fertilizing potential of acrosome-defective sperm following microsurgical injection into eggs. Gamete Res 1988;19:329–337.
14. Lanzendorf SE, Maloney MK, Veeck LL, Slusser J, Hodgen GD. A preclinical evaluation of pronuclear formation by microinjection of human spermatozoa into human oocytes. Fertil Steril 1988;49:835–842.

15. Palermo G, Joris H, Devroey P, Van Steirteghem AC. Pregnancies after intracytoplasmic sperm injection of single spermatozoon into an oocyte. Lancet 1992;340:17–18.
16. Van Steirteghem AC, Nagy Z, Joris H, Liu J, Staessen C, Smitz J, Wisanto A, Devroey P. High fertilization and implantation rates after intracytoplasmic sperm injection. Hum Reprod 1993;8:1061–1066.
17. Oehninger S, Mahony M, Ozgur K, Kolm P, Kruger T, Franken D. Clinical significance of human sperm-zona pellucida binding. Fertil Steril 1997;67:1121–1127.
18. Mercan R, Oehninger S, Muasher SJ, Toner JP, Mayer J, Lanzendorf SE. Impact of fertilization history and semen parameters on ICSI outcome. J Assist Reprod Genet 1998;15:39–45.
19. Miller KF, Falcone T, Goldberg JM, Attaran M. Previous fertilization failure with conventional IVF is associated with poor outcome of ICSI. Fertil Steril 1998;69:242–245.
20. Bar-Hava I, Ashkenazi J, Shelef M, Schwartz A, Brenguaz M, Feldberg D, Orvieto R, Ben-Rafael Z. Morphology and clinical outcomes of embryos after IVF are superior to those after ICSI. Fertil Steril 1997;68:653–657.
21. Hsu M-I, Mayer J, Aronshon M, Lanzendorf S, Muasher S, Oehninger S. Embryo implantation in IVF and ICSI: Impact of the number of embryos transferred, morphology grade and cleavage status. Fertil Steril 1999;72:679–685.
22. Oehninger S, Kruger TF, Simon T, Jones D, Mayer JF, Lanzendorf S, et al. A comparative analysis of embryo implantation potential in patients with severe teratozoospermia undergoing in-vitro fertilization with a high insemination concentration or intracytoplasmic sperm injection. Hum Reprod 1996;11: 1086–1089.
23. Yang D, Shahata A, Al-Bader M, Al-Natsha SD, Al-Flamerzia, Al-Shawaf T. Intracytoplasmic sperm injection improving embryo quality: Comparison of the sibling oocytes of non-male-factor couples. J Reprod Genet 1996;13:351–355.
24. Alvarez JG, Touchstone JC, Blasco JC, Storey BT. Spontaneous lipid peroxidation and production of hydrogen peroxide and superoxide in human spermatozoa. Superoxide dismutase as major enzyme protectant against oxygen toxicity. J Androl 1987;8:338–348.
25. Atiken RJ, Clarkson JS. Cellular basis of defective sperm function and its association with the genesis of reactive oxygen species by human spermatozoa. J Reprod Fertil 1987;81:456–469.
26. Macas E, Imthum B, Boros M, Rosselli M, Maurer-Major E, Keller PJ. Impairment of the developmental potential of frozen-thawed human zygotes obtained after ICSI. Fertil Steril 1998;69:630–635.
27. Al-Hasani S, Ludwig M, Gagsteiger F, Kupker W, Sturn R, Yilmaz A, Bauer O, Diedrich K. Comparison of cryopreservation of supernumerary pronuclear human oocytes obtained after intracytoplasmic sperm injection (ICSI) and after conventional in-vitro fertilization. Fertil Steril 1996;11:604–607.
28. Hoover L, Baker A, Check JH, Lurie D, Summers D. Clinical outcome of cryopreserved human pronuclear stage embryos resulting from intracytoplasmic sperm injection. Fertil Steril 1997;67: 621–624.
29. Kowalik A, Palermo GD, Barmat L, Veeck L, Rimarachin J, Rosenwaks Z. Comparison of clinical outcome after cryopreservation of embryos obtained from intracytoplasmic sperm injection and in vitro fertilization. Hum Reprod 1998;13:2848–2851.
30. Gianaroli L, Fiorentino A, Magli MC, Ferraretti AP, Montanaro N. Prolonged sperm-oocyte exposure and high sperm concentration affect human embryo viability and pregnancy rate. Hum Reprod 1996;11: 2507–2511.
31. Tournaye H, Liu J, Nagy Z. Intracytoplasmic sperm injection (ICSI): the Brussels experience. Reprod Fertil Dev 1995;7:269–279.
32. Persson JW, Peters GB, Saunders DM. Genetic consequences of ICSI. Hum Reprod 1996;11:921–924.
33. Aboulghar MA, Mansour RT, Serour GI, Amin YM, Kamal A. Prospective controlled randomized study of in vitro fertilization versus intracytoplasmic sperm injection in the treatment of tubal factor infertility with normal semen parameters. Fertil Steril 1996;66:753–756.
34. Van Steirteghem A, De Vos A, Staessen C, Verheyen G, Aytoz A, Bonduelle M, et al. Is ICSI the ultimate ART procedure? In: Kempers RD, Cohen J, Haney AF, Younger JB, eds. Fertility and Reproductive Medicine, Elsevier, New York, NY, 1998, pp. 27–38.
35. Aboulghar MA, Monsour RT, Serour GI. Intracytoplasmic sperm injection in nonmale factor patients? In: Kempers RD, Cohen J, Haney AF, Younger JB, eds. Fertility and Reproductive Medicine. Elsevier, New York, NY, 1998, pp. 475–482.
36. Silber SJ, Ord T, Balmaceda J, Patrizio P, Asch R. Congenital absence of the vas deferens. N Engl J Med 1990;323:1788–1792.

37. Tournaye H, Devroey P, Liu J, Nagy Z, Lissens W, Van Steirteghem A. Microsurgical epididymal sperm aspiration and intracytoplasmic sperm injection: a new effective approach to infertility as a result of congenital absence of the vas deferens. Fertil Steril 1994;61:1045–1051.

38. Rosenlund B, Westlander G, Wood M, Lundin K, Reismer E, Hillensjo T. Sperm retrieval and fertilization in repeated percutaneous epididymal sperm aspiration. Hum Reprod 1998;13:2805–2807.

39. Nudell DM, Conaghan J, Pedersen R, Givens CR, Schriock ED, Turek PJ. The mini-micro-epididymal sperm aspiration for sperm retrieval: a study of urological outcomes. Hum Reprod 1998;13:1260–1265.

40. Aboulghar MA, Mansour RT, Serour GI, Fahmy I, Kamal A, Tawab NA, Amin YM. Fertilization and pregnancy rates after intracytoplasmic sperm injection using ejaculate semen and surgically retrieved sperm. Fertil Steril 1997;68:108–111.

41. Schoysman R, Vanderzwalmen P, Nijs M, Segal L, Segal-Bertin G, Geerts L, et al. Pregnancy after fertilisation with human testicular spermatozoa. Lancet 1993;342:1237.

42. Devroey P, Liu J, Nagy Z, Goossens A, Tournaye H, Camus M, et al. Pregnancies after testicular sperm extraction and intracytoplasmic sperm injection in non-obstructive azoospermia. Hum Reprod 1995;10: 1457–1460.

43. Silber SJ, Van Steirteghem AC, Liu J, Nagy Z, Tournaye H, Devroey P. High fertilization and pregnancy rate after intracytoplasmic sperm injection with spermatozoa obtained from testicle biopsy. Hum Reprod 1995;10:148–152.

44. Mansour R, Aboulghar M, Serour G, Fahmi I, Ramzy A, Amin Y. Intracytoplasmic sperm injection using microsurgically retrieved epididymal and testicular sperm. Fertil Steril 1996;65:566–572.

45. Abuzeid MI, Sasy MA, Salem H. Testicular sperm extraction and intracytoplasmic sperm injection: a simplified method for treatment of obstructive azoospermia. Fertil Steril 1997;68:328–333.

46. Madgar I, Hourvitz A, Levron J, Seidman DS, Shulman A, Raviv GG, et al. Outcome of in vitro fertilization and intracytoplasmic injection of epididymal and testicular sperm extracted from patients with obstructive and nonobstructive azoospermia. Fertil Steril 1998;69:1080–1084.

47. Friedler S, Raziel A, Soffer Y, Strassburger D, Komarovsky D, Ron-El R. Intracytoplasmic injection of fresh and cryopreserved testicular spermatozoa in patients with nonobstructive azoospermia: a comparative study. Fertil Steril 1997;68:892–897.

48. Allan JA, Cotman AS. A new method for freezing testicular biopsy sperm: three pregnancies with sperm extracted from cryopreserved sections of seminiferous tubule. Fertil Steril 1997;68:741–744.

49. Nagy ZP, Verheyen G, Tournaye H, Devroey P, Van Steirteghem AC. An improved treatment procedure for testicular biopsy specimens offers more efficient sperm recovery: case series. Fertil Steril 1997;68: 376–379.

50. Crabbe E, Verheyen G, Silber S, Tournaye H, Van de Velde H, Goossens A, Van Steirteghem A. Enzymatic digestion of testicular tissue may rescue the intracytoplasmic sperm injection cycle in some patients with non-obstructive azoospermia. Hum Reprod 1998;13:2791–2796.

51. Reubinoff BE, Abeliovich D, Werner M, Schenker JG, Safran A, Lewin A. A birth in non-mosaic Klinefelter's syndrome after testicular fine needle aspiration, intracytoplasmic sperm injection and preimplantation genetic diagnosis. Hum Reprod 1998;13:1887–1892.

52. Ogura A, Yanagimachi R. Round spermatid nuclei injected into hamster oocytes form pronuclei and participate in syngamy. Biol Reprod 1993;48:219–225.

53. Ogura A, Yanagimachi R, Usui N. Behavior of hamster and mouse round spermatid nuclei incorporated into mature oocytes by electrofusion. Zygote 1993;1:1–8.

54. Ogura A, Matsuda J, Asano T, Suzuki O, Yanagimachi R. Mouse oocytes injected with cryopreserved round spermatids can develop into normal offspring. J Assist Reprod Genet 1996;13:431–434.

55. de Kretser DM, Kerr JB. The cytology of the testis. In: Knobil E, Neill JD, eds. The Physiology of Reproduction, vol 1. Raven, New York, NY, 1994, pp. 1177–1290.

56. Bernabeu R, Cremades N, Takahashi K, Sousa M. Successful pregnancy after spermatid injection. Hum Reprod 1998;13:1898–1900.

57. Fishel S, Green S, Bishop M, Thornton S, Hunter A, Fleming S, Al-Hassan S. Pregnancy after intracytoplasmic injection of spermatid. Lancet 1995;345:1641–1642.

58. Tesarik J, Rolet F, Brami C, Sedbon E, Thorel J, Tibi C, Thebault A. Spermatid injection into human oocytes. II. Clinical application in the treatment of infertility due to non-obstructive azoospermia. Hum Reprod 1996;11:780–783.

59. Antinori S, Versaci C, Dani G, Antinori M, Pozza D, Selman HA. Fertilization with human testicular spermatids: four successful pregnancies. Hum Reprod 1997;12:286–291.

60. Vanderzwalmen P, Zech H, Birkenfeld A, Yemini M, Bertin G, Lejeune B, et al. Intracytoplasmic injection of spermatids retrieved from testicular tissue: influence of testicular pathology, type of selected spermatids and oocyte activation. Hum Reprod 1997;12:1203–1213.

61. Araki Y, Motoyama M, Yoshida A, Kim S-Y, Sung H, Araki S. Intracytoplasmic injection with late spermatids: a successful procedure in achieving childbirth for couples in which the male partner suffers from azoospermia due to deficient spermatogenesis. Fertil Steril 1997;67:559–561.

62. Antinori S, Versaci C, Dani G, Antinori M, Selman HA. Successful fertilization and pregnancy after injection of frozen-thawed round spermatids into human oocytes. Hum Reprod 1997;12:554–556.

63. Tesarik J, Mendoza C. Spermatid injection into human oocytes. I. Laboratory techniques and special features of zygote development. Hum Reprod 1996;11:772–779.

64. Nagy ZP, Joris H, Liu J, Staessen C, Devroey P, Van Steirteghem AC. Intracytoplasmic sperm injection of 1-day old unfertilized human oocytes. Hum Reprod 1993;8:2180–2184.

65. Sjogren A, Lundin K, Hamberger L. Intracytoplasmic sperm injection of 1 day old oocytes after fertilization failure. Hum Reprod 1995;10:974–975.

66. Lundin K, Sjogren A, Hamberger L. Reinsemination of one-day-old oocytes by use of intracytoplasmic sperm injection. Fertil Steril 1996;66:118–121.

67. Bussen S, Mulfinger L, Sutterlin M, Schleyer M, Kress W, Steck T. Dizygotic twin pregnancy after intracytoplasmic sperm injection of 1 day old unfertilized oocytes. Hum Reprod 1997;12:2560–2562.

68. Ezra Y, Simon A, Laufer N. Defective oocytes: a new subgroup of unexplained infertility. Fertil Steril 1992;58:24–27.

69. Almeida PA, Bolton VN. Immaturity and chromosomal abnormalities in oocytes that fail to develop pronuclei following insemination in vitro. Hum Reprod 1993;8:229–232.

70. Plachot M, de Grouchy J, Junca A-M, Mandelbaum J, Salat-Baroux J, Cohen J. Chromosome analysis of human oocytes and embryos: does delayed fertilization increase chromosome imbalance? Hum Reprod 1988;3:125–127.

71. Verlinsky Y. Preimplantation genetic diagnosis. J Assist Reprod Genet 1996;13:87–89.

72. Harper JC. Preimplantation diagnosis of inherited disease by embryo biopsy: an update of the world figures. J Assist Reprod Genet 1996;13:90–95.

73. Gitlin SA, Gibbons WE. Reducing contaminant DNA and preimplantation genetic diagnosis. Assisted Reprod Rev 1995;5:97–101.

74. Chen C. Pregnancy after human oocyte cryopreservation. Lancet 1986;2:884–886.

75. van Uem JFHM, Siebzehnrubl EF, Schuh B, Kock R, Trotnow S, Lang N. Birth after cryopreservation of unfertilized oocytes. Lancet 1987;1:752.

76. Porcu E, Fabbri R, Seracchioli R, Ciotti PM, Magrini O, Flamigni C. Birth of a healthy female after intracytoplasmic sperm injection of cryopreserved human oocytes. Fertil Steril 1997;68:724–726.

77. Tucker M. Successful human egg freezing-technique and clinical implications. The Embryologists' Newsletter, Fall, 1997, pp. 1–16.

78. Polak de Fried E, Notrica J, Rubinstein M, Morazzi A, Gomez Gonzalez M. Pregnancy after human donor oocyte cryopreservation and thawing in a patient with ovarian failure. Fertil Steril 1998;69:555–557.

79. Johnson MH, Pickering SJ, George MA. The influence of cooling on the properties of the zona pellucida of the mouse oocyte. Hum Reprod 1998;3:383–387.

80. Kazem R, Thompson LA, Srikantharajah A, Laing MA, Hamilton MPR, Templeton A. Cryopreservation of human oocytes and fertilization by two techniques: in vitro fertilization and intracytoplasmic sperm injection. Hum Reprod 1995;10:2650–2654.

81. Toth TL, Baka SG, Veeck LL, Jones HW, Muasher S, Lanzendorf SE. Fertilization and in vitro development of cryopreserved human prophase I oocytes. Fertil Steril 1994;61:891–894.

82. Flood JT, Chillik CF, Van Uem JFHM, Iritani A, Hodgen GD. Ooplasmic transfusion: prophase germinal vesicle oocytes made developmentally competent by microinjection of metaphase II egg cytoplasm. Fertil Steril 1990;53:2049–2054.

83. Cohen J, Scott R, Schimmel T, Levron J, Willadsen S. Birth of infant after transfer of anucleate donor oocyte cytoplasm into recipient eggs. Lancet 1997;350:186.

84. Cohen J, Scott R, Alikani M, Schimmel T, Munne S, Levron J, et al. Ooplasmic transfer in mature human oocytes. Mol Hum Reprod 1998;4:269–280.

8

The Production of Viable Human Blastocysts

The Evolution of Sequential Culture Systems

Thomas B. Pool, PHD *and Joseph E. Martin,* MD

CONTENTS

INTRODUCTION
THE TRANSITION TO SEQUENTIAL MEDIA
SEQUENTIAL CULTURE SYSTEMS
CONCLUDING REMARKS
THE FUTURE
REFERENCES

INTRODUCTION

In October, 1970, in Detroit, Michigan, USA, during the Harold C. Mack Symposium on the Biology of Fertilization and Implantation, the world first learned from Professor Robert G. Edwards of the feasibility of producing human blastocysts in vitro. The published account of this work, which appeared the following year in *Nature (1)*, documented that out of six embryos cultured, two developed into rudimentary blastocysts with low cell number, whereas two others developed through typical morulae into fully expanded blastocysts. Not only is this work of historic significance to experimental developmental biologists and clinical scientists alike, but it was also technically prophetic as well, because these embryos were produced using not a single culture medium, but a two-step sequence of media or a "sequential culture system." More specifically, in vitro fertilization (IVF) was accomplished in "Bavister's medium" *(2)*, a modified Tyrode's solution containing bovine serum albumin (BSA) that was shown previously to be successful for IVF of hamster oocytes *(3; see* Chapter 2), and embryonic growth was attained in Ham's F10 *(4)* supplemented either with human or fetal calf serum (FCS). Earlier attempts to fertilize human oocytes in a chemically complex media had been much less successful *(5)*. Thus, the initial system for human blastocyst production in culture was a sequential one that employed a simple solution in the first culture interval to meet the specific nutritional requirements of fertilization, followed by a chemically complex medium for the second culture interval, aimed at supporting embryonic growth.

From: *Contemporary Endocrinology: Assisted Fertilization and Nuclear Transfer in Mammals*
Edited by: D. P. Wolf and M. Zelinski-Wooten © Humana Press Inc., Totowa, NJ

It is ironic, therefore, that the better part of the three decades have passed since this report first appeared, with scientists showing little to no interest in pursuing human blastocyst production with sequential media. Instead, embryo culture technology over the past 10 years has focused on using the simultaneous culture of embryos with a feeder layer of somatic cells in co-culture, a technique developed many years ago in tissue culture facilities attempting to propagate either primary cell cultures or other fastidious cell lines in vitro. More recently, however, programs of assisted reproduction have become able to routinely produce viable human blastocysts in vitro following IVF using commercially-available media without the need for whole serum or somatic cell support (*see* Gardner *[5]*, Gardner and Lane *[6]*, and Pool et al. *[7]* for reviews). The key to doing so has been to employ new generations of sequential media, those that are designed to support the nutritional requirements of embryos at particular stages of pre-implantation development.

The goal of this chapter is to summarize the scientific work leading to contemporary sequential culture systems, to identify the components found in media used for the first and second culture intervals, to describe the most successful systems in use today, and to evaluate critically the formulations of these systems by examining the results obtained to date.

Why Blastocyst Culture and Transfer in Assisted Reproductive Technologies (ART)?

The explosion in both interest and success with human blastocyst culture has precipitated a plethora of works enumerating both the indications/applications of blastocyst transfer to ART and the potential pitfalls. Details of both perspectives are given in an excellent debate series *(8-11)* and the reader is referred to these works for comprehensive considerations of the practice. There is an emerging consensus from the literature that the major advantages of blastocyst production and transfer in human ART include:

1. Temporal and spatial synchronization of embryo and uterus at the time for transfer *(6)*;
2. A reduction in the incidence of high-order multiple gestation *(6-19)*;
3. The opportunity to select better embryos for transfer *(6,14)*; and
4. The potential to perform genetic screening, such as preimplantation genetic diagnosis (PGD), in conjunction with ART *(6,14)*.

Additionally, Gardner and Lane *(6)* have suggested that the routine propagation of human blastocysts may facilitate the application of metabolic selection methods that they have developed and applied successfully in the mouse *(19)*.

Limitations to Improving Culture Conditions

There is much less agreement to date on the pitfalls of blastocyst transfer, although many of the potential problems have been summarized recently by Tsirigotis *(8)*. In evaluating the possible applications of human blastocyst transfer in assisted reproduction, Bavister and Boatman *(12)* described a major concern held by all programs engaged in blastocyst production and transfer, namely, the failure of a particular culture system to support growth to the blastocyst stage in vitro of an embryo completely capable of forming a viable fetus in vivo. The capacity of a culture medium/system to produce outcomes in vitro equivalent to those that would have been obtained in vivo for a given embryo is an impossible one to measure scientifically, for obvious reasons. In general, the development and optimization of human embryo culture media have been thwarted by a number of problems, including the lack of a large number of developmentally synchronous embryos for experimentation and the unavailability of an appropriate and affordable animal model for basic investigation. Further, ethical, moral, and legal constraints prevent the generation and destruction of normal human embryos for biochemical and molecular analyses needed to assess the requirement and roles of many medium components, alone and in combination. From a practical perspective, there is no research facility worldwide that is sanctioned or prepared to utilize the scientific method in a rigorous manner so that the experimental testing of a hypothesis can be initiated without regard to the answer being positive or negative. In a sense, experimentation with human embryos destined for transfer to patients is always slanted to produce an improved outcome. In strict experimental science, a clean answer to the question posed is the valued result, regardless if the answer is given by negative outcomes. By extension, we cannot strictly investigate the effects of culture perturbations at one stage of development in the human and measure a possible downstream effect by embryo transfer without some indication, perhaps in a tangential animal model, that the effect is at least harmless if not positive. Of course, the "gold standard" for clinical investigation is the prospective, randomized trial, initiated with enough subjects calculated to provide statistical power even if no difference in treatment is detected. But the magnitude and diversity of variation in the characteristics of age and diagnosis, in endocrine status, in genetics, in physiological status, and in drug responsiveness alone in patients generating embryos makes such a trial a theoretical entity. Even within a single patient, both the genetic variation and the developmental plasticity demonstrated by a cohort of embryos is remarkable. The evaluation of the effect of changing the composition or even the temporal application of a given medium becomes a statistical argument, one in which the failure of a competent embryo to reach the blastocyst stage owing to medium insufficiency will go undetected. Biological, ethical, legal, and logistic constraints to research with human embryos ensure such an outcome and the pursuit of improved culture media and conditions for human embryogenesis in vitro remains an inexact science at best.

THE TRANSITION TO SEQUENTIAL MEDIA

Blastocyst Production Using A Single Culture Medium

The standard approach to fertilizing human oocytes and to culturing human embryos in vitro for the vast majority of the 20-year history of clinical ART has been to use a single culture medium. Although the source and concentration of protein supplementation has varied between programs and is often altered between insemination and culture phases within the same program, a single-medium formulation has been utilized throughout. This strategy was based on the ubiquitous clinical practice of transferring cleavage-stage embryos to the uterus on d 2 or d 3 after oocyte retrieval. It also failed to recognize the dynamic physiology of preimplantation embryos. The earliest efforts to produce viable human blastocysts for transfer demonstrated this concept clearly.

Bolton et al. *(20)* tested the hypothesis that it is more physiologically appropriate for blastocysts to be transferred to the uterus than cleavage-stage embryos, recognizing that it is likely possible to better select embryos for transfer after activation of the embryonic genome following the eight-cell stage. To test this, a study was initiated in which the embryos of patients under 35 years of age, with tubal occlusion as the sole source of infertility, were grown for either 2 or 5 d prior to transfer of a maximum of three embryos. The culture medium utilized for embryo culture was Earle's balanced salt solution (EBSS) supplemented with heat-inactivated patient serum (21). The transfer of cleavage-stage embryos on d 2 resulted in a pregnancy rate of 24% per embryo transfer, a livebirth rate of 16% per transfer, and an implantation rate of 9%. Of those embryos cultured for 5 d, 70% reached the morula stage and 40% became blastocysts. The pregnancy and livebirth rates per transfer, however, were 10% and 10%, respectively, with an implantation rate of 7%. The initial hypothesis was rejected given these data, but the authors were careful to conclude that improvements in culture media could change this conclusion in the future. Lastly, they suggested that even with lower pregnancy rates, a role for blastocyst generation and transfer could be envisaged in conjunction with preimplantation genetic diagnosis.

Huisman et al. (22) similarly examined the effect of 2, 3, or 4 d of embryo culture prior to transfer, using as a culture medium a mixture of EBSS and Ham's Nutrient Mixture F-10 in a ratio of 17:3. This investigation is remarkable in several ways. First, it lent itself well to valid statistical scrutiny because it involved both a large number of embryos, almost 6,000, and a large number of transfers (2306). No other investigation on the effect of culture interval has, to date, duplicated the magnitude of this study. Secondly, the investigators tracked embryonic developmental rates throughout the study and, thus, were able to analyze pregnancy outcome and implantation rates both globally per transfer day and as a function of embryonic growth rates. When both the pregnancy and implantation rates were compared globally, without considering embryonic growth rate, no differences were seen statistically between 2, 3, and 4 d of culture. Thus, these outcomes, like those of the study by Bolton et al. (20), would suggest no advantage for extended culture in clinical ART. However, consideration of implantation rates as a function of embryonic growth rates on d 2, 3, and 4 of transfer were both significant and instructive. The percentage of embryos that maintained either a normal or advanced developmental rate on d 2 and 3 was similar (60.5 and 54.2%, respectively). The percentage of embryos showing normal or advanced development by d 4 fell precipitously to 18.4%. Although only 1/5 of embryos cultured for 4 d showed normal or accelerated growth, they produced a 41% implantation rate upon transfer compared to a significantly reduced rate of 11% for growth-retarded embryos transferred on d 4. Implantation rates for normally-developing embryos transferred on d 2 and 3 were significantly lower at 18.2 and 19.2%, respectively. From this investigation, it is clear that a distinct advantage to implantation is imparted by transferring later-stage embryos that have maintained a normal developmental rate in vitro. Of equal clarity though is the finding that four out of five embryos fail to demonstrate a normal developmental rate in vitro using the culture conditions and/or medium employed. The value of these data to future developments in culture optimization was considerable as they supported the use of growth rate, earlier in embryogenesis, as a marker for viability at a later stage. As will be seen, this is one of the philosophical principles of sequential culture, namely, to optimize growth and metabolism by matching medium components to the physiological need of an embryo at each particular stage of development. As those needs change, the environment must also change.

Blastocyst Production with Somatic Cells: Lessons From Co-Culture

It is not the intent of this chapter to review the voluminous literature concerning both the development of co-culture and its applications to human ART. For this, the reader is referred to the works of Bongso et al. *(23)*, Menezo et al. *(24,25)*, and Weimer et al. *(26)*. That the practice of co-culture has had a pivotal influence upon many programs to pursue the transfer of later-stage embryos is certain (*see* Chapter 16), although this method has not been without its detractors *(27,28)*. Nonetheless, it is co-culture that first facilitated the routine production of viable blastocysts for transfer in humans *(24)*. That somatic cells of varying origins could modulate the chemistry of culture medium in a way favorable to embryogenesis in vitro was reported worldwide. Additionally, through the facilitation of blastocyst production via co-culture, both basic knowledge regarding blastocyst physiology and practical methods, such as blastocyst freezing, were obtained *(14)*. But another dogmatic statement can be made as well: the method was adopted into clinical practice widely without a scientific explanation of the mechanism by which co-culture exerts an effect on the culture environment and the embryo. The pressure for immediate enhancement of outcome has fostered the incorporation of a number of practices into clinical IVF, such as assisted hatching, solely as phenomena without a demonstrated underlying mechanism, and the use of co-culture is no exception. In reality, given the competitive influences upon ART programs, it is no surprise that co-culture became a mainstay in the clinical setting. What is startling, however, is the little experimental interest shown by academic centers performing human ART in defining the science behind co-culture, although a moratorium on funding such work, at least in the United States, has contributed significantly to this situation.

Although this paucity of mechanistic data remains for human embryo culture, several investigations into the chemical modulation of culture medium by bovine oviductal epithelial cells have provided valuable glimpses into the specific manner in which co-culture exerts an influence on embryogenesis. Rieger et al. *(29)* compared the effects of either co-culture or medium alone, conditioned previously by a monolayer of oviductal epithelial cells, on the development and metabolism of bovine embryos. It was seen that co-cultured embryos reached the 16-cell, morula, and blastocyst stages 24 h earlier than did those produced with conditioned medium and did so with significantly more cells in the blastocysts, a finding reported previously by Trounson et al. *(30)*. Of particular interest, the metabolism of glucose was significantly higher by embryos in conditioned medium and occurred earlier, between the 4- and 16-cell stages, than in co-cultured embryos. Further, the concentration of glucose was significantly lower and that of lactate significantly higher in co-culture medium than in conditioned medium. The authors derived an important conclusion from their data: the lower number of cells in the blastocysts grown in conditioned medium suggests that the delay in development between the 4-cell and 16-cell stages is associated with decreases in subsequent developmental potential of the embryo. Therefore, the theme that perturbations in early stages of development give rise to reduced implantation capacity surfaces once again, but from a different experimental paradigm. Additionally, the significance of the first culture interval in the formulation of contemporary sequential culture systems is, again, emphasized.

The finding of Rieger et al. *(29)* that the reduced glucose levels and elevated lactate concentrations are produced by co-culture was confirmed by Edwards et al. *(31)*, who studied not only bovine oviductal epithelial cells, but also 3T3 mouse fibroblasts and Buffalo rat liver cells. That these alterations in metabolite concentrations are related mechanistically to enhanced embryonic growth of bovine embryos was tested directly by modifying the concentrations of glucose, lactate, and pyruvate in synthetic oviduct fluid (SOF) to match those produced by co-culture. Significantly more embryos grown in this modified synthetic medium reached the blastocyst stage than did those grown in SOF containing the same concentrations of these compounds found in tissue culture medium (TCM)-199 in which no somatic cells were grown. Although blastocyst production was good at a lactate concentration of greater than 0.82 mM, blastocyst cell number was low until the concentration was raised to 3.3 mM, supporting the additional conclusion that morphological criteria alone cannot be used to judge blastocyst development. This is another concept that recurs throughout the experimental literature leading to sequential culture systems, unless one can count cell number, determining the viability of a given blastocyst by morphological criteria alone is impossible. In addition to showing that somatic cells lower glucose and elevate the concentrations of lactate and pyruvate in medium, Edwards et al. *(31)* also demonstrated that the concentrations of some nonessential amino acids were not depleted from the medium, but were instead elevated. As will be discussed later, this modification of culture medium by co-culture cells is also important in facilitating healthy embryogenesis.

Despite the fact that co-culture has been widely held as an effective practice to promote embryonic growth in vitro, there are a number of concerns regarding the use of this method for clinical IVF. These have been summarized recently *(7)* and include:

1. Optimization of the culture environment for co-culture cells innately produces a suboptimal environment for embryos, one that must be paradoxically corrected by the somatic cells for the benefit of the embryos;
2. The addition of a separate layer of technology is both time demanding and expensive *(27)*; and
3. The use of heterologous sources of somatic cells potentially introduces infectious agents into the culture environment that ultimately may infect a resulting fetus, the mother or both.

That innovations and improvements to simpler culture systems have now paralleled or exceeded the outcomes produced previously with co-culture has convinced one of the pioneers of co-culture and culture medium technology in general, Yves Menezo, to declare that the time has come to switch from co-culture to sequential defined media for the growth of embryos destined for transfer at the blastocyst stage *(14)*.

Experimental Evidence Suggesting How Sequential Media Should Be Formulated

PREIMPLANTATION STAGES

The use of the term "preimplantation" to define that period of embryonic development from fertilization to intercalation of the embryo into the uterine endometrium is certainly accurate, however, it has also lulled us into perceiving that "preimplantation" also denotes a singular physiological state. Data from a wide variety of mammalian embryonic systems clearly support the notion that the preimplantation period is divisible into discrete stages with specific characteristics. Leese *(32)* indicates that preimplantation development may conveniently be divided into two phases, early and late. The early embryo is undifferentiated, nonvascularized, shows no net growth, is controlled by maternal RNA, and is largely insensitive to exogenous hormones and growth factors. By comparison, the late preimplantation embryo shows net growth, is under genomic regulation, differentiates trophoblast and inner cell mass, and responds to extracellular modulators of growth, such as hormones and growth factors (*see* Chapter 2). Although we agree completely with this assessment, we find it helpful to refine these periods with additional criteria that

Table 1
Characteristics of Preimplantation Stages During Human Embryogenesis

	Preimplantation Stage		
	1	*2*	*3*
Form of genetic regulation	Maternal (translational)	Genomic (transcriptional)	Genomic (transciptional)
Preferred energy source	Lactate/pyruvate	Glucose	Glucose
Form of cell cycle regulation	Intrinsic	Extrinsic (autocrine)	Extrinsic (paracrine)
Amino acid requirement	Simple (osmolyte)	Complex	Complex

relate simplistically to the nutritional requirements that have been established in a number of experimental settings. Table 1 shows that one might divide the preimplantation period into three stages, based solely upon a characterization of the source of genetic regulation, predominate energy source utilized, the manner in which growth is regulated during the cell cycle, and the amino acid requirement. In reality, this classification scheme does not differ significantly from the ideas of Leese because he carefully categorizes metabolic control of the embryo into intrinsic and extrinsic levels *(32)*. Some of the key evidence supporting the concept of discrete physiological stages within the preimplantation period are given later as these are the scientific rudiments that underscore the construction of sequential media.

ENERGY SOURCES

The inclusion of glucose in IVF media in concentrations ranging from 2.5–10.0 mM is not one driven from an experimentally established need, but rather is a remnant of the "borrowing" of somatic cell medium formulations for embryo culture that has occurred historically *(see* Pool et al. *[7])*for a review). Although Brinster *(33)* showed that energy sources other than glucose were required during mouse embryogenesis over 30 years ago, the inclusion of high concentrations of glucose in embryo culture-medium formulations has persisted. In 1988, Schini and Bavister *(34)* demonstrated that the 2-cell block to development in vitro in the hamster embryo could be alleviated by eliminating glucose and inorganic phosphate from the culture medium. Further work by this group showed that oxygen consumption was lowered by the presence of both glucose and inorganic phosphate in culture medium, but that it was restored by eliminating either metabolite alone or in combination. That this may impinge upon the generation of ATP and that a minimum level of ATP in oocytes and resulting embryos is strongly correlated with viability in humans *(35)* are indicative that selecting both the appropriate forms and concentrations of energy substrates in culture media is crucial. The changing requirements of preimplantation embryos for energy substrates in the human has been firmly established by Hardy *(36)*. She measured the uptake of various metabolites, including glucose, by human embryos in vitro and recorded a preferential uptake of pyruvate during cleavage stages followed by a sharp rise in glucose utilization during the blastocyst stage. The direct experimentation on human embryos in culture by Conaghan et al. *(37)* established that pyruvate, but not glucose, is required during early embryogenesis. In fact, omission of glucose in the early interval resulted in slightly more embryos reaching the

8-cell stage, as well as significantly more trophectodermal cells forming in resulting blastocysts. A beneficial effect of completely removing glucose from culture media during early stages of the preimplantation period has now been demonstrated in a wide array of mammalian species *(7)*. A detailed consideration of the experimentation that has brought about changes in the energy substrates used in IVF media has been published recently by Graham and Pool *(38)*.

No study to date in humans has demonstrated a need for any glucose in the early culture interval, a point that will be considered in detail later in this chapter. As stated earlier, the concentration of glucose in most embryo culture media has been from 2.5–10 mM. Thompson et al. *(39)*, however, have conducted one of the few dose-response studies on the effects of glucose on mammalian embryos and has shown that development is impaired in bovine embryos at concentrations above 1.5 mM. This threshold has not been tested in other species to our knowledge, but measurements of the concentrations of glucose and other metabolites in human oviducts and uterus as a function of stage of the menstrual cycle have been made by Gardner et al. *(40)*. Whereas the concentration of glucose was high in the oviducts during the follicular and luteal phase, it was low (0.5 mM) during midcycle, specifically cycle days 12 through 16, the time corresponding to when the embryo is in the oviduct in vivo. Although the absolute value may have little meaning, because it was determined by analyzing only six samples, it does support the idea that glucose concentrations are dramatically lower at the site of early embryogenesis during midcycle in vivo than they are earlier or later in the oviduct and throughout the cycle in the uterus. The collective data on the effects of glucose during preimplantation embryogenesis support the concept that glucose is not needed in culture media that are used during the early culture interval. The data from both Thompson et al. *(39)* and Gardner et al. *(40)* suggest that a reduced level of glucose, perhaps under 1.5 mM as seen in sheep, can be tolerated during the first culture interval, but no data suggest it is required or improves outcome. Work by Behnke (*see* Pool et al. *[7]*), Quinn *(41)*, Rawlins et al. *(42)*, Graham et al. *(43)*, Lee et al. *(44)*, and Pool et al. *(7)* has shown improvements in embryogenesis and in pregnancy rates in humans using culture medium devoid of glucose during the earliest preimplantation stage.

AMINO ACIDS

The significant and changing requirement for amino acids over the preimplantation stages of development have been brought to light primarily by work from two investigators; David Gardner, formerly of Monash University and now with the Colorado Center for Reproductive Medicine, and Barry Bavister at the University of Wisconsin–Madison. These investigators and their colleagues have employed two distinct approaches to studying the requirement for amino acids, but both have arrived at similar conclusions regarding which amino acids are crucial. They may even now agree on the mechanism of action by amino acids in embryonic blastomeres, as will be discussed later in this chapter.

Bavister and McKiernan *(45)* have measured the ability of single amino acids to support growth of hamster embryos, referencing the measured performance to that obtained when glutamine was used as the sole nitrogen source in culture. The amino acids that were able to support the growth of significantly more embryos to later stages when added alone were taurine, glycine, serine, asparagine, aspartic acid, histidine, lysine, and proline. Not only was it shown that not all amino acids have growth-promoting activity, but

also that certain amino acids, such as cystine, tyrosine, valine, isoleucine, and phenylala-
nine actually inhibited embryogenesis. This is of particular interest because classical
studies of amino acid requirements showed that animal and human cell lines, whether
derived from normal or from malignant tissue, require cystine and tyrosine, and upon
their omission, cells degenerate and die *(46)*. Once again, the imposition of somatic cell
nutritional requirements upon embryonic blastomeres is not only unwarranted, but is
potentially harmful. Subsequent work by Lane and Gardner *(47)* have demonstrated con-
clusively that, with respect to amino acids, this is the case in mouse embryos.

Studies of the effects of single amino acids, however, may not be without serious
limitations. For example, Van Winkle and Dickinson *(48)* measured changes in the free
amino acid content of mouse embryos grown in vitro from the 2-cell to the blastocyst
stage, comparing them to those of d 4 blastocysts produced in vivo. Not only were there
significant differences seen between the in vitro- and in vivo-derived blastocysts, but
attempts to correct the changes by supplementing culture medium with a single amino
acid often resulted in an alteration in the free content of several amino acids. This, in fact,
was the rule when five different amino acids were added, one at a time. Thus, the behavior
of free amino-acid pools in embryos may be akin to that of an over-stuffed pillow, where
pushing down a lump in one region is greeted by the appearance of two new lumps
elsewhere on the pillow. Gardner and his group, however, potentially avoided this pitfall
by studying the effects of amino acids in groups, specifically the essential and nonessential groups of Eagle *(46)*. This is an exhaustive body of work conducted with mouse
embryos over several years, but it is well-summarized in Lane and Gardner *(47)*. In these
studies, the nonessential amino acids plus glutamine were tested for growth-promoting
capacity against both the essential amino acids and all 20 amino acids (essentials and
nonessentials plus glutamine) in both the early and the late culture intervals. This work
established that the highest rate of development was achieved when nonessential amino
acids plus glutamine were included in the first culture interval, prior to the 8-cell stage,
and all 20 amino acids were included in the second interval, from 8-cell stage onward.
An additional finding was that neither blastocyst formation nor hatching were reliable in
vitro markers of viability, as evidenced by corrletation studies with pregnancy rates following embryo transfer (ET). As a consequence, they are also poor markers of the suit-
ability of a particular culture system for IVF/ET. This study sets a new benchmark for
all that follow: improvements to culture systems must be documented by enhanced outcomes following embryo transfer. A failure to follow through with viability studies, as
difficult as they may be, is a major weakness of many of the published studies regarding
enhancements to the culture environment.

Although informative in many respects, the use of groups of amino acids for eluci-
dating embryonic requirements is also not without potential problems. First, the concentrations of amino acids in these groups were formulated to approximate the protein
composition of cultured human cells. It is totally unclear what relevance, then, studying
amino acids in the amounts found in cell protein in human cell lines has upon mouse
embryogenesis. Secondly, smaller subsets or even single amino acids may be seen to
produce the same biological effect as these larger groups. Although the commercial
availability of essential and nonessential amino acids makes them convenient groupings
for study, this convenience may actually introduce an unnecessary degree of complexity
to culture media. Lastly, although the amino acid taurine is not without considerable

effect upon embryogenesis, it is not included in either the essential or nonessential group. However, it should be noted that taurine was included in the first generation of sequential culture media (G1), destined for use in human IVF, that were fashioned from these mouse data *(64)*.

GLUTAMINE

Glutamine is included in the formulation of a number of embryo culture media although a justification for doing so is often lacking. This may be overstated in rodent and other animal studies, but is clearly the case for human embryo culture medium. Recent work by Devreker et al. *(49)* looked specifically at the effects of 1 m*M* glutamine upon human preimplantation development and concluded that its inclusion resulted in more morulae and blastocysts. Unfortunately, little light was actually shed on this subject since the investigation only measured the effects of glutamine in EBSS, failing to evaluate it in conjunction with other amino acids, and did not include the results of embryo transfer as an assessment of embryonic viability. Furthermore, the embryos were placed into this medium after first being grown in medium containing whole patient serum. All in all, this collection of conditions make the data difficult to evaluate. Although the study suggests that a well-designed investigation is warranted, the requirement for glutamine in human embryogenesis currently remains to be demonstrated.

THE ROLE OF AMINO ACIDS IN EARLY DEVELOPMENT

What has been made very clear by the foregoing work on amino acids is that a) only a subset of amino acids is required during the initial preimplantation stage, and b) the complexity of the requirement increases in the later preimplantation stages. A complex requirement is easy to understand later in development given that an efficient protein synthetic capacity, under genomic direction, is needed to support actual embryonic growth. But what functions are served by amino acids at the early stage where intracellular amino acid pools are large, yet no overt growth occurs? Bavister and McKiernan *(45)* proposed a hypothetical model whereby amino acids shuttle into and out of oocytes/ embryos, exporting protons in the process and, thus, function as modulators of intracellular pH (pHi). This novel mechanism does not require a complex array of amino acids and, in fact, was described solely utilizing the two amino acids present in the reproductive tract at high concentrations, glycine and taurine. The hypothesis that amino acids buffer intracellular pH has recently been tested in the mouse embryo, where it was seen that a group of amino acids could prevent experimentally induced intracellular acidification up to the 4-cell stage, an effect that was not observed from the 8–16-cell stage onwards *(50)*. These experiments were conducted using groups of amino acids, specifically Eagle's nonessential amino acids with glutamine, essential amino acids with glutamine, and essential amino acids without glutamine. The ability of either taurine or glycine to buffer intracellular pH, either alone or in combination, was not tested. There is no reason to assume, however, that a single amino acid with the appropriate pK's could not provide adequate buffer capacity to early preimplantation stage embryos. Both taurine and glycine have very low (~2–3) and very high (~9) pK's at pH 6.0–7.0 *(45)*.

Amino acids such as taurine and glycine share another significant physical property: both can function as organic osmolytes during early development. Dawson et al. *(51)* have summarized the paradox regarding osmolality and early development. As they indicate, the osmotic pressure exerted by mouse oviductal fluid has been calculated to be high, above 340 mOsM, but experimental evidence reveals that mouse zygotes fail to develop in culture when osmotic pressure exceeds 300 mOsM. However, inclusion of an organic osmolyte, one permeable to the developing embryo, will facilitate development at higher osmotic pressures. That glycine can serve a protective function from inorganic compounds during early mouse embryogenesis was first reported by Van Winkle et al. *(48)*, but Dawson and co-workers *(51)* provided strong experimental support to the hypothesis by demonstrating that early mouse embryos, in fact, accumulate glycine as a function of the osmolarity of the medium. A similar role for taurine has been demonstrated in the mouse embryo *(48)*. Taurine is a well known osmoregulator in a number of cell types *(52)*. The addition of taurine to culture medium is beneficial to development in a number of species, including the hamster *(45)*, mouse *(48)*, pig *(53)*, and cow *(54)*. Dumoulin et al. *(55)* using unfertilized human oocytes and human embryos from the 2- to 8-cell stage, showed that radioactive taurine, preloaded into cells by a 4-h incubation, was retained under hypo-osmotic conditions and released in hyperosmotic media. Two suggestions were made by this group: 1) taurine is released by embryos when they have to adjust their cell volume, such as in conditions of osmotic imbalance induced by poor culture conditions or during cell division; and 2) culture in medium lacking taurine leads to taurine depletion of embryos, thus causing more reliance upon inorganic osmotic regulators.

One final possibility as to the function served by taurine during early embryogenesis has been suggested by Li et al. *(56)* in the rabbit. They compared the effects of catalase, superoxide dismutase (SOD), and taurine as potential antioxidants in macromolecule-free culture of rabbit zygotes. The inclusion of either SOD or taurine, but not catalase, resulted in significantly more embryos reaching the blastocyst stage and a significant increase in cell number of blastocysts. Although compelling, no direct evidence was given in this investigation to show that any of the compounds were functioning as antioxidants, thus this function for amino acids in early development remains only theoretical.

MACROMOLECULES AND GROWTH FACTORS

Culture media for human IVF have been supplemented with a wide array of macromolecules, largely from whole serum derived from diverse sources (*see* Pool et al. *[7]* for a review). Both the undefined nature of whole serum and the batch to batch variability its use imparts to culture media are legendary, not to mention the potential concerns for infectious disease. One of the major advantages of adopting a sequential approach to embryo culture is that whole serum is not required to reach advanced stages of embryogenesis in vitro *(5)* and viable blastocysts can be produced with a defined protein or protein fractions. The role that proteins fulfill in sequential culture, and both the qualitative and quantitative nature of macromolecular supplementation during extended embryo culture, have not been addressed. We wish to raise several points regarding this issue:

1. Although the simplest approach for the production of viable blastocysts is the best approach, a classical tenet of William of Occham, it is still possible that a macromolecular requirement evolves with time during embryogenesis, one that is not fully satisfied with albumin or globulins,
2. The predominate form of macromolecule in the reproductive tract is not albumin, as is widely held, but rather glycoproteins in the form of mucopolysaccharide, glycosaminoglycans, and assorted mucins.
3. As we have indicated previously *(7,57,58)*, one should not overlook the physical role that macromolecules, particularly those listed previously, play in the culture environment.

Envisioning the tubal ampulla as containing a chemically ideal solution is a far cry from reality and thus the physiology that has been described from ideal solutions is not reflective of the physiology of the tube. The practice of conducting a tubal inventory of soluble components, essentially describing a "chemical anatomy," and drawing "physiological" conclusions from these components by assuming the chemistry of ideal solutions without regard to the profound biological effects these compounds might produce via physical modulation of tubal solvent properties, is simply bad science. In fact, we suggest that investigators refrain from the popular tendency to deem one version of a medium "physiological" and another version "nonphysiological" or even "artifactual" as has occurred. Our factual understanding of the mechanisms of human preimplantation embryogenesis is currently too infantile to do otherwise.

That a distinct requirement for growth factors evolves as a hallmark of later preimplantation stages is suggested by investigations in mice (discussed later) and cattle (*see* Chapter 2). Lighten et al. *(59)* have examined the expression of mRNA for the insulin-like growth factors (insulin, IGF-1, IGF-2) and their receptors (insulin receptor, IGF1R, IGF2R) in human oocytes and preimplantation embryos. Only IGF-2 is expressed in oocytes and embryos although transcripts for all three receptors are present. The authors indicate that this situation is analogous to that in the mouse where expression of IGF-2 by embryos has an autocrine effect upon embryogenesis. Further, they suggest that IGF-1 may be expressed by the reproductive tract, thus influencing embryogenesis in a paracrine manner as has been reported for the mouse. This hypothesis was tested recently by the same group *(60)* and mRNA transcripts of IGF-1 were detected at midcycle in the human Fallopian tube. This growth factor was found in tubal fluid at a concentration of 8 nM and in that of the uterus at 10.9 nM. Inclusion of IGF-1 in culture medium from d 2–6 resulted in significant increases in the percentage of embryos reaching blastocyst and in the cellularity of the inner cell mass. The certainty of these observations was assured through the use of elegant control experiments. Specifically, the presence of the IGF-1 receptor in blastocysts was confirmed with immunohistochemistry using a monoclonal antibody to IGF-1 receptor. Additionally, the biological effect of enhanced blastocyst formation in the presence of IGF-1 was completely inhibited in the presence of the same antibody. It is this level of investigation that is sorely needed to provide concrete data on specific growth factor requirements during embryogenesis. A recent review by Kane et al. *(61)* examines in critical detail the issue of growth factors during embryogenesis and the attendant pitfalls of these investigations.

SEQUENTIAL CULTURE SYSTEMS

Sequential Culture in an Animal Model

Credit for the current popularity of sequential culture systems deservedly belongs to Dr. David K. Gardner. As early as 1994, he recognized that optimal development requires different levels of metabolites and amino acids on successive days of development and even proposed a perfusion culture system to achieve this goal *(5)*. Not only did his laboratory group elucidate many of the specifics of these changing requirements, but they also demonstrated in 1997 *(47)* the optimal way in which these could be applied in the mouse to facilitate the production of viable blastocysts without whole serum or co-culture.

There were other groups, however, that were testing similar ideas in other animal models at about the same time. That sequential culture could produce results only previously experienced with either organ culture or co-culture was demonstrated in 1995 using pig embryos as a model. Pollard et al. *(62)* showed a significant increase in the percentage of embryos that hatched in vitro by growing them first in a simple medium lacking glucose followed by culture in a complex medium, a modified Minimum Essential Medium. This sequential regimen was superior to leaving embryos in either the simple medium throughout, the complex medium throughout, or to culture in a simple medium supplemented with whole serum. It was also at about this same time that sequential culture was extended to human ART.

Sequential Culture Systems for Human Embryos and the Outcomes From Blastocyst Transfer

MEDI-CULT

Although Gardner is responsible for popularizing the sequential approach for the culture of human embryos, the initial prospective clinical trial of transferring advanced embryos produced sequentially was conducted by Forsdahl et al. *(63)* from Norway in 1994. This group cultured embryos for the first 2 d in Medi-Cult Universal IVF Medium and then in Medi-Cult M3 medium for the duration (Medi-Cult, Copenhagen, Denmark). Embryo transfer on d 4 or d 5 produced a "normal" pregnancy rate of 59% (n = 23) and 48% (n = 13) respectively, compared to 31% (n = 31) on d 3. Both d 4 and d 5 transfers raised the implantation rate to approx 40% compared to 18% observed for d 3 transfers. This sequential system clearly produced improved outcomes in this limited trial, but the media represent the extremes of typical single media used for clinical IVF; a simple salt solution with glucose followed by a very complex medium that actually was optimized for the clonal, anchorage-dependent growth of somatic cells. That such high implantation rates were achieved indicates that, even though the media were not formulated based on experiments in embryonic systems, a sequential system was still superior to the use of a single, simple medium.

G1/ G2 AND SUBSEQUENT MODIFICATIONS

The first report of livebirth resulting from production of a blastocyst with the sequential media G1 and G2, with the "G" signifying "growth," was from Barnes et al. *(64)* in 1995. The healthy female infant was truly a technological marvel because the case involved the transfer of a single, early-stage blastocyst resulting from immature oocyte retrieval, in vitro maturation (IVM), fertilization via intracytoplasmic sperm injection (ICSI), and embryonic growth in the sequential media G1/G2. This paper also was the first to include the specific composition of G1 and G2, and demonstrated that Gardner had incorporated the metabolite concentrations he had earlier reported for human oviducts into the formulas, using low glucose (0.5 mM), and high lactate (21 mM) in G1, compared to high glucose (3.15 mM) and lower lactate (11.74 mM) in G2. Further, he included Eagle's nonessential amino acids plus glutamine and taurine in G1, switching to both essential and nonessential amino acids plus glutamine in G2, as suggested from growth studies in the mouse embryo. Also included in both media was inorganic phosphate, whereas ethylenediaminetetracetic acid (EDTA) was included solely in G1. In both G1 and G2, the protein source was BSA.

Two reports, both evaluating the efficacy of transferring blastocysts produced sequentially, appeared simultaneously in January of 1998. In one report, Gardner et al. *(15)* compared implantation rates produced by two unrelated treatment strategies, namely the transfer of artificially-hatched, d 3 embryos produced by culture in Ham's F-10 containing 15% fetal cord serum vs the transfer of blastocysts on d 5 produced sequentially in G1 and G2 media. Although the trial was small (d 3, n = 15; d 5, n = 8), the increased implantation rate resulting from d 5 transfer vs d 3 transfer (45.5 vs 21%) reached statistical significance. Included in this report was an evaluation of the necessity of G1 in the first culture interval. This was tested by culturing 63 zygotes in Ham's F-10 for the first 3 d followed by 48 h of culture in G2 and comparing growth on d 5 to 38 embryos that had been grown in G1 for the first 3 d, followed by 48 h growth in G2. Of the embryos cultured in G1/G2 sequentially, 66% reached blastocyst by d 5 compared to only 38% for those grown sequentially in Ham's F-10/G2. It was unfortunate that an equivalent evaluation of the necessity for G2 was not conducted by including the reciprocal arm of sequential G1/Ham's F-10 in the study.

Although the authors made a compelling case that blastocyst transfer is an appropriate way to reduce multiple gestation while maintaining a high pregnancy rate *(15)*, their conclusion that sequential, physiologically-based, serum-free culture media can be used to produce highly viable human blastocysts was not substantiated by their data. This is because in 6 of the 8 transfers involving blastocysts, embryos derived from both sequential arms of the study were included for transfer, making the contribution from each arm to implantation and pregnancy impossible to decipher. Obviously, Ham's F-10 containing 15% fetal cord serum can hardly be considered either physiologically-based for embryos or serum-free.

The second investigation by Jones et al. *(16)* detailed the evolution of a successful culture system for blastocyst production and viability. This was accomplished by comparing several media (Gardner's G1, Gardner's G2, and IVF-50 medium, a modified human tubal fluid (HTF) containing 10 mg/mL of human serum albumin (HAS), produced by Scandinavian IVF Science AB [Gothenburg, Sweden]) in various sequential strategies. The value of regrouping faster developing embryos at various times during culture and of refeeding embryos from d 5–7 was also studied. These variables were combined in different ways to produce 8 protocols that ultimately were tested for their ability to produce blastocysts and continuing pregnancies. Protocols 1 through 7 employed G1/G2 sequentially with either BSA or HSA as the protein source. A total of two continuing pregnancies were achieved in 17 transfers from these combined protocols. Protocol 8, however, replaced G1 medium with IVF-50 medium. Additionally, embryos were refed with fresh G2 medium on d 5 of culture. A total of 13 continuing pregnancies out of 34 transfers was achieved, representing a continuing pregnancy rate of 38.2%. It must be re-emphasized, however, that media and supplements were not the only variables tested in this work. The most successful strategy, protocol 8, also included grouping embryos on d 3, regrouping them on d 5, and completely removing the zona pellucida of blastocysts by digestion with pronase prior to transfer.

Most recently, Gardner and his colleagues from Englewood, CO conducted a prospective randomized trial of blastocyst transfer vs the transfer of d 3 embryos, as an extension of their earlier work *(17)*. Outcomes from transfers of embryos produced by 3 d of culture in Ham's F-10, containing 15% fetal cord serum, again were compared to those resulting from the transfer of blastocysts produced sequentially with modified G1 and G2 media (G1.2 and G2.2). Although the pregnancy rates for d 3 and d 5 transfers did not differ (66 and 71%, respectively), the number of embryos required to produce pregnancy did (3.7

and 2.2, respectively), confirming that high pregnancy rates can be achieved with a concomitant reduction in multiple pregnancy through the transfer of blastocysts. Further, the question of whether or not serum-free sequential media produced the blastocysts that ultimately implanted was removed in the experimental design. Unfortunately, the authors elected not to fully disclose the specifics of the media formulations used, for "commercial reasons."

P-1/ BLASTOCYST MEDIUM

Barry Behr and co-workers from Stanford University have employed a sequential culture strategy consisting of P-1 medium (7) for the first culture interval and Blastocyst Medium, a modification of Ham's F-10 medium from Irvine Scientific, Inc. (Santa Ana, CA) for the second culture interval (13). Synthetic Serum Substitute (58) was used as the protein supplement for both media at a concentration of 10% (v/v), which corresponds to a total protein concentration of 6 mg/mL. P-1 medium is a modification of HTF medium (65) that lacks both glucose and inorganic phosphate and is supplemented with sodium citrate and the amino acid taurine. HTF was modified in accordance with the data of Schini and Bavister (34) in the hamster embryo regarding the beneficial effects of removing glucose and inorganic phosphate and from the data of Bavister and McKiernan (45) regarding taurine. The use of P-1 medium for the culture of embryos for 3 d has resulted in significantly enhanced clinical pregnancy rates (7,42–44). Barrett et al. (66) compared P-1 to HTF in a trial involving 218 patients and found that the pregnancy rate in the P-1 group was 16% higher than that of the HTF group ($p = 0.013$). It should be emphasized that P-1 medium was formulated specifically to meet requirements of the first culture interval and that the name refers to "Preimplantation Stage 1" from Table 1.

In a preliminary study designed to measure blastocyst production with this system (18), a total of 838 supernumerary embryos grown in P-1 medium for 3 d were transferred to Blastocyst Medium for an additional 2 d. Overall, 53.5% reached the expanded blastocyst stage by 120 h of culture. No effect was seen of reducing oxygen concentration to 5% in both culture intervals compared to 5% CO_2 in air. Initial experience with cryopreservation of blastocysts produced by this system followed by thaw and transfer yielded 7 pregnancies out of 16 transfers. Using this same culture system, we have since confirmed that blastocysts produced with this system show both high survival (>90%) and viability (40% clinical pregnancy rate; 25% implantation rate) upon thaw and transfer (unpublished results).

Behr et al. (personal communication) have also conducted a trial of transfer of fresh blastocysts produced by P-1/Blastocyst Medium at Stanford University. They have enrolled over 60 patients in the trial, age range 30–40.5 yr (average 36 yr), and have used as inclusion criteria those IVF patients that have at least three 8-cell embryos by d 3 of culture. The pregnancy rate per retrieval was 73% and the implantation rate was 51%. More recently, Milki et al. (67) have shown that the transfer of two blastocysts produced by this system resulted in pregnancy rates equivalent to the transfer of three blastocysts while reducing the multiple gestation rate, indicating that their culture system behaves qualitatively similar to G1.2/G2.2. In fact, the high implantation and pregnancy rates seen with blastocyst transfers by da Motta et al. (68) provides evidence, they conclude, for the benefits of extending human embryo culture with P-1 and Blastocyst Medium for all normally fertilized embryos in vitro. A summary of the application of sequential culture systems for preimplantation embryogenesis during IVF in humans is given in Table 2.

Table 2
Evolution of the Use of Sequential Culture Media for Preimplantation Embryogenesis in Humans

Year	Investigators	Media	Amino acids	P_i	Energy source	Protein source	Duration of culture
1971	Steptoe et al. (1)	Bavister's	None	Yes	g,p,l[a]	BSA	12–15 h
		Ham's F10	Complex	Yes	g,p calf serum	20% fetal	123 h
1994	Forsdahl et al. (63)	Universal IVF[b]	None	Yes	g,p	Not given	48 h
		M3[b]	Complex	Yes	g,p,gln	Not given	48–72 h
1995	Barnes et al. (64)	G1 (Gardner)	Nonessential	Yes	p,l, low g	BSA	68 h
		G2 (Gardner)	Complex	Yes	g,p,l	BSA	42 h
1997	Behr (13)	P1[c]	Taurine	No	p,l	SSS[d]	72 h
		Blastocyst[c]	Complex	Yes	g,p	SSS	48–72 h
1998	Jones et al. (16)	IVF-50[d]	None	Yes	g,p,l	HSA	72 h
		G2 (Gardner)	Complex	Yes	g,p,l	HSA	48–96 h
1998	Gardner et al. (17)	Ham's F10	Complex	Yes	g,p	15% fetal cord serum	15–18 h
		G1.2[d]	Nonessential	Low	p,l, low g	HSA	~48–54 h
		G2.2[d]	Complex	Yes	g,p,l	HSA	48 h

[a] Glucose, pyruvate, lactate.
[b] Medi-Cult, Inc.
[c] Irvine Scientific, Inc.
[d] Scandinavian IVF Science AB.

CONCLUDING REMARKS

Are There Unifying Principles for Sequential Culture?

In this chapter, we have concentrated on those systems that have produced, through blastocyst transfer, both pregnancy and livebirth. Other strategies exist and, no doubt, will shed new light on the biology of human blastocysts, once they have been tested for the ability to generate viable embryos by transfer. Obviously, the data to date from outcomes produced in humans using sequential culture systems are rudimentary, but clearly support the conclusion forwarded by Menezo et al. (14) that this is the approach of choice for achieving this goal. But as can be seen from the preceding descriptions of various culture systems, there is no consensus on which components are essential to each sequential medium. This in part is owing to the way in which the systems were developed. In some, the media were modified from those used successfully in animal models. In others, the formulae were based upon media developed initially for somatic cells. Another pronounced influence on some medium designers is that the components be "physiological;" in this context meaning that they have been found as naturally occurring substances in the oviduct. Although a chemical inventory of the oviduct provides a convenient starting point for medium design, it by no means defines optimal conditions and can even be quite misleading. The healthy oviduct is a patent conduit housing a chemical environment whose composition is determined not only by the transporting and synthetic activities of the tubal epithelium, but also by the chemistry of the peritoneal cavity at the distal end and the chemistry of the uterus and even the vagina at the proximal end. Therefore, to assume that all compounds in the oviduct are used by developing embryos is a leap that should be avoided in the absence of hard-won data.

A better alternative is to determine the essentials of medium composition by an analysis of outcome, thus letting results dictate medium design. Until in vitro correlates of blastocyst viability are established unambiguously by experimentation, the outcomes of choice are implantation rate and clinical pregnancy rate. No doubt these measures are contaminated by factors such as variability in the clinical skills of ET and the strategy and method of hormonal support following transfer, as well as patient compliance. Nonetheless, all one has to do is review the exhaustive analysis conducted by Lane and Gardner *(47)* on the development of sequential media in the mouse to realize that the in vitro measures that seem intuitively to be predictive of viability of an embryo upon transfer, such as percentage of blastocysts formed and hatching, in fact, have no predictive value whatsoever. This underscores the importance of letting results be the guide rather than intuition or a preconception of what is physiological.

As preliminary as it might be, the question still arises: Are there any clear-cut "rules" or requisites for each culture interval that are emerging from the current outcome data?

THE FIRST CULTURE INTERVAL

The following characteristics of culture media used for the first culture interval (d 1–3) are associated with the production of viable blastocysts in sequential culture:

1. Elimination of glucose or reduction of glucose to 0.5 mM. There currently is no evidence that including glucose at any concentration during the first culture interval contributes to development. This may be a situation, such as that described by Thompson et al. *(39)* for sheep embryos, where glucose above a certain level impairs growth. Below this level, growth progresses normally whether glucose is present in small amounts or totally absent. There is no need to include glucose in the insemination medium in the absence of glutamine, EDTA, and a complex array of amino acids. Glucose is not required for fertilization in the human, at least in a simple medium such as P-1 *(7,38)*. The survival of sperm for 24 or 48 h in culture may be higher in the presence of glucose, but it remains unclear how or if extended survival relates to fertilization.
2. The inclusion of lactate (10.5 mM, L-form) and pyruvate (0.33 mM).
3. The inclusion of the amino acid taurine. Addition of nonessential amino acids plus taurine is compatible with subsequent blastocyst production, but as yet has not been demonstrated to be a requisite for humans as it appears to be for the mouse.
4. The inclusion of a protein source.

THE SECOND CULTURE INTERVAL

The following conditions are associated with viable blastocyst production in the second culture interval (d 4, 5 and perhaps 6).

1. Restoration of glucose levels to at least 2.5 mM.
2. The inclusion of a complex array of amino acids (essential and nonessential amino acids).
3. The inclusion of pyruvate (at least 0.1 mM).
4. The inclusion of a protein source.

From these two short lists, it is evident that many components appear in medium formulations for human embryo culture that have yet to be demonstrated experimentally as a requirement for the production of viable blastocysts. These include glutamine, cheators (EDTA), antioxidants, nucleic acid precursors, fatty acids, and vitamins. Data certainly exist supporting the inclusion of components such as these in culture media for animal embryos, but not for human embryos. The current lack of a suitable animal model for human embryos makes extrapolation from the animal to the human speculative at best.

THE FUTURE

The ability to produce viable human blastocysts through the use of sequential culture systems is a reality, and one compelling to all centers of assisted reproduction owing to the commercial availability of these media. It would seem that the future of clinical IVF is clear; production of later-stage embryos, transfer of fewer blastocysts, higher implantation rates, and a lower rate of multiple pregnancy. But is the ultimate optimization of clinical IVF, the maximization of the incidence of pregnancy from this technology, going to come from late-stage transfers? Maybe, but perhaps not. The history of the adoption of the basic methods of IVF and embryo culture from the research setting to the clinical setting has been one of expediency. Restraints on research with human embryos, lack of funding for this research, and lack of a suitable model system, as well as the demand for technology from prospective patients, have all been used to justify this urgency, but expediency still best characterizes the process. As this chapter has attempted to demonstrate, it has taken 25 years for culture technology to catch up to the applications of IVF in the clinical environment. Invariably, expediency trades time for thoroughness, a situation from which clinical IVF has not been exempted. In the rush to find methods that will produce later-stage embryos, much basic biology has been overlooked. Recently, the human embryo has been reconsidered by Edwards and Beard *(69)* in light of the genetic and developmental mechanisms that are known to function in other mammalian embryos. In particular, the role that polarity in the oocyte plays, along with the other mechanisms defined from mammalian systems that govern cell determination, in establishing viability in human embryos has been considered. From this, it is seen that human embryos are likely not different from other mammalian embryos in that blastocysts form as a result of genetic and morphogenic mechanisms that function in the earliest stages of embryogenesis. It is quite possible that in our zeal to make blastocysts, we are overlooking opportunities to intervene while these mechanistic events are operational. As Edwards and Beard *(69)* suggest, perhaps we should be looking earlier at human embryos, not later as is the trend. One thing is certain: different versions of culture media, and their clinical applications, will come and go. However, in our generation and for many to come, the biology of the human embryo will not change and it is the clear elucidation of this biology, not by conjecture but by experimental evidence, that will illuminate the path into the future.

REFERENCES

1. Steptoe PC, Edwards RG, Purdy J. Human blastocysts grown in culture. Nature 1971;229:132–133.
2. Edwards RG, Bavister BD, Steptoe PC. Early stages of fertilization *in vitro* of human oocytes matured *in vitro*. Nature 1969;221:632–635.
3. Bavister BD. Environmental factors important for *in vitro* fertilization in the hamster. J Reprod Fert 1969;18:544–545.
4. Ham RG. An improved nutrient solution for diploid Chinese hamster and human cell lines. Exp Cell Res 1963;29:515–526.
5. Gardner DK. Mammalian embryo culture in the absence of serum or somatic cell support. Cell Biol Intl 1994;18:1163–1179.
6. Gardner DK, Lane M. Culture and selection of viable human blastocysts: a feasible proposition for human IVF? Hum Reprod Update 1997;3:367–382.

7. Pool TB, Atiee SH, Martin JE. Oocyte and embryo culture. Basic concepts and recent advances. In: May JV, ed. Assisted Reproduction: Laboratory Considerations. Infert Reprod Med Clinics North Am. W.B. Saunders, Philadelphia, PA, 1998;9:181–203.
8. Tsirigotis M. Blastocyst stage transfer: pitfalls and benefits. Hum Reprod 1998;13:3285–3295.
9. Gardner D, Schoolcraft W. No longer neglected: the human blastocyst. Hum Reprod 1998;13:3289–3292.
10. Desai NN. The road to blastocyst transfer. Hum Reprod 1998;13:329–3294.
11. Quinn P. Some arguements on the pro side. Hum Reprod 1998;13:3294,3293.
12. Bavister BD, Boatman DE. The neglected human blastocyst revisited. Hum Reprod 1997;12:1607–1609.
13. Behr B. Blastocyst culture without co-culture: role of embryo metabolism. J Asst Reprod Genet 1997; 14(Suppl):13S.
14. Menezo Y, Hamamah S, Hazout A, Dale B. Time to switch from co-culture to sequential defined media for transfer at the blastocyst stage. Hum Reprod 1998;13:2043–2044.
15. Gardner DK, Vella P, Lane M, Wagley L, Schlenker T, Schoolcraft WB. Culture and tranfer of human blastocysts increases implantation rates and reduces the need for multiple embryo transfers. Fertil Steril 1998;69:84–88.
16. Jones GM, Trounson AO, Gardner DK, Kausche A, Lolatgis N, Wood C. Evolution of a culture protocol for successful blastocyst development and pregnancy. Hum Reprod 1998;13:169–177.
17. Gardner DK, Schoolcraft WB, Wagley L, Schlenker T, Stevens J, Hesla J. A prospective randomized trial of blastocyst culture and transfer in in-vitro fertilization. Hum Reprod 1998;13:3434–3440.
18. Behr B, Pool TB, Milki AA, Moore D, Gebhardt J, Dasig D. Preliminary clinical experience with human blastocyst development *in vitro* without co-culture. Hum Reprod 1999;14:454–457.
19. Lane M, Gardner DK. Selection of viable mouse blastocysts prior to transfer using metabolic criterion. Hum Reprod 1996;11:1975–1978.
20. Bolton VN, Wren ME, Parsons JH. Pregnancies after in vitro fertilization and transfer of human blastocysts. Fertil Steril 1991;55:830–832.
21. Bolton VN, Hawes SM, Taylor CT, Parsons JH. Development of spare human preimplantation embryos in vitro: an analysis of the correlations among morphology, cleavage rates, and development to the blastocyst. J In Vitro Fert Embryo Transfer 1989;6:30–35.
22. Huisman G, Alberda A, Leerentveld R, Verhoeff A, Zeilmaker G. A comparison of in vitro fertilization results after embryo transfer after 2,3, and 4 days of embryo culture. Fertil Steril 1994;61:970–971.
23. Bongso A, Ng SC, Sathananthan H, Ng PL, Rauff M, Ratnam SS. Improved quality of human embryos when co-cultured with human ampullary cells. Hum Reprod 1989;4:706–713.
24. Menezo Y, Hazout A, Dumont M, Herbaut N, Nicollet B. Coculture of embryos on Vero cells and transfer of blastocysts in humans. Hum Reprod 1992;7(Suppl 1):101–106.
25. Menezo Y, Nicollet B, Herbaut N, Andre D. Freezing cocultured human blastocysts. Fertil Steril 1992; 58:977–980.
26. Weimer KE, Cohen J, Amborski G, Wright G, Wiker S, Munzakazi L, Godke RA. In vitro development and implantation of human embryos following culture on fetal bovine uterine fibroblast cells. Hum Reprod 1989;4:595–600.
27. Bavister BD. Co-culture for embryo development: is it really necessary? Hum Reprod 1992;7:1339–1341.
28. Van Blerkom J. Development of human embryos to the hatched blastocyst stage in the presence of a monolayer of Vero cells. Hum Reprod 1993;8:1525–1539.
29. Rieger D, Grisart B, Semple E, Van Langendonckt A, Betteridge K, Dessey F. Comparison of the effects of oviductal cell co-culture and oviductal cell-conditioned medium on the development and metabolic activity of cattle embryos. J Reprod Fertil 1995;105:91–98.
30. Trounson A, Pushett D, Maclellan LJ, Lewis I, Gardner DK. Current status of IVM/IVF and embryo culture in humans and farm animals. Theriogenology 1994;41:57–66.
31. Edwards L, Batt P, Gandolfi F, Gardner D. Modifications made to culture medium by bovine oviduct epithelial cells: changes to carbohydrates stimulate bovine embryo development. Mol Reprod Dev 1997; 46:146–154.
32. Leese H. Metabolic control during preimplantation mammalian development. Hum Reprod Update 1995;1:63–72.
33. Brinster RL. Studies on the development of mouse embryos in vitro. II. The effect of energy sources. J Exp Zool 1965;158:59–68.
34. Schini S, Bavister BD. Two-cell block to development of cultured hamster embryos is caused by phosphate and glucose. Biol Reprod 1988;39:1183–1192.

35. Van Blerkom J, Davis PW, Lee J. ATP content of human oocytes and developmental potential and outcome after in-vitro fertilization and embryo transfer. Hum Reprod 1995;10:415–424.
36. Hardy K. Development of human blastocysts in vitro. In: Bavister BD, ed. Preimplantation Embryo Development. Springer-Verlag, New York, NY, 1993, pp. 184–199.
37. Conaghan J, Handyside A, Winston R, Leese H. Effects of pyruvate and glucose on the development of human preimplantation embryos in vitro. J Reprod Fert 1993;99:87–95.
38. Graham M, Pool T. Evolution of energy substrates in the culture of human embryos. Assist Reprod Rev 1997;8:65–68.
39. Thompson JG, Simpson AC, Pugh PA, Tervit HR. Requirement for glucose during in vitro culture of sheep preimplantation embryos. Mol Reprod Dev 1992;31:253–257.
40. Gardner D, Lane M, Calderon H, Leeton J. Environment of the preimplantation human embryo in vivo: metabolite analysis of oviduct and uterine fluids and metabolism of cumulus cells. Fertil Steril 1996;65: 349–353.
41. Quinn P. Enhanced results in mouse and human embryo culture using a modified human tubal fluid medium lacking glucose and phosphate. J Asst Reprod Genet 1995;12:97–105.
42. Rawlins RG, Pool T, Fahy M, Sant'Anna, Wood-Molo M, Binor Z, Radwanska E. Improved clinical pregnancy rates for IVF/ET using glucose- and phosphate-free HTF medium (P1) compared to HTF medium. J Asst Reprod Genet 1997;14(Suppl):133S.
43. Graham MC, Lewis V, Partridge A, Phipps WR. Glucose-free medium improves embryo growth in vitro. J Soc Gynecol Invest 1997;4 (Suppl):176a,1997.
44. Lee MA, Cardone VRS, Hardy RI, et al. Comparison of sibling oocytes in a glucose-free culture media system (P1) with a conventional (B2) and a short term co-culture system [abstract P-244]. In: Abstracts of the Fifty-Second Annual Meeting of the American Society for Reproductive Medicine, Boston, MA, 1996, p. S206.
45. Bavister BD, McKiernan SH. Regulation of hamster embryo development in vitro by amino acids. In: Bavister BD, ed. Preimplantation Embryo Development. Springer-Verlag, New York, NY, 1993, pp. 57–72.
46. Eagle H. Amino acid metabolism in mammalian cell cultures. Science 1959;130:432–437.
47. Lane M, Gardner D. Differential regulation of mouse embryo development and viability by amino acids. J Reprod Fert 1997;109:153–164.
48. Van Winkle L, Dickinson H. Differences in amino acid content of preimplantation mouse embryos that develop in vitro versus in vivo: in vitro effects of five amino acids that are abundant in oviductal secretions. Biol Reprod 1995;52:96–104.
49. Devreker F, Winston R, Hardy K. Glutamine improves human preimplantation development in vitro. Fertil Steril 1998;69:293–299.
50. Edwards LJ, Williams DA, Gardner DK. Intracellular pH of the mouse preimplantation embryo: amino acids act as buffers of intracellular pH. Hum Reprod 1998;13:3441–3448.
51. Dawson KM, Collins JL, Baltz JM. Osmolarity-dependent glycine accumulation indicates a role for glycine as an organic osmolyte in early preimplantation mouse embryos. Biol Reprod 1998;59:225–232.
52. Huxtable RJ. Physiological actions of taurine. Physiol Rev 1992;72:101–163.
53. Petters RM, Wells KD. Culture of pig embryos. J Reprod Fertil Suppl 1993;48:61–73.
54. Liu Z, Foote RH. Development of bovine embryos in KSOM with added superoxide dismutase and taurine and with five and twenty percent O_2. Biol Reprod 1995;53:786–790.
55. Dumoulin JCM, van Wissen LCP, Menheere PPCA, Michiels AHJC, Geraedts JPM, Evers JLH. Taurine acts as an osmolyte in human and mouse oocytes and embryos. Biol Reprod 1997;56:739–744.
56. Li J, Foote RH, Simkin M. Development of rabbit zygotes cultured in protein-free medium with catalase, taurine or superoxide dismutase. Biol Reprod 1993;48:33–37.
57. Pool TB, Martin JE. High continuing pregnancy rates after in vitro fertilization-embryo transfer using medium supplemented with a plasma protein fraction containing alpha- and beta-globulins. Fertil Steril 1994;61:714–719.
58. Weathersbee PS, Pool TB, Ord T. Synthetic serum substitute (SSS): a globulin-enriched protein supplement for human embryo culture. J Asst Reprod Genet 1995;12:354–360.
59. Lighten A, Hardy K, Winston R, Moore G. Expression of mRNA for the insulin-like growth factors and their receptors in human preimplantation embryos. Mol Reprod Dev 1997;47:134–139.
60. Lighten A, Moore G, Winston R, Hardy K. Routine addition of human insulin-like growth factor-I ligand could benefit clinical in-vitro fertilization culture. Hum Reprod 1998;13:3144–3150.
61. Kane M, Morgan P, Coonan C. Peptide growth factors and preimplantation development. Hum Reprod Update 1997;3:137–157.

62. Pollard JW, Plante C, Leibo SP. Comparison of development of pig zygotes and embryos in simple and complex culture media. J Reprod Fert 1995;103:331–337.

63. Forsdahl F, Bertheussen K, Bungum LJ, Bungum MH, Willumsen J, Maltau JM. A study on extended culture time with embryo replacement at the morula and blastocyst stage. Hum Reprod Suppl 1994;9: 142–143.

64. Barnes FL, Crombie A, Gardner DK, Kausche A, Lacham-Kaplan O, Suikkari A, et al. Blastocyst development and birth after in-vitro maturation of human primary oocytes, intracytoplasmic sperm injection and assisted hatching. Hum Reprod 1995;10:3243–3247.

65. Quinn P, Kerin J, Warnes G. Improved pregnancy rate in human in vitro fertilization with the use of a medium based on the composition of human tubal fluid. Fertil Steril 1985;44:493–498.

66. Barrett, Penzias AS, Powers RD. P1/SSS embryo culture medium yields higher pregnancy rate than HTF/Plasmanate in IVF/ET [abstract P-084]. In: Abstracts of the Fifty-Third Annual Meeting of the American Society for Reproductive Medicine, Cincinnati, OH, 1997, p. S132.

67. Milki AA, Fisch JD, Behr B. Two blastocyst transfer has similar pregnancy rates and a decreased multiple gestation rate compared to three blastocyst transfer. Fertil Steril 1999; (in press).

68. da Motta ELA, Alegretti JR, Baracat EC, Olive D, Serafini PC. High implantation and pregnancy rates with transfer of human blastocysts developed in preimplantation stage one and blastocyst media. Fertil Steril 1998;70:659–663.

69. Edwards RG, Beard HK. Oocyte polarity and cell determination in early mammalian embryos. Mol Hum Reprod 1997;3:863–905.

9

Embryo Transfer

A Concise and Practical Summary of the Techniques

Kenneth A. Burry, MD

CONTENTS

INTRODUCTION

The goal of the assisted reproductive technologies, ARTs, is to provide infertile couples with a high live birth rate of normal babies. The process needs to be cost-effective for both the couple and for the healthcare system, and in order for this to happen, it is essential to maintain a low rate of multiple pregnancies. The transfer of one or two high-quality embryos is the only way to achieve a high pregnancy rate without the risk of a high order (more than 2) multiple pregnancy.

Over the 20 years since the birth of the first in vitro-conceived baby, success rates have significantly improved; however, there still exists nearly a 10-fold difference in pregnancy outcomes among clinics. Multiple factors influence the outcome of ARTs: age of the female partner, etiology of infertility, type and response to ovarian stimulation, quality of gametes and resulting embryos, uterine environment, and the skill and experience of the laboratory and clinicians. Embryo culture protocols, embryo-transfer technique and timing, number of embryos transferred, and embryo cryopreservation technology significantly impact the outcome of the ARTs.

The embryo transfer is seemingly simple, yet it is arguably the most important step in the ARTs; thus, meticulous attention should be paid to this procedure. This chapter will

From: *Contemporary Endocrinology: Assisted Fertilization and Nuclear Transfer in Mammals*
Edited by: D. P. Wolf and M. Zelinski-Wooten © Humana Press Inc., Totowa, NJ

focus on embryo transfer, especially the timing, technique, and number of embryos to transfer. Evaluation of the female partner prior to in vitro fertilization (IVF) and the evaluation and management of the patient at the time of and after transfer will also be discussed.

EVALUATION OF THE FEMALE PARTNER PRIOR TO IN VITRO FERTILIZATION

The interval prior to an ovarian-stimulation cycle is an opportunity for couples to ensure a healthy start to their pregnancy. Prevention and identification of disease is the primary goal of modern medicine, and screening, in this application, includes Hepatitis A, B, and C, and HIV of both the woman and her partner. If these infectious screening tests are positive then an appropriate infectious disease consult is warranted. Some states even forbid ART procedures in couples who are positive for any of these conditions. Screening for immunity to childhood diseases is routinely done; if a woman is nonimmune to Rubella and/or Varicella, then immunization is offered. Prenatal vitamins or vitamins with adequate folic acid should be taken prior to pregnancy to reduce the incidence of birth defects. Because both ovarian response to gonadotropins and uterine receptivity are adversely affected by smoking, cessation of smoking should be completed prior to ovarian stimulation. Feichtinger and colleagues (1) conducted a meta-analysis to establish the influence of smoking on the clinical pregnancy rate. They concluded that smoking significantly decreased the chance of success. El-Nemr and coworkers (2) found that women under the age of 36 who smoked had significantly higher basal follicle stimulating hormone (FSH) concentrations. Consequently, they required a higher gonadotropin dose for ovarian stimulation but fewer oocytes were retrieved as compared to nonsmokers.

Anatomical screening of the uterine cavity should be a routine part of the pre-procedure evaluation and may be accomplished by hysterosalpingography, hysteroscopy, or saline infusion sonography. The hysterosalpingogram carries the advantage of providing information about patency of the fallopian tube. Because IVF is a treatment for all causes of infertility, knowledge of oviduct patency is useful if ovarian stimulation is less than adequate, thereby precluding oocyte retrieval. If there is patency of at least one oviduct then, in some cases, AI may be offered in canceled IVF cycles. Some clinics perform a luteal-phase endometrial biopsy on older women in order to assess potential defects. Potter and coworkers (3) believe that an endometrial biopsy is especially important in women 40 years and older. Women using oocyte donation had a higher risk of out-of-phase endometrium despite receiving higher doses of progesterone. The variability between pathologists in assessing endometrial histology makes the endometrial biopsy of little value, therefore, it is not routinely used.

The identification of a hydrosalpinx is an important screening test because its presence has a negative effect on pregnancy outcome. Zeyneloglu and colleagues (4) reported a 50% reduction in the clinical pregnancy rate and more than a twofold increase in spontaneous abortions when a hydrosalpinx was identified. The surgical removal of a hydrosalpinx prior to proceeding to IVF is an option that may improve implantation and pregnancy outcomes. However, even when removed, hydrosalpinges may have a permanent adverse effect on ovarian function and oocyte quality. Freeman and coworkers (5) observed a lower implantation rate and an increase in arrested embryo growth even after surgical treatment. Other investigators (6) recommend aspiration of hydrosalpinges at the time

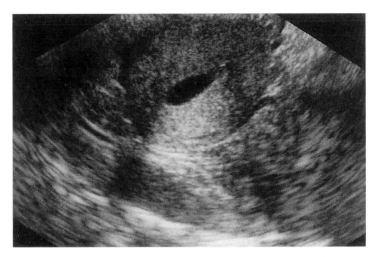

Fig. 1. Sagittal section through a normal uterus after 4 mL sterile saline was infused. Note the smooth contours of the uterine walls. With ultrasound, the entire cavity can be evaluated during the examination.

of oocyte retrieval as an acceptable alternative to surgery. Transvaginal aspiration of a hydrosalpinx is a reasonable option when the hydrosalpinx becomes clinically obvious during the stimulation protocol. Although some authors *(7)* feel that hydrosalpinges visible by ultrasound are solely responsible for the impaired outcome, Sowter and colleagues *(8)* reported that distal occlusion of the oviducts, even when there is no fluid distention, is associated with a significant reduction in embryo implantation. The mechanism by which a hydrosalpinx causes poor implantation rates is unclear, because the presence of hydrosalpinx fluid in culture has no major negative effect on blastocyst development or on in vitro implantation on an artificial endometrium *(9)*.

Hysteroscopy can be done in the office to directly evaluate the uterine cavity. Operative hysteroscopy is used for the direct removal of polyps, for lysis of adhesions, and the resection of submucosal myomas. Saline infusion sonography (SIS) is also a simple way to assess the uterine cavity in the office setting (Fig. 1) because it is minimally invasive and can be done at the time of a trial or mock transfer. Measurement of cervical length and uterine depth can be accomplished by ultrasound and an embryo-transfer catheter can be visualized within the fundus of the uterus (Fig. 2). The procedure is performed by inserting 4–10 mL of sterile saline into the uterine cavity, thereby allowing filling defects to be identified with uterine distention. (Fig. 3) Intramural myomas that are not detected on physical examination and not seen by hysterosalpingography or hysteroscopy may be detected by ultrasound. A trial transfer at the time of SIS is also helpful in predicting the difficult transfer and anticipating the specific catheter or technique required at the time of embryo transfer.

EVALUATION OF THE FEMALE PARTNER DURING STIMULATION

Ovarian stimulation is an important factor affecting the outcome of the ART cycle and should result in the development of a reasonable number of mature oocytes. In fact, the number of oocytes retrieved may be a predictor of a successful outcome. Many clinics will cancel a cycle if fewer than six follicles ($\geq$16 mm) develop. Ovarian hyperstimulation syndrome (OHSS) is a risk when serum estradiol levels are too high, due to development

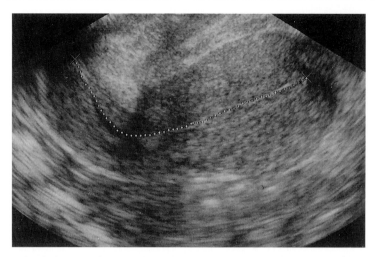

Fig. 2. Transvaginal ultrasound evaluation of cervical length and depth of the fundus. The cervix is to the left and the uterine fundus is to the right. The dotted line is the measurement. This may be done prior to a trial transfer and saline infusion sonogram (SIS). Re-evaluation at the time of transfer may be done because the uterine size can change under the influence of estrogen and progesterone.

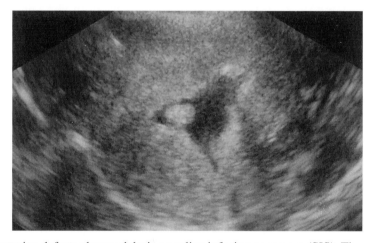

Fig. 3. Intrauterine defects observed during a saline infusion sonogram (SIS). These proved to be uterine polyps, which were successfully removed, allowing the patient to proceed with IVF.

of an unusually high number of large (>15 mm) follicles. The risk of OHSS is small when a pregnancy does not occur, but rising human chorionic gonadotropin (hCG) levels during early pregnancy may increase the risk of this syndrome. Furthermore, endometrial receptivity may be altered when the estrogen levels are highly elevated. In these cases, all resulting embryos may be cryopreserved and the embryo transfer may be deferred to a later time when the uterine environment is optimal *(10)*. Maternal age is associated with a decline in ovarian reserve and consequently poorer outcomes. Ovarian reserve can be assessed by a clomiphene citrate challenge test (*see* Chapter 5). Typically, a serum FSH is measured on d 3 of a cycle. The woman is then given 100 mg of clomiphene citrate on d 5–9, and a second serum FSH is measured on d 10. The acceptable level of FSH will depend on the assay and should be determined by individual clinics. If either the d 3 or d 10 concentration of FSH is above a predetermined threshold, then ovarian reserve is inadequate for ovarian stimulation and oocyte donation should be considered. Many clinics modify their stimulation protocols in women 35 years and older by increasing the amount of exogenous gonadotropin administered and by the use of microdose leuprolide acetate.

THE "MANAGED" ET CYCLE

The endometrium of the recipient must be synchronized with that of an oocyte donor in order to receive embryos at an appropriate time for implantation. This is accomplished by first using a gonadotropin releasing hormone (GnRH) analog such as leuprolide acetate for at least 10 d. Micronized estradiol, estradiol patches, or injectable estrogen in increasing doses are administered to the recipient while the donor is being stimulated with gonadotropins. After the donor receives hCG preceding oocyte retrieval, the recipient begins injections of progesterone in oil to create a secretory endometrium in anticipation of an embryo transfer, similar to the protocol below.

Embryo thaw and transfer (ET&T) for frozen embryo transfer (FET) of cryopreserved embryos can be accomplished in natural cycles, stimulated cycles and in artificial cycles with similar success (11). Various protocols for estrogen and progesterone stimulation have been utilized for synchronization and artificial cycles. Gonadotropin downregulation has been incorporated into some protocols, but is not required for a successful outcome (12). Micronized estradiol may be used orally in an increasing dose over 2 wk. A typical protocol involves 5 d of estradiol, 2 mg per day, beginning on d 3 of menses or after suppression with leuprolide acetate, followed by 4 d of 2 mg twice a day, then three doses of 2 mg daily for 5 d. Endometrial response is evaluated by ultrasound to measure thickness and to assess morphology. If the endometrium is deemed adequate, (9 mm thickness and a tri-laminar appearance; see Chapter 6), then the estradiol dose can be reduced to 2 mg twice a day and progesterone is administered (50–100 mg in oil I.M. daily) through the first 12 wk of pregnancy. The window of time for an embryo transfer depends on the duration of progesterone administration (13) and the stage of embryo development. Eight-cell embryos are successfully transferred on d 18–19 of an artificial cycle, whereas blastocysts are transferred 2–3 d later.

QUALITY AND NUMBER OF EMBRYOS TO TRANSFER

A determination of the exact number of embryos for transfer is problematic, but is ideally based on embryo quality and implantation efficiency. Unfortunately, assessment of embryo quality is difficult because objective markers are notoriously inaccurate. An unacceptably high number of multiple pregnancies is evidence of the difficulties encountered in embryo quality selection. Triplet and higher-order multiple pregnancies are associated with increased morbidity and mortality and cost health care systems millions of dollars (14). There is a growing consensus worldwide that clinics should not transfer more than two embryos because of this increased risk (15–19). In some countries, legislative action limits the number of embryos that can be transferred. Possible exceptions to this policy are in cases of advanced maternal age (20), and intracytoplasmic sperm injection (ICSI) where implantation rates are markedly reduced. One suggestion is to increase the number of embryos transferred by one for each 5-yr incremental increase in maternal age after age 35 (21). The Belgium experience (22) suggests that the implantation capacity of ICSI-produced embryos is lower irrespective of embryo morphology.

The best predictor of pregnancy, albeit difficult to assess, is embryo quality *(23)*. Culture media and conditions have changed significantly over the past 20 years and a sequential exposure of embryos to media of increasing complexity is now fashionable (*see* Chapter 8). The transfer of early-stage embryos until recently was more successful *(24)*. The assessment of embryo quality in early-stage embryos is subjective and without a high predictive value for implantation. Therefore, several embryos, usually four but sometimes more, were transferred. The early experiences resulted in a low pregnancy rate but paradoxically a high rate of multiple pregnancy, including high-order (more than twins) multiple pregnancies. The ability to select high-quality embryos allows the transfer of one or two without adversely affecting pregnancy rates. Embryos that progress to the expanded blastocyst stage by d 5 or 6 have defined themselves as being high quality. Extended culture to the blastocyst stage results in the "deselection" of embryos that fail to progress (*see* Chapter 8). Moreover, culturing for a longer time allows other interventions such as preimplantation genetic diagnosis (PGD; *see* Chapter 7). This may be of benefit to certain couples and may improve the chance of pregnancy in patients with an otherwise poor prognosis *(25)*. Biopsy of blastomeres can be done for PGD on d 3 when the embryo reaches the 8-cell stage, and the results can be available by d 5–6 when the normal embryos are transferred *(26)*.

WHEN TO TRANSFER EMBRYOS

Embryos have been transferred on every day of the IVF cycle from the pronuclear or zygote stage (d 1) through to the hatching or hatched blastocyst (d 5–7). Recent reports suggest that pronuclear or zygote stage transfer can result in acceptable pregnancy rates, however, up to six embryos were transferred *(27)*. The experience of extending embryo culture to allow the transfer of embryos on d 3 was encouraging and had little impact on the laboratory because co-culture or sequential media exposure was not involved. The outcome of transferring on d 3 was an increase in implantation and pregnancy rate *(28, 29)*. The ability to culture embryos for an even longer period of time has resulted in an improvement of the assessment of embryo quality, by factors such as cleavage rate and ability to develop into blastocysts. Initially, no differences were reported in outcomes of transferring embryos on d 2, 3, or 4; however, a significant decline in pregnancy rates was noted when embryos, cultured in a system suboptimal for blastocyst development, were transferred on d 5 *(30)*. Earlier studies suggested progressively better outcomes with later transfers and that a transfer after 4 d in culture gave embryologists the ability to better recognize embryos with a higher implantation potential *(31)*. Delaying transfer also results in embryo self-selection because developmental arrest or fragmentation of poorer embryos occurs with extended culture.

Newly developed media, which can support embryo development to the blastocyst stage without need for a co-culture system, have further aided in the selection of quality embryos for transfer *(32,33; see* Chapter 8). When embryos progress to an expanded blastocyst stage (d 5–6), only one or two need to be transferred. The outcome is a higher pregnancy rate (>40%) relative to transfer on d 3 (<30%) with a reduction in the incidence of multiple pregnancy, especially the high-order multiple pregnancies, which are nearly eliminated *(34)*. Hatched blastocysts or blastocysts that have had the zona removed can implant and produce normal pregnancies *(35,36)*. The ability to achieve high pregnancy rates without establishing high-order multiple pregnancies addresses the worldwide concerns about cost and morbidity mentioned previously.

During an ET&T or FET cycle, cryopreserved embryos are thawed at various times prior to their transfer depending on the stage at which they were frozen. As seen with fresh embryo transfers, the appearance of high-quality embryos is most predictive of implantation and successful pregnancy outcomes *(37)*. Of course, embryos that continue to develop in culture post-thaw may have higher implantation efficiencies *(38)*, especially if they progress to the blastocyst stage. Cryopreserved blastocysts are usually transferred on the day of thaw, however, there is as yet such a limited experience that an implantation efficiency cannot be cited.

EVALUATION AND MANAGEMENT AT THE TIME OF TRANSFER

There are many protocols for pre-medication in anticipation of an embryo transfer ranging from no treatment to the use of a variety of drugs including: nonsteroidal anti-inflammatory agents, antibiotics, corticosteroids, and sedatives such as Valium. Most experience, because of the use of unique drugs or drug combinations, is anecdotal. Non-steroidal anti-inflammatory agents are well-tolerated and may reduce prostaglandin-related uterine contractions. However, immunosuppression with corticosteroids probably adds little benefit to early implantation *(39)*. Genital infections such as Chlamydia are associated with a decrease in implantation *(40)* and ongoing pregnancy rates, *(41)* thus tetracycline class antibiotics have been used. Francin and coworkers *(42)* observed a reduction in pregnancy rates when culture of the catheter tip post-transfer was positive for bacterial growth. The predominant organism identified was *Escherichia coli*, which was observed in 64% of the cultures. In these women, a broad spectrum penicillin would be the antibiotic of choice. A woman's vulnerability to stress may be associated with a lower pregnancy rate; possibly, mild sedation may be helpful in these cases *(43)*. The routine use of heparin is controversial and currently under review. It appears as if there is little if any benefit from its use and serious complications have been reported *(44)*. The laboratory protocols for handling embryos on the day of transfer are also variable and their outcomes are equally anecdotal. Media used for the transfer usually contain protein, especially from serum, e.g., synthetic serum substitute (SSS, Irvine Scientific, Santa Ana, California), an enriched fraction of serum containing albumin and globulins. There is a report of an anaphylactic reaction associated with the use of bovine serum albumin (BSA) during an embryo transfer *(45)*.

Increased implantation and pregnancy rates have been associated with assisted hatching (AH), but this is not a universal experience *(46,47)*. AH may improve pregnancy and implantation rates in women with a poor prognosis of pregnancy, such as advanced maternal age (>38 yr) or three or more failed cycles of IVF *(48)* and the procedure has been used with variable success on cryopreserved embryos or in older women *(49,50)*. However, AH probably does not improve outcomes in couples with an initially good prognosis *(51)*. Typically, high-quality embryos are not hatched because there is a risk of damage owing to exposure to acidified Tyrodes medium. As previously mentioned, the use of extended culture techniques that allow embryos to progress to expanded blastocysts seems the most promising recent advance in the ARTs. This procedure allows the transfer of one or two embryos resulting in a high pregnancy rate and lower risk for a multiple pregnancy beyond twins. However, a potential risk associated with the ARTs is an increase in the risk of monozygotic twins *(52)*. This may especially be true when transferring embryos at the blastocyst stage. AH of blastocysts may reduce this risk and some programs routinely enzymatically remove or weaken the zona pellucida prior to transfer *(53)*.

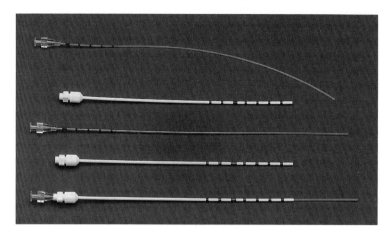

Fig. 4. Examples of Soft-Pass® (Cook Ob-Gyn, Spencer, IN) embryo transfer catheters, which can be after-loaded and have inner catheters with soft tips. The middle catheter is similar except it has a metal stylet that extends to near the end of the outer catheter. This allows easier passage of the inner catheter through the outer catheter when an after-loading technique for transfer is used. The bottom picture demonstrates the combination of inner and outer catheters.

Improved techniques of loading embryos in the catheter have contributed to the successful delivery of embryos. The method of hydraulic loading while still displacing a minimal amount of fluid has resulted in less embryo retention and loss during the transfer. A successful method of loading embryos is to use a TB syringe, completely filled with media, for instance TALP-HEPES with 0.3% human serum albumin (HSA). The catheter is then attached to the syringe and medium is flushed through the length of the system making sure that it is free of air bubbles. The embryos are transferred to a dish containing TALP-HEPES with 75% SSS and then aspirated into the catheter making sure that the total aspirated volume does not exceed 0.03 cc. Numerous types of catheter systems have been successfully used for embryo transfer, ranging from the basic Tom Cat® (Sherwood Medical, St. Louis, MO) to complex coaxial systems with guide wires for negotiating through a difficult cervix. The use of catheters with softer materials should result in less endometrial trauma, which may be associated with better outcomes. Examples of embryo transfer catheters in which there is a stiff outer sheath and a soft inner catheter are illustrated (Fig. 4). To make the inner catheter easier to advance through the outer catheter, there is the option of a metal stylet.

Prior to embryo transfer, the patient is placed in the dorsal lithotomy position and the table is adjusted to make her comfortable. The environment should be as quiet as possible and stimuli such as bright lights should be minimized. Adequate visualization of the cervix is required so an appropriate size speculum should be used. A tenaculum may be applied to the cervix if needed; usually a local anesthetic is unnecessary. Many practitioners use betadyne or other cleansing agents without a problem; however, the use of culture media to wipe away cervical mucus and vaginal secretions seems more appropriate and carries the theoretical benefit of avoiding cytotoxic, and therefore embryotoxic, agents. Removal of excess cervical mucus from the external os is recommended because catheters contaminated with mucus have been associated with retained embryos (54,55). The addition of ultrasound observation during the transfer also results in confirmed placement of the embryos in the fundus. The length of the cervix and the depth of the uterine cavity should be reassessed by ultrasound immediately before the transfer because the hormonal milieu of ovarian hyperstimulation may result in a change of these measurements as compared to the screening evaluation. Some clinicians use ultrasound to assess uterine contractions; if observed, they may have a negative impact on pregnancy outcome *(56)*. The use of ultrasound during the embryo transfer can avoid sub-endometrial and tubal transfers *(57)*. Prior to loading the embryos into the catheter, an attempt to pass the catheter through the cervix can be made. If there is no resistance, the catheter can be loaded and the transfer completed with ultrasound guidance. To determine whether to use the catheter as one unit or to after-load the embryos, one can assess if there is resistance to the catheter passing through the cervix. If resistance is experienced, then an after-loading technique can be used. The after-loading technique is accomplished by placing the outer sheath of the catheter beyond the point of resistance so that the softer inner catheter can easily pass into the uterine cavity to within 1 cm of the fundus. Placing the tip of the inner catheter at this depth avoids the risk of endometrial trauma at the uterine fundus. Attempts should be made to avoid passing the stiffer outer catheter into the uterine cavity in order to minimize trauma to the endometrium. Difficult transfers or transfers in which the uterine fundus is touched by the catheter can cause uterine contractions that are capable of relocating intrauterine embryos *(58)*. Fibrin sealants have been used to prevent relocation of embryos, potentially reducing the risk of expulsion or ectopic pregnancy *(59)*. Another potential advantage of extended embryo culture and transfer of embryos on d 5–6 is that the endogenous progesterone concentration is higher, resulting in fewer uterine contractions. In any case, after the transfer, the catheter is checked for retained embryos. Fortunately, the immediate retransfer of retained embryos does not appear to compromise outcome *(54)*. Retained embryos are not a frequent complication, occurring in approx 1% of transfers. Traumatic transfers may be associated with bleeding and blood on the outside of the transfer catheter, and are associated with a decrease in implantation and clinical pregnancy rates *(60)*. One group has used a CO_2 pulsed flexible hysteroscope to perform a direct intra-endometrial transfer of d 2 embryos with limited success *(61)*. It is unlikely that operative transfer of embryos will replace the transcervical catheter because of the increased trauma associated with hysteroscopy.

POST-TRANSFER MANAGEMENT

Options for the activity level of women after the transfer of embryos has ranged from strict bed rest in the Trendelenberg position to immediate normal activity. Sharif and coworkers *(62)* reported their experience with over 1000 cycles and concluded that bed rest was not necessary following embryo transfer. Woolcott and Stanger *(63)* studied the effect of standing shortly after embryo transfer to see if there were any adverse affect on the position of the embryos. Using ultrasound, they tracked the embryo-associated air bubble and found no movement in over 94% of their transfers. Most clinics advise rest for a short period of time, 20–60 min, followed by minimal to moderate activity. Strenuous exercise is generally not recommended; however, this is based on hypothetical opinion and not on controlled studies.

Hormonal supplementation to support a shortened luteal phase following the ovarian stimulation protocol is often used. Women who are the recipients of oocyte donation or ET&T using artificial cycles will need hormonal support throughout the first trimester of pregnancy. There are various protocols for luteal support using either oral, vaginal, or parenteral routes for progesterone administration. Supplemental hCG is also used, either alone or in combination with progesterone. Whether or not hormonal supplementation is beneficial to pregnancy outcome in nonartificial cycles remains controversial.

Pregnancy testing can be done 10 d after transfer of d 5–6 embryos. However, if supplemental injections of hCG are given then a false-positive pregnancy test may result. Serial hCG concentrations, usually 2 d apart, are measured to assess the viability of the early pregnancy as well as the incidence of abnormal or multiple pregnancies. The risk of a spontaneous abortion is related to the age of the woman; however, ectopic pregnancies are no more frequent than the normal population incidence. If more than one or two embryos are transferred, the couple can be evaluated for a high-order multiple pregnancy and counseled on selective reduction if the need arises.

SUMMARY

The ideal embryo transfer results in the birth of one normal baby. Limiting the number of embryos transferred to those with the highest implantation potential is an important advancement in our ability to meet this goal. Extended culture techniques in which embryos progress to the blastocyst stage support the transfer of one or two high-quality embryos while maintaining high pregnancy rates. Improvements in catheter design allowing for less endometrial disruption and uterine contractions have also contributed to better outcomes. Hydraulic loading of embryos and the use of ultrasound for accurate placement of the catheter tip may also improve success. The embryo transfer is seemingly simple, yet it is arguably the most important step in the ARTs; thus, meticulous attention should be paid to this procedure.

REFERENCES

1. Feichtinger W, Papalambrou K, Poehl M, Krischker U, Neumann K. Smoking and *in vitro* fertilization: a meta-analysis. J Assist Reprod Genet 1997;14(10):596–599.
2. El-Nemr A, Al-Shawaf T, Sabatini L, Wilson C, Lower AM, Grudzinskas JG. Effect of smoking on ovarian reserve and ovarian stimulation in *in vitro* fertilization and embryo transfer. Hum Reprod 1998; 13(8):2192–2198.
3. Potter DA, Witz CA, Burns WN, Brzyski RG, Schenken RS. Endometrial biopsy during hormone replacement cycle in donor oocyte recipients before *in vitro* fertilization-embryo transfer. Fertil Steril 1998;70(2):219–221.
4. Zeyneloglu HB, Arici A, Olive DL. Adverse effects of hydrosalpinx on pregnancy rates after *in vitro* fertilization-embryo transfer. Fertil Steril 1998;70(3):492–499.
5. Freeman MR, Whitworth CM, Hill GA. Permanent impairment of embryo development by hydrosalpinges. Hum Reprod 1998;13(4):983–986.
6. Van Voorhis BJ, Sparks AET, Syrop CH, Stovall DW. Ultrasound-guided aspiration of hydrosalpinges is associated with improved pregnancy and implantation rates after *in vitro* fertilization cycles. Hum Reprod 1998;13(3):736–739.
7. de Wit W, Gowrising CJ, Kuik DJ, Lens JW, Schats R. Only hydrosalpinges visible on ultrasound are associated with reduced implantation and pregnancy rates after *in vitro* fertilization. Hum Reprod 1998; 13(6):1696–1701.
8. Sowter MC, Akande VA, Williams JA, Hull MG. Is the outcome of *in vitro* fertilization and embryo transfer treatment improved by spontaneous or surgical drainage of a hydrosalpinx? Hum Reprod 1997; 12(10):2147–2150.
9. Strandell A, Sjogren A, Bentin-Ley U, Thorburn J, Hamberger L, Brannstrom M. Hydrosalpinx fluid does not adversely affect the normal development of human embryos and implantation *in vitro*. Hum Reprod 1998;13(10):2921–2925.

10. Queenan JT Jr, Veeck LL, Toner JP, Oehninger S, Muasher SJ. Cryopreservation of all prezygotes in patients at risk of sever hyperstimulation does not eliminate the syndrome, but the chances of pregnancy are excellent with subsequent frozen-thaw transfers. Hum Reprod 1997;12(7):1573–1576.

11. Tanos V, Friedler S, Zajicek G, Neiger M, Lewin A, Schenker JG. The impact of endometrial preparation on implantation following cryopreserved-thawed-embryo transfer. Gynecol Obstet Invest 1996;41(4): 227–231.

12. Simon A, Hurwitz A, Zentner BS, Bdolah Y, Laufer N. Transfer of frozen-thawed embryos in artificially prepared cycles with and without prior gonadotrophin-releasing hormone agonist suppression: a prospective randomized study. Hum Reprod 1998;13(10):2712–2717.

13. Prapas Y, Prapas N, Jones EE, Duleba AJ, Olive DL, Chatziparasidou A, Vlassis G. The window for embryo transfer in oocyte donation cycles depends on the duration of progesterone therapy. Hum Reprod 1998;13(3):720–723.

14. Callahan TL, Hall JE, Ettner SL, Christiansen CL, Greene MF, Crowley WF Jr. The economic impact of multiple-gestation pregnancies and the contribution of assisted-reproduction techniques to their incidence. N Engl J Med 1994;331(4):244–249.

15. Tasdemir M, Tasdemir I, Kodama H, Fukuda J, Tanaka T. Two instead of three embryo transfer in *in vitro* fertilization. Hum Reprod 1995;10(8):2155–2158.

16. Roest J, van Heusden AM, Verhoeff A, Mous HV, Zeilmaker GH. A triplet pregnancy after *in vitro* fertilization is a procedure-related complication that should be prevented by replacement of two embryos only. Fertil Steril 1997;67(2):290–295.

17. Murdoch A. Triplets and embryo transfer policy. Hum Reprod 1997;12(11 Suppl):88–92.

18. Templeton A, Morris JK. Reducing the risk of multiple births by transfer of two embryos after *in vitro* fertilization. N Engl J Med 1998;339(9):573–577.

19. Fujii S, Fukui A, Yamaguchi E, Sakamoto T, Sato S, Saito Y. Reducing multiple pregnancies by restricting the number of embryos transferred to two at the first embryo transfer attempt. Hum Reprod 1998; 13(12):3550–3554.

20. Hu Y, Maxson WS, Hoffman DI, Ory SJ, Eager S, Dupre J, Lu C. Maximizing pregnancy rates and limiting higher-order multiple conceptions by determining the optimal number of embryos to transfer based on quality. Fertil Steril 1998;69(4):650–657.

21. Minaretzis D, Harris D, Alper MM, Mortola JF, Berger MJ, Power D. Multivariate analysis of factors predictive of successful live births in *in vitro* fertilization (IVF) suggests strategies to improve IVF outcome. J Assist Reprod Genet 1998;15(6):365–371.

22. Grimbizis G, Vandervorst M, Camus M, Tournaye H, Van Steirteghem A, Devroey P. Intracytoplasmic sperm injection, results in women older than 39, according to age and the number of embryos replaced in selective or non-selective transfers. Hum Reprod 1998;13(4):884–889.

23. Schwartz LB, Chiu AS, Courtney M, Krey L, Schmidt-Sarosi C. The embryo versus endometrium controversy revisited as it relates to predicting pregnancy outcome in *in vitro* fertilization-embryo transfer cycles. Hum Reprod 1997;12(1):45–50.

24. Quinn P, Stone BA, Marrs RP. Suboptimal laboratory conditions can affect pregnancy outcome after embryo transfer on day 1 or 2 after insemination *in vitro*. Fertil Steril 1990;53(1):168–170.

25. Gianaroli L, Magli MC, Munne S, Fiorentino A, Montanaro N, Ferraretti AP. Will preimplantation genetic diagnosis assist patients with a poor prognosis to achieve pregnancy? Hum Reprod 1997;12(8): 1762–1767.

26. Grifo JA, Giatras K, Tang YX, Krey LC. Successful outcome with day 4 embryo transfer after preimplantation diagnosis for genetically transmitted diseases. Hum Reprod 1998;13(6):1656–1659.

27. Scott LA, Smith S. The successful use of pronuclear embryo transfers the day following oocyte retrieval. Hum Reprod 1998;13(4):1003–1013.

28. Dawson KJ, Conaghan J, Ostera GR, Winston RM, Hardy K. Delaying transfer to the third day postinsemination, to select non-arrested embryos, increases development to the fetal heart stage. Hum Reprod 1995;10(1):177–182.

29. Carrillo AJ, Lane B, Pridman DD, Risch PP, Pool TB, Silverman IH, Cook CL. Improved clinical outcomes for *in vitro* fertilization with delay of embryo transfer from 48 to 72 hours after oocyte retrieval: use of glucose- and phosphate-free media. Fertil Steril 1998;69(2):329–334.

30. Goto Y, Kanzaki H, Nakayama T, Takabatake K, Himeno T, Mori T, Noda Y. Relationship between the day of embryo transfer and the outcome in human *in vitro* fertilization and embryo transfer. J Assist Reprod Genet 1994;11(8):401–404.

31. Huisman GJ, Alberda AT, Leerentveld RA, Verhoeff A, Zeilmaker GH. A comparison of *in vitro* fertilization results after embryo transfer after 2,3, and 4 days of embryo culture. Fertil Steril 1994;61(5):970–971.
32. Gardner DK, Lane M. Culture and selection of viable blastocysts: a feasible proposition for human IVF? Hum Reprod Update 1997;3(4):367–382.
33. Jones GM, Trounson AO, Gardner DK, Kausche A, Lolatgis N, Wood C. Evolution of a culture protocol for successful blastocyst development and pregnancy. Hum Reprod 1998;13(1):169–177.
34. Gardner DK, Vella P, Lane M, Wagley L, Schlenker T, Schoolcraft WB. Culture and transfer of human blastocysts increases implantation rates and reduces the need for multiple embryo transfers. Fertil Steril 1998;69(1):84–88.
35. Fong CY, Bongso A, Ng SC, Anandakumar C, Tounson A, Ratnam S. Ongoing normal pregnancy after transfer of zona-free blastocysts: implications for embryo transfer in the human. Hum Reprod 1997;12(3):557–560.
36. Jones GM, Trounson AO, Lolatgis N, Wood C. Factors affecting the success of human blastocyst development and pregnancy following in vitro fertilization and embryo transfer. Fertil Steril 1998;70(6):1022–1029.
37. Kondo I, Suganuma N, Ando T, Asada Y, Furuhashi M, Tomoda Y. Clinical factors for successful cryopreserved-thawed embryo transfer. J Assist Reprod Genet 1996;13(3):201–206.
38. Van der Elst J, Van den Abbeel E, Vitrier S, Camus M, Devroey P, Van Steirteghem AC. Selective transfer of cryopreserved human embryos with further cleavage after thawing increases delivery and implantation rates. Hum Reprod 1997;12(7):1513–1521.
39. Mottla GL, Smotrich DB, Gindoff PR, Stillman RJ. Increasing clinical pregnancy rates after IVF/ET. Can immunosuppression help? J Reprod Med 1996;41(12):889–891.
40. Witkin SS, Sultan KM, Neal GS, Jeremias J, Grifo JA, Rosenwaks Z. Unsuspected Chlamydia trachomatis infection and *in vitro* fertilization outcome. Am J Obstet Gynecol 1994;164:1767–1770.
41. Witkin SS, Kligman II, Grifo JA, Rosenwaks Z. Chlamydia trachomatis detected by polymerase chain reaction in cervices of culture-negative women correlates with adverse *in vitro* fertilization outcome. J Infect Dis 1995;17:1657–1659.
42. Fanchin R, Harmas A, Benaoudia F, Lundkvist U, Olivennes F, Frydman R. Microbial flora of the cervix assessed at the time of embryo transfer adversely affects *in vitro* fertilization outcome. Fertil Steril 1998;70(5):866–870.
43. Facchinetti F, Matteo ML, Artini GP, Volpe A, Genazzani AR. An increased vulnerability to stress is associated with a poor outcome of *in vitro* fertilization-embryo transfer treatment. Fertil Steril 1997;67(2):309–314.
44. Pregnancy-related death associated with heparin and aspirin treatment for infertility, 1996. MMWR Morb Mortal Wkly Rep 1998;47(18):368–371.
45. Wehner-Caroli J, Schreiner T, Schippert W, Lischka G, Fierlbeck G, Rassner G. Anaphylactic reaction to bovine serum albumin after embryo transfer. Fertil Steril 1998;70(4):771–773.
46. Chao KH, Chen SU, Chen HF, Wu MY, Yang YS, Ho HN. Assisted hatching increases the implantation and pregnancy rate of *in vitro* fertilization (IVF)-embryo transfer (ET), but not that of IVF-tubal ET in patients with repeated IVF failures. Fertil Steril 1997;67(5):904–908.
47. Lanzendorf SE, Nehchiri F, Mayer JF, Oehninger S, Muasher SJ. A prospective, randomized, double-blind study for the evaluation of assisted hatching in patients with advanced maternal age. Hum Reprod 1998;13(2):409–413.
48. Magli MC, Gianaroli L, Ferraretti AP, Fortini D, Aicardi G, Montanaro N. Rescue of implantation potential in embryos with poor prognosis by assisted zona hatching. Hum Reprod 1998;13(5):1331–1335.
49. Bider D, Livshits A, Yonish M, Yemini Z, Mashiach S, Dor J. Assisted hatching by zona drilling of human embryos in women of advanced age. Hum Reprod 1997;12(2):317–320.
50. Meldrum DR, Wisot A, Yee B, Garzo G, Yeo L, Hamilton F. Assisted hatching reduces the age-related decline in IVF outcome in women younger than age 43 without increasing miscarriage or monozygotic twinning. J Assist Reprod Genet 1998;15(7):418–421.
51. Hurst BS, Tucker KE, Awoniyi CA, Schlaff WD. Assisted hatching does not enhance IVF success in good-prognosis patients. J Assist Reprod Genet 1998;15(2):62–64.
52. Wenstrom KD, Syrop CH, Hammitt DG, Van Voorhis BJ. Increased risk of monochorionic twinning associated with assisted reproduction. Fertil Steril 1993;60(3):510–514.
53. Fong CY, Bongso A, Ng SC, Kumar J, Trounson A, Ratnam S. Blastocyst transfer after enzymatic treatment of the zona pellucida: improving *in vitro* fertilization and understandng implantation (In Process Citation). Hum Reprod 1998;13(10):2926–2932.

54. Nabi A, Awonuga A, Birch H, Barlow S, Stewart B. Multiple attempts at embryo transfer: does this affect *in vitro* fertilization treatment outcome? Hum Reprod 1997;12(6):1188–1190.

55. Awonuga A, Nabi A, Govindbhai J, Birch H, Stewart B. Contamination of embryo transfer catheter and treatment outcome in *in vitro* fertilization. J Assist Reprod Genet 1998;15(4):198–201.

56. Fanchin R, Righini C, Olivennes F, Taylor S, de Ziegler D, Frydman R. Uterine contractions at the time of embryo transfer alter pregnancy rates after *in vitro* fertilization. Hum Reprod 1998;13(7):1968–1974.

57. Woolcott R, Stanger J. Potentially important variables identified by transvaginal ultrasound-guided embryo transfer. Hum Reprod 1997;12(5):963–966.

58. Lesny P, Killick SR, Tetlow RL, Robinson J, Maguiness SD. Embryo transfer: can we learn anything new from the observation of junctional zone contractions? Hum Reprod 1998;13(6):1540–1546.

59. Feichtinger W, Strohmer H, Radner KM, Goldin M. The use of fibrin sealant for embryo transfer: development and clinical studies. Hum Reprod 1992;7(6):890–893.

60. Goudas VT, Hammitt DG, Darnario MA, Session DR, Singh AP, Dumesic DA. Blood on the embryo transfer catheter is associated with decreased rate of embryo implantation and clinic pregnancy with the use of *in vitro* fertilization-embryo transfer. Fertil Steril 1998;70(5):878–882.

61. Itskovitz-Eldor J, Filmar S, Manor D, Stein D, Lightman A, Kol S. Assisted implantation: direct intra-endometrial embryo transfer. Gynecol Obstet Invest 1997;43(2):73–75.

62. Sharif K, Afnan M, Lashen H, Elgendy M, Morgan C, Sinclair L. Is bed rest following embryo transfer necessary? Fertil Steril 1998;69:478–481.

63. Woolcott R, Stanger J. Ultrasound tracking of the movement of embryo-associated air bubbles on standing after transfer. Hum Reprod 1998;13(8):2107-2109.

10

Cryopreservation of Mammalian Embryos, Gametes, and Ovarian Tissues

Current Issues and Progress

William F. Rall, PHD

INTRODUCTION

The ground-breaking report by Chris Polge and his colleagues in 1949 *(1)* on the protective action of glycerol during the freezing of fowl spermatozoa was immediately recognized as enabling technology for controlling the reproduction of animals. This was confirmed by the rapid development and application of procedures for cryopreserving bull and human spermatozoa *(2,3)*. Cryopreserved spermatozoa have made important contributions to efforts to improve the genetic characteristics of domestic livestock, treat infertility in humans, and conserve unique animal models and endangered species. Similar progress followed the first reports of successful freezing of mouse embryos in 1972 by Whittingham, Leibo and Mazur *(4)*, and Wilmut *(5)*. A large number of protocols for embryo cryopreservation have been described using many cryoprotective agents and diverse cooling and warming conditions. Unfortunately, progress in developing procedures for cryopreserving mammalian oocytes and ovarian tissue has been much slower. Recent advances in the development of ultra-rapid cooling procedures for oocytes suggest that practical application may occur soon. Comprehensive reviews of the history, theory, and protocols for cryopreservation of spermatozoa, oocytes, and embryos are available elsewhere *(6–9)*.

This chapter will discuss current issues related to the application of cryobiology to the control of reproduction of mammals:

From: *Contemporary Endocrinology: Assisted Fertilization and Nuclear Transfer in Mammals*
Edited by: D. P. Wolf and M. Zelinski-Wooten © Humana Press Inc., Totowa, NJ

1. Review issues related to the long-term storage of cells, gametes, and embryos at low temperatures;
2. Discuss promising developments in ultra-rapid cryopreservation procedures; and
3. Review the status of the cryopreservation of mammalian embryos, spermatozoa, oocytes, and ovarian tissue.

LONG-TERM STORAGE OF CRYOPRESERVED CELLS

Most attention to cryopreservation is devoted to the development of simple, effective procedures for cooling to and warming from the storage temperature. Little attention has been given to the challenges of long-term storage conditions. Several important issues concerning low temperature storage have been raised in recent years.

There is no convincing scientific evidence that viability changes during storage of cryopreserved embryos and cells at temperatures of −130°C or lower. The complete solidification of cell suspensions during cooling is thought to play an important role in eliminating most chemical and physical mechanisms of injury during the storage period. Cryopreservation of cell suspensions using low concentrations of cryoprotectants (<3 molar) and conventional controlled cooling yields two solids, crystals and glasses. The suspension separates into a mixture of pure ice in the solution surrounding the cells and a concentrated residual solution within the cell and between the ice crystals (10). The concentrated residual solution and the dehydrated cytoplasm transform into glassy solids during cooling to the storage temperature by a process called vitrification (11). "Vitrified" cell suspensions also solidify during cooling but differ from that of frozen suspensions by the absence of ice crystals (12). The combination of complete solidification and low temperature reduces the diffusion of potential chemical reactants and increases the thermodynamic equilibrium constant of all chemical reactions. These changes in the cell suspension prevent normal chemical reactions from degrading the cells during storage. Limited chemical reactions are likely prerequisites for long-term suspended animation of cells.

Five threats or hazards are thought to be capable of compromising cells during low-temperature storage. First, the viability and genetic stability of cells can be altered by exposure to ionizing radiation. Injury may result from photophysical damage to macromolecules (e.g., DNA breaks) or the formation of free radicals (13). These changes would accumulate during storage at low temperature owing to the lack of biological repair mechanisms. Experimental irradiation of frozen cells results in genetic changes and the primary target is reportedly the nucleus (14). Fortunately, experimental studies indicate that normal terrestrial background radiation and cosmic rays do not pose a major threat during long-term storage of cryopreserved mouse embryos (15). Exposure to the equivalent of 2,000 years of simulated background radiation at −196°C yielded no detrimental effect on viability of the embryos or obvious genetic mutation. Because the mechanism of radiation damage is a consequence of the physical-chemical properties of frozen aqueous solutions, this conclusion ought to apply to all cryopreserved biological cells during storage at temperatures below the solidification temperature of cell suspensions (<−150°C).

A second, more likely, threat to the viability of cells during storage is a failure to ensure a continuous storage temperature of −130°C or lower. Uncontrolled warming and prolonged exposure to temperatures between −90 and −40°C may place embryos and cells at risk of injury due to devitrification and recrystallization of ice within and outside the cells (11,16). The safest storage conditions would be to place the cells in a hermetically-sealed container (e.g., plastic straw heat sealed at both ends) and place the container in a liquid-nitrogen refrigerator submerged in liquid nitrogen (−196°C). A high level of quality control is essential to ensure continued optimum storage conditions. Ideally, refrigerators should be placed in a secure location with some samples from each donor in a backup refrigerator at a remote location managed by another organization. All refrigerators should be equipped with controls that allow automatic and manual filling with liquid nitrogen. Refrigerators should be inspected daily and filled at least weekly. Additional precautions include redundant electronic alarms that continuously monitor refrigerator temperature and liquid-nitrogen level and a call list of personnel trained to respond to all alarm conditions.

A third threat to embryos and cells during storage is contamination by contact with liquid nitrogen containing viruses, bacteria, fungi, or other pathogens. Considerable evidence from the fields of virus banking *(17,18)*, blood transfusion *(19–21)*, dermatology *(22,23)*, and food processing *(24)* demonstrates that liquid nitrogen may harbor virus and microbial pathogens and cross-contaminate material during storage. The recovery of infective viruses from liquid nitrogen also suggests that personnel managing cell and embryo repositories may be at risk. It is prudent that precautions are taken to minimize risks. All liquid-nitrogen refrigerators containing clinical material should be assumed to contain contaminated liquid nitrogen. Liquid nitrogen used for laboratory processes should be obtained from supply tanks and not storage refrigerators. The containers of embryo and cell suspensions should be hermetically sealed and the outside surfaces should be decontaminated before cryopreservation and immediately after thawing. Finally, some consideration should be given to sample storage in liquid-nitrogen vapor. However, vapor storage is not advisable for plastic straws and other small sample configurations because their low thermal mass places cell suspensions at high risk of transient warming when refrigerators are opened.

A fourth hazard is the explosion of sample containers after the storage period owing to improper sealing or the use of containers incapable of hermetic sealing. A leaky sample container permits liquid nitrogen to enter and come into direct contact with the embryo or cell suspension. The rate and amount of liquid nitrogen entering a container varies depending on several factors. These include the volume of the air space (or bubbles) in the container, the effective diameter and length of the "hole" in the seal, and the length of time in storage. The physical process leading to liquid nitrogen inside the container is related to the development of a partial vacuum in the air space within the container. This can be estimated using the ideal gas law, $PV = nRT$, where P, V, and T are, respectively, the pressure, volume, and absolute temperature (°K) of gas in the container when it is "sealed" before cooling. n and R are, respectively, the number of moles of gas molecules and the gas constant. The vacuum forms primarily during cooling from room temperature (293°K) to the temperature of boiling liquid nitrogen (77°K). Inspection of the gas equation indicates that, if the volume and number of moles of gas molecules remain constant during cooling in liquid nitrogen, the pressure (P) of the gas in the container must be only 26% (77/293) of that before cooling. This simplified analysis means that the liquid nitrogen is actually sucked into the container during storage.

A fifth hazard is damage to the zona pellucida during cooling to and warming from the storage temperature that is usually manifested as a crack or tear in the zona pellucida as though cut with a sharp blade. Sometimes, the cell mass also is cut. One explanation for this damage is fracturing of the solidified cell suspension and tissues due to large thermal gradients when cooled and warmed at low temperatures *(25–28)*. Thermally-induced fracturing is a well-known property of solidified samples and is extensively documented for ice blocks *(29)* and glasses *(30,31)*. Experimental data indicates that the incidence of fracture depends on complex factors that include the size of the sample, choice of sample container, and the cooling and warming conditions. Both frozen and vitrified embryo suspensions are subject to fracture during the cooling and/or warming steps. The highest rates of zona fracture were associated with the use of glass containers (vials or tubes), rapid cooling, and warming at temperatures below −100°C (especially direct immersion in liquid nitrogen or a water bath). The lowest rates of damage were obtained when zonae were warmed slowly between −196° and −100°C in 0.25-mL plastic straws by holding the straw in room temperature air for at least 10 s before immersion in a water bath *(25)*.

Many other causes have been proposed for the appearance of cracks in the zona pellucida of embryos and other biological material following cryopreservation. These include interactions between embryos and the meniscus or surface of air bubbles, composition of the cryoprotectant solution, irradiation of straws, and the nucleation or movement of air bubbles during freezing or thawing *(32–35)*. The relative importance and mechanisms of these factors are not well-understood compared to that of thermally induced fracture.

One important conclusion from our current understanding of the stability of cryopreserved embryos and cells in liquid nitrogen is that, barring a refrigerator failure or the other considerations and hazards listed previously, cryopreserved living cells ought to remain viable for centuries or even a millennium.

RECENT DEVELOPMENTS
IN THE VITRIFICATION OF OOCYTES AND EMBRYOS

Current vitrification procedures often use 0.25 mL plastic insemination straws as the sample container. Embryo and cell suspensions placed in these straws can be cooled rapidly, but the highest cooling rates are limited to about 50°C/s. Ultra-rapid cooling (>150°C/s) may be useful for mammalian and insect cells and embryos with a high sensitivity to chilling injury, such as, Drosophila embryos, cleavage-stage bovine embryos, in vitro-produced bovine morulae, and all preimplantation stages of porcine embryos. Increasing the cooling rate is usually achieved by reducing the sample size and increasing heat transfer. The potentially beneficial effects of ultra-rapid cooling for the vitrification of bovine embryos were demonstrated in a recent report *(36)*. Bovine oocytes were placed on an electron microscope grid in a thin film of vitrification solution and cooled rapidly by direct immersion into partially-solidified liquid nitrogen (−210°C). Development of thawed oocytes to blastocysts was significantly improved over that reported previously using conventional slow-freezing or straw-vitrification procedures (respectively, 30 and 3%).

Two recent reports of novel procedures for ultra-rapid cooling of cell suspensions may further simplify vitrification procedures for mammalian oocytes and embryos. The first is the "Open Pulled Straw" (OPS) vitrification method *(37)*. The novel feature of this method is the use of a plastic capillary tube as the sample container. The capillaries are prepared by heating a 0.25-mL plastic insemination straw and pulling it to half its original diameter (available commercially from Demtek A/S, DK-8200 Aarhus N, Denmark). This provides a simple, convenient container for embryos that allows extremely high rates of cooling and warming by direct immersion, respectively, in liquid nitrogen and room temperature medium (ca. 350°C/s). The utility of the OPS method has been demonstrated using cleavage-stage bovine embryos and mature oocytes, which exhibit high sensitivity to chilling injury *(38)*. The success of OPS vitrification depended on the developmental stage of the embryos *(39)*. Low rates of survival (assessed by in vitro development of thawed embryos to blastocysts) were obtained when embryos were vitrified after 1 d of culture (31%). However, survival gradually increased to 90% as the number of days of culture before vitrification increased to seven. Furthermore, three pregnancies were obtained from vitrified blastocysts produced from oocytes that were also vitrified before in vitro fertilization (IVF) and culture. OPS vitrification of cleavage-stage bovine embryos and mature oocytes yielded the highest post-thaw rate of embryo development in vitro reported to date.

Another approach to ultra-rapid cooling is to reduce the size and thermal mass of the sample by eliminating the sample container. High rates of in vitro and in vivo survival have been obtained by simply expelling small drops (5–20 μL) of vitrification solution containing mouse embryos directly into liquid nitrogen *(40,41)*. One disadvantage of this approach is the difficulty of collecting, storing, and handing many small drops in liquid nitrogen. Some of these handling problems have been recently solved by the use of a 0.3–1-mm diameter nylon loop (CryoLoop, Hampton Research, Laguna Niguel, CA) to support a small drop of cryoprotectant containing embryos during the cooling, storage, and warming steps *(42)*. The basic approach is similar to methods used in handling protein crystals during low temperature storage and crystallography studies *(43,44)*. Embryos are equilibrated in standard vitrification solutions and then placed in a drop (or thin film) suspended on the CryoLoop. The CryoLoop is then immersed in liquid nitrogen. High rates of in vitro and in vivo development of one and two-cell hamster embryos were reported following vitrification using this "container-less" technique.

One common feature of these ultra-rapid cooling procedures is a low incidence of zona fracture. This may reflect the small diameter and thermal masses of the suspension and container, properties that limit thermal fracture by reducing temperature gradients across the suspensions during cooling and warming. Unfortunately, these and most ultra-rapid cooling procedures suffer from the lack of a sealed container to prevent possible contamination by contact with liquid nitrogen containing viral, bacteria, fungal, or other pathogens. Recently, Vajta and his colleagues *(45)* suggested that contamination might be eliminated by applying sterile conditions during the cooling and warming steps, and sealing the OPS capillary in a 0.5-mL plastic insemination straw during storage in liquid nitrogen. They proposed filter sterilization of liquid nitrogen using a 0.2 μm-pore size filter would eliminate potential microbial contaminants. Although it is likely that filtering can remove most bacteria, fungi, and their spores from contaminated liquid nitrogen, there is no experimental evidence that viruses can be eliminated by filtering. One way of eliminating contamination is to use another inert refrigerant that is inherently capable of being sterilized. For example, Drosophila embryos have been successfully vitrified on electron microscope grids cooled in $<-170°C$ liquid propane *(46)*.

CURRENT STATUS OF THE CRYOPRESERVATION OF MAMMALIAN EMBRYOS, GAMETES, AND OVARIAN TISSUE

Mammalian Embryos

Since the first report of live-born young from cryopreserved mouse embryos, similar success has been reported for 21 additional mammalian species (Table 1). Excellent

Table 1
Mammalian Species Yielding Normal Offspring Following
the Transfer of Cryopreserved Embryos to Foster Mothers

Species	Year	Reference
Mouse	1972	(4)
Cattle	1973	(55)
Rabbit	1974	(56)
Sheep	1974	(57)
Rat	1975	(58)
Goat	1976	(59)
Horse	1982	(60)
Eland	1983	(61)
Human	1984	(62)
Baboon	1984	(63)
Marmoset	1986	(64)
Cynomolgus macaque	1987	(65)
Cat	1988	(66)
Rhesus macaque	1989	(67)
Pig	1989	(68)
Red deer	1991	(69)
Wapiti	1991	(70)
Hybrid macaque	1992	(71)
Swamp buffalo	1993	(72)
Fallow deer	1994	(73)
Hamster	1999	(74)
Mongolian gerbil	1999	(75)

general reviews are available on basic and applied aspects of the cryobiology of mammalian embryos (9,47–49).

Usually, the optimum conditions for embryo cryopreservation exhibit much lower species variation than those for mammalian spermatozoa. However, two factors, developmental stage and species, influence two important intrinsic cryobiological properties. First, the permeability of embryos to cryoprotectants often increases during embryonic development from zygote to blastocyst, and may vary for embryos from different species at the same embryonic stage (50). One consequence of these differences is the need to choose a cryoprotectant as well as equilibration and dilution conditions consistent with the embryo's permeability properties. Second, embryos from at least two species, cattle and pig, are reported to exhibit a high sensitivity to cooling to 0°C during development, respectively, from zygote to early morulae or expanded blastocysts. Such chilling injury is thought to be associated with the dark cytoplasmic lipid droplets in these embryos that persist to later developmental stages in suboptimal in vitro culture systems (51,52).

Most research and application of embryo cryopreservation have concentrated on three species: mice, cattle, and human. Mouse and cattle receive the greatest attention and have yielded tens of thousands of live offspring. The number of offspring produced from cryopreserved embryos of other mammalian species is much lower. Optimization of cryopreservation and embryo-transfer procedures for mice and cattle currently permits remarkably high overall rates of development. For example, in a direct comparison of controlled slow freezing and vitrification procedures using 8-cell mouse embryos, 75% of frozen and 64% of vitrified embryos developed into normal late-stage fetuses and live-born pups

Table 2
Mammalian Species Yielding Normal Offspring
Following Artificial Insemination with Cryopreserved Spermatozoa

Domesticated
Cattle, Sheep, Horse, Pig, Goat, Water buffalo, Rabbit, Cat, Dog, Domestic ferret, Mouse.
Primates
Human, Chimpanzee, Cynomolgus macaque, Marmoset, Gorilla.
Deer
Axis deer, Eld's deer, Fallow deer, Red deer, Reindeer, Wapiti, White-tailed deer, Pere David's deer.
Felids
Cheetah, Leopard cat, Ocelot.
Other
Bighorn sheep, Bison, Gaur, Addax, Damas gazelle, Mohor gazelle, Scimitar-horned oryx, Blackbuck, Black-footed ferret, Siberian polecat, Arctic fox, Red fox, Wolf, Giant panda.

following thawing and transfer to recipient females *(53)*. Similarly high pregnancy rates ranging from 55–70% are reported in commercial embryo transfer of thawed bovine embryos *(54)*. The overall efficiency of embryo cryopreservation is lower for other species listed in Table 1. In some species, only one or a handful of offspring has been born.

Mammalian Spermatozoa

Since the first report of live-born young from cryopreserved cattle spermatozoa, similar success has been reported for at least 41 additional mammalian species (Table 2). Excellent general reviews are available on basic and applied aspects of the cryobiology of mammalian spermatozoa *(76,77)* and current progress for several mammalian species *(78–82)*.

Although effective cryopreservation procedures have been reported for a number of species, mammalian spermatozoa provide the best example of the limits to predictive cryobiology. From a cryobiologist's point of view, the general properties of spermatozoa ought to be very favorable for successful cryopreservation. They are small cells, exhibit a high permeability to water and cryoprotectant, and have a low water content. Analysis of the osmotic behavior of spermatozoa during freezing using Mazur's thermodynamic model predicts no special precautions except possibly for a requirement of high rates of cooling *(83)*. Unfortunately the predicted optimum cooling rates have been approx two orders of magnitude higher than the empirically observed optimums *(84)*.

Practical experience indicates that special properties of sperm and other factors complicate the application of sperm cryopreservation to many mammalian species. First, sperm are a highly differentiated cell with evidence of structural and functional compartmentalization *(78)*. There is some evidence of differential sensitivity of these compartments and associated cell membranes to osmotic and toxic stresses during the process of cryopreservation *(85–87)*. Second, spermatozoa of many species are subject to injury during rapid cooling at subambient temperatures *(88)*. Prior equilibration with special additives, such as egg yolk, and slow cooling may reduce injury to acceptable levels *(89)*. Other complicating factors include heterogeneity in the properties of individual sperm in a suspension, the unknown functions of seminal plasma components and the need to preserve motility and associated metabolism. Finally, perhaps the most important complication is that the relative importance of these special properties often varies between species and even between individuals within a species.

These important cellular properties and considerations confound efforts to predict optimum procedures from measurements and estimates of the osmotic behavior of sperm. This may reflect important differences in the cryobiological properties of the individual compartments of the sperm cell and require compromises in the cryopreservation conditions to both minimize overall cryoinjury and optimize overall survival of each compartment. As in many human endeavors, one size rarely fits all.

Despite these difficulties, empirical approaches have yielded high levels of success for the human, most economically important domesticated livestock and some laboratory and companion mammals. Usually, about half the sperm population survives after thawing. Any decrease in the fertility of thawed sperm suspensions can be compensated by inseminating females with higher numbers of sperm. The number of thawed spermatozoa inseminated is often adjusted to 5–10-fold higher than that used for fresh spermatozoa (77).

Comparisons of species effects on the efficiency of sperm cryopreservation are not possible because only a single offspring has been produced for many species listed in Table 2. The usual strategy for developing a cryopreservation procedure for spermatozoa from a new species is to select a successful protocol for a taxonomically-related species ("model species") and empirically modify it until acceptable post-thaw motility and then fertility is obtained (90).

Mammalian Oocytes

The cryopreservation of mammalian oocytes would greatly assist the application of several reproductive biotechnologies, such as in vitro production of embryos (54), treatment of infertility (91), cloning (92), and gene banking (90). Because immature oocytes at the germinal vesicle (GV) stage are often difficult to mature in vitro and most applications require mature oocytes, oocyte cryopreservation efforts have focused on the metaphase II (MII) stage. Several features of mature oocytes may present problems during cryopreservation. First, mature oocytes are among the largest cells in mammals and their spherical geometry yields a low surface area to volume ratio. Both properties act to limit the permeation of cryoprotectants and water into and out of the oocyte (48). Second, mature oocytes of most mammals arrest with chromosomes aligned on the MII spindle, cortical granules positioned immediately adjacent to the plasma membrane, and cytoskeletal elements associated with the spindle and cortical regions. Maintenance of these cytological features until the time of fertilization is required for normal developmental processes. Unfortunately, many reports indicate that these and other features are changed by cooling to subambient temperatures or equilibration with cryoprotective solutes (93,94).

Despite these difficulties, considerable progress has been made in the past decade on the cryopreservation of mouse oocytes. Thousands of normal late-stage fetuses and offspring have been produced from cryopreserved mouse oocytes following IVF and embryo transfer. The efficiency of the process is high and rates of development to normal pups after slow freezing and vitrification procedures are reportedly similar to that using control oocytes (95,96). This result has been confirmed in two recent reports that further suggest a small but significant detrimental effect of the presence of sodium in cryoprotectant solutions (97,98). Unfortunately, the beneficial effect of replacing sodium with choline is based on in vitro development of thawed oocytes to blastocysts after IVF.

Full confirmation of a beneficial effect of reducing sodium concentrations during oocyte cryopreservation awaits further studies of in vivo development following embryo transfer.

Progress in developing reliable oocyte cryopreservation procedures for other species remains elusive. Most of the research has concentrated on mature oocytes of two species, cattle and human. Until recently, the percentage of thawed bovine oocytes yielding blastocysts and calves following IVF, in vitro culture, and embryo transfer has been low (respectively, 2–12% and 1–2%; *99–101*). Recent reports provide new optimism that improvements of the conditions of in vitro fertilization and culture and the use of ultra-rapid cooling procedures may significantly increase the efficiency of oocyte cryopreservation for bovine and other species *(36,39)*.

The first report of the successful cryopreservation of mature (MII) human oocytes resulting in a normal pregnancy and birth *(102)* was followed shortly after by two additional reports *(103,104)*. Human oocyte cryopreservation was not adopted into routine clinical practice because of low post-thaw survival, low rates of fertilization, and concerns of cytological damage *(105,106)*. A recent study report suggests that intracytoplasmic sperm injection (ICSI) may overcome some of the problems associated with hardening of the zona pellucida during cryopreservation and increase the rate of fertilization of cryopreserved oocytes *(107)*. Clinical trials of oocyte cryopreservation using improved slow freezing procedures and ICSI have yielded normal births, but the low numbers of oocytes and patients preclude an accurate assessment of improvements in efficiency over that of IVF *(91,108)*.

Cryopreservation of immature germinal vesicle (GV) oocytes may eliminate some risks of irreversible damage to the metaphase spindle and other cytological features of mature oocytes *(109,110)*. A major impediment to immature oocyte cryopreservation is the lack of effective procedures for in vitro maturation, with the possible exception of the mouse *(111)*. Mouse oocytes at the GV stage have been successfully cryopreserved by slow-freezing procedures and reportedly develop and fertilize in vitro at rates similar to those of control oocytes *(112)*. However, the rate of post-implantation mortality of embryos produced using cryopreserved GV oocytes was about double that of controls. The lower developmental competence of GV oocytes presumably reflects nonoptimal conditions for in vitro maturation, fertilization, and/or culture *(113)*. Similar studies in cattle have yielded calves from cryopreserved GV oocytes *(101,114)*, but the efficiency of the process was low. There is one report in the human of the successful cryopreservation of an immature oocyte and the birth of a normal baby *(91,115)*.

Ovarian Tissue

Cryopreservation of ovarian tissue offers a simple method for storing gametes *(116, 117)*. Ovarian tissue is a rich source of primordial follicles that are remarkably resistant to the stress of cryopreservation. The resistance of primordial follicles to cryoinjury is probably related to their small size, mitotic quiescence, and low metabolic activity. Indeed, the first report of the successful restoration of fertility of mice in 1960 used relatively simple cryopreservation procedures *(118)*, before our current understanding of the mechanisms of cryoinjury and cryoprotection and 12 years before the first successful transfer of cryopreserved mouse embryos. Transplantation of fresh and cryopreserved ovarian tissue is an established procedure in the mouse for research and practical applications *(119–121)*. Cryopreserved ovarian tissue has also restored fertility following autologous transplantation in only one other species, the sheep *(122,123)*.

Cryopreserved ovarian tissue from cats, marmosets, African elephants, and the human has been reported to yield morphologically normal antral follicles following transplantation to immunodeficient mice *(124–127)*. However, none of the antral follicles present at the time of cryopreservation developed after thawing indicating a high susceptibility of these larger structures to cryoinjury. It is interesting to note that a variable latency period was required before new antral follicles were recruited from primordial follicles in transplanted ovarian tissue.

Clinical applications of ovarian tissue cryopreservation are limited by several considerations. First, the risks of transplantation (especially viral infection, immunosuppression, and rejection) will probably limit clinical uses to autologous transplantation. One proposed application of ovarian tissue cryopreservation, restoration of fertility following chemo- or radiation therapy for malignant cancer, is complicated by the risk of contamination of ovarian grafts with malignant cells *(128)*. Second, whole ovaries are too large to be cryopreserved with current cryopreservation technology. Immediate prospects are that wedges (about 2 cm^2 in area) or strips (about 1×10 mm) of ovarian cortex, known to be rich in primordial follicles, will be the most practical candidates for cryopreservation. One consequence is that the number of primordial follicles transplanted will be limited and fertility may be transient (<2 yr) unless sufficient numbers of grafts are preserved for multiple transplants. Recipients may exhibit signs of ovarian failure. For example, sheep receiving bilateral autografts of thawed ovarian tissue exhibited elevated levels of follicle stimulating hormone (FSH), a common sign that ovarian failure is incipient *(123)*. Third, many risks and ethical dilemmas associated with transplantation of cryopreserved ovarian tissue would be minimized if in-vitro maturation and embryo-production procedures can be optimized. The ability to recruit human primordial follicles and grow them in vitro to developmentally competent, mature oocytes is a formidable challenge. Current procedures in the mouse have been inefficient and have yielded few pups *(111)*.

SUMMARY

The cryopreservation and banking of gametes, embryos, and ovarian tissue provides a powerful method to control animal reproduction. The benefits of germ plasm cryopreservation originate from its ability to arrest all biological processes and place cells into a state of suspended animation for any desired period of time.

Considerable progress has been made in applying sperm and embryo cryopreservation to mammalian species. The difficulty in applying sperm and embryo cryopreservation to species not listed in Tables 1 and 2 likely results from an inadequate understanding of the reproductive physiology of other species (e.g., uncertainty of when and where to deposit the spermatozoa during artificial insemination). In some species, the specific cryobiological properties of the spermatozoa and embryos may require significant modifications of the cryopreservation procedures. Recent progress in developing alternative cryopreservation procedures (vitrification, ultra-rapid cooling) may assist in those instances.

The cryopreservation of MII mouse oocytes has been optimized and is ready for application. Unfortunately, oocyte cryopreservation is still inefficient or ineffective for other mammalian species. Some progress has been made in improving the survival of vitrified cattle oocytes using ultra-rapid cooling methods.

Ovarian tissue can be successfully cryopreserved using simple freezing procedures provided that the size of the specimen is small enough to minimize concentration gradients between the outer and innermost cells. Recent research indicates that antral follicles do not survive cryopreservation, but primary follicles tolerate cryopreservation. Transplantation of cryopreserved mouse ovarian tissue has restored fertility of ovariectomized recipients. Clinical applications of ovarian cryopreservation are limited by the usual risks of transplantation and probably be restricted to autologous transplantation.

REFERENCES

1. Polge C, Smith AU, Parkes AS. Revival of spermatozoa after vitrification and dehydration at low temperatures. Nature 1949;164:666.
2. Polge C, Rowson LEA. Fertilizing capacity of bull spermatozoa after freezing to −79°C. Nature 1952; 169:626–627.
3. Bunge RG, Keettel WC, Sherman JK. Clincial use of frozen semen. Fertil Steril 1954;5:520–529.
4. Whittingham DG, Leibo SP, Mazur P. Survival of mouse embryos frozen to −196 and −269°C. Science 1972;178:411–414.
5. Wilmut I. The effect of cooling rate, warming rate, cryoprotective agent and stage of development on survival of mouse embryos during freezing and thawing. Life Sci 1972;11:1071–1079
6. Mazur P. The role of intracellular freezing in the death of cells cooled at supraoptimal rates. Cryobiology 1977;14:251–272.
7. Mazur P. Stopping biological time: the freezing of living cells. Ann NY Acad Sci 1988;541:514–531.
8. Schiewe MC. The science and significance of embryo cryopreservation. J Zoo Wildlife Med 1991;22: 6–22.
9. Rall WF. Cryopreservation of oocytes and embryos: methods and applications. Anim Reprod Sci 1992; 28:237–245.
10. Rall WF, Mazur P, Souzu H. Physical-chemical basis of the protection of slowly frozen human erythrocytes by glycerol. Biophysical J 1978;23:101–120.
11. Rall WF, Reid DS, Polge C. Analysis of slow-warming injury of mouse embryos by cryomicroscopical and physio-chemical methods. Cryobiology 1984;21:106–121.
12. Rall WF, Fahy GM. Ice-free cryopreservation of mouse embryos at −196°C by vitrification. Nature 1985;313:573–575.
13. Becker D, Sevilla MD. The chemical consequences of radiation-damage to DNA. Adv Rad Biol 1993; 17:121–180.
14. Kaplan MI, Morgan WF. The nucleus is the target for radiation induced chromosomal instability. Radiat Res 1998;150:382–390.
15. Glenister PH, Whittingham DG, Lyon MF. Further studies on the effect of radiation during the storage of frozen 8-cell mouse embryos at −196°C. J Reprod Fertil 1984;70:229–234.
16. Simione FP. Key issues relating to the genetic stability and preservation of cells and cell banks. J Parenter Sci Technol 1992;46:226–232.
17. Schaffer TW, Everett J, Silver GH, Came PE. Biohazard: virus-contaminated liquid nitrogen. Science 1976;192:25–26.
18. Schaffer TW, Everett J, Silver GH, Came PE. Biohazard potential: recovery of infectious virus from the liquid nitrogen of a virus repository. Health Lab Sci 1976;13:23–24.
19. Tedder RS, Zuckerman MA, Goldstone AH, Hawkins AE, Fielding A, Briggs EM, et al. Hepatitis-B transmission from contaminated cryopreservation tank. Lancet 1995;346:137–140.
20. Fountain DM, Schulz MC, Higgins N, Benjamin RJ. Microbial contamination of liquid nitrogen storage tanks. Transfusion 1996;36(Suppl):S175–S175.
21. Fountain D, Ralston M, Higgins N, Gorlin JB, Uhl L, Wheeler C, Antin JH, Churchill WH, Benjamin RJ. Liquid nitrogen freezers: a potential source of microbial contamination of hematopoietic stem cell components. Transfusion 1997;37:585–591.
22. Jones SK, Darville JM. Transmission of virus-particles by cryotherapy and multi-use caustic pencils: a problem to dermatologists. Brit J Dermatol 1989;121:481–486.
23. Jones SK, Darville JM, Burton JL. Viruses, skin-lesions, and liquid-nitrogen. Lancet 1995;345:1369.
24. Berry ED, Dorsa WJ, Siragusa GR, Koohmaraie M. Bacterial cross-contamination of meat during liquid nitrogen immersion freezing. J Food Protect 1998;61:1103–1108.
25. Rall WF, Meyer TK. Zonae fracture damage to mammalian embryos during cryopreservation and its avoidance. Theriogenology 1989;31:683–692.

26. Kasai M, Zhu SE, Pedro PB, Nakamura K, Sakurai T, Edashige K. Fracture damage of embryos and its prevention during vitrification and warming. Cryobiology 1996;33:459–464.
27. Pegg DE, Wusteman MC, Boylan S. Fractures in cryopreserved elastic arteries. Cryobiology 1997;34:183–192.
28. Goffin Y, Grandmougin D, Van Hoeck B. Banking cryopreserved heart valves in Europe: assessment of a 5-year operation in an international tissue bank in Brussels. Eur J Cardiothorac Surg 1996;10:505–512.
29. Gold LW. Formation of cracks in ice plates by thermal shock. Nature 1961;192:130–131.
30. Adams LH, Williamson ED. Annealing of glass. J Franklin Inst 1920;190:597–631.
31. Kroener C, Luyet BJ. Formation of cracks during the vitrification of glycerol solutions and the disappearance of cracks during rewarming. Biodynamica 1966;10:47–52.
32. Takeda T. Effect of thawing procedures on damage to zonae pellucidae of bovine ova frozen in plastic straws. Theriogenology 1987;27:284 (Abstract).
33. Shaw JM, Diotallevi L, Trounson A. Ultrarapid embryo freezing: effect of dissolved-gas and pH of the freezing solutions and straw irradiation. Hum Reprod 1988;3:905–908.
34. Kojima T, Hashimoto K, Ito S, Hori Y, Tomizuka T, Oguri N. Protection of rabbit embryos against fracture damage from freezing and thawing by encapsulation in calcium alginate gel. J Exp Zool 1990;254:186–191.
35. Gao DY, Lin S, Watson PF, Critser JK. Fracture phenomena in an isotonic salt solution during freezing and their elimination using glycerol. Cryobiology 1995;32:270–284.
36. Martino A, Songsasen N, Leibo SP. Development into blastocysts of bovine oocytes cryopreserved by ultra-rapid cooling. Biol Reprod 1996;54:1059–1069.
37. Vajta G, Booth PJ, Holm P, Greve T, Callesen H. Successful vitrification of early stage in vitro produced embryos with the open pulled straw (OPS) method. Cryo-Letters 1997;18:191–195.
38. Pollard JW, Leibo SP. Chilling sensitivity of mammalian embryos. Theriogenology 1994;41:101–106.
39. Vajta G, Holm P, Kuwayama M, Booth PJ, Jacobsen H, Greve T, Callesen H. A new way to avoid cryoinjuries of mammalian ova and embryos: the OPS vitrification. Mol Reprod Dev 1998;51:53–58.
40. Landa V, Tepla O. Cryopreservation of mouse 8-cell embryos in microdrops. Folia Biol (Praha) 1990;36:153–158.
41. Landa V, Slezinger MS. Production of transgenic mice from DNA-injected embryos cryopreserved by vitrification in microdrops. Folia Biol (Praha) 1992;38:10–15.
42. Lane M, Bavister BD, Lyons EA, Forest KT. Container less vitrification of mammalian oocytes and embryos: adapting a proven method for flash-cooling protein crystals to the cryopreservation of live cells. Nature Biotechnol 1999;17:1234–1236.
43. Teng TY. Mounting of crystals for macromolecular crystallography in a free-standing thin film. J Appl Cryst 1990;23:387–391.
44. Rogers DW. Practical Cryocrystallography. Methods Enzymol 1997;276:183–202.
45. Vajta G, Lewis IM, Greve T, Callesen H. Sterile application of the open pulled straw (OPS) vitrification method. Cryo-letters 1998;19:389–392.
46. Steponkus PL, Meyers SP, Lynch DV, Gardner L, Bronshteyn V, Leibo SP, Rall WF, Pitt RE, Lin TT, MacIntyre RJ. Cryopreservation of Drosophila melanogaster embryos. Nature 1990;345:170–172.
47. Rall WF. Factors affecting the survival of mouse embryos cryopreserved by vitrification. Cryobiology 1987;24:387–402.
48. Mazur P. Equilibrium, quasi-equilibrium and nonequilibrium freezing of mammalian embryos. Cell Biophys 1990;17:53–92.
49. Glenister PH, Rall WF. Cryopreservation and rederivation of embryos and gametes. In: Jackson I, Abbott C, eds. Mouse Genetics and Transgenics: A Practical Approach. Oxford University, Oxford, UK, 1999, pp. 27–59.
50. Leibo SP. Cryobiology: preservation of mammalian embryos. In: Evans JW, Hollander A, eds. Genetic Engineering of Animals. Plenum, New York, NY, 1986, pp. 251–272.
51. Leibo SP, Martino A, Kobayahi, Pollard JW. Stage-dependent sensitivity of oocytes and embryos to low temperatures. Anim Reprod Sci 1996;42:45–53.
52. Massip A, Mermillod P, Dinnyes A. Morphology and biochemistry of in vitro-produced bovine embryos: implications for their cryopreservation. Hum Reprod 1995;10:3004–3011.
53. Dinnyes A, Wallace GA, Rall WF. Effect of genotype on the efficiency of mouse embryo cryopreservation by vitrification or slow freezing methods. Mol Reprod Dev 1995;40:429–435.
54. Hasler JF. Current status and potential of embryo transfer and reproductive technology in dairy cattle. J Dairy Sci 1992;75:2857–2879.

55. Wilmut I, Rowson LE. Experiments on the low-temperature preservation of cow embryos. Vet Rec 1973;92:686–690 .

56. Bank H, Maurer RR. Survival of frozen rabbit embryos. Exp Cell Res 1974;89:188–196.

57. Willadsen SM, Polge C, Rowson LE, Moor RM. Deep freezing of sheep embryos. J Reprod Fertil 1976;46:151–154.

58. Whittingham DG. Survival of rat embryos after freezing and thawing. J Reprod Fertil 1975;43:575–578.

59. Bilton RJ, Moore NW. In vitro culture, storage and transfer of goat embryos. Aust J Biol Sci 1976; 29:125–129.

60. Yamamoto Y, Oguri N, Tsutsumi Y, Hachinohe Y. Experiments in the freezing and storage of equine embryos. J Reprod Fertil Suppl 1982;32:399–403.

61. Dresser BL, Pope CE, Kramer L, Kuehn G, Dahlhausen RD, Maruska EJ, et al. Birth of bongo antelope (Tragelaphus euryceros) to eland antelope (Traurotragus oryx) and cryopreservation of bongo embryos. Theriogenology 1985;23:190.

62. Zeilmaker GH, Alberda AT, van Gent I, Rijkmans CM, Drogendijk AC. Two pregnancies following transfer of intact frozen-thawed embryos. Fertil Steril 1984;42:293–296.

63. Pope CE, Pope VZ, Beck LR. Live birth following cryopreservation and transfer of a baboon embryo. Fertil Steril 1984;42:143–145.

64. Summers PM, Shepard AM, Taylor CT, Hearn JP. The effects of cryopreservation and transfer on embryonic development in the common marmoset monkey, Callithrix jacchus. J Reprod Fertil 1987; 79:241–250.

65. Balmaceda JP, Heitman TO, Garcia MR, Pauerstein CJ, Pool TB. Embryo cryopreservation in cyno-mologus monkeys. Fertil Steril 1986;45:403–406.

66. Dresser BL, Gelwicks EJ, Wachs KB, Keller GL. First successful transfer of cryopreserved feline (Felis catus) embryos resulting in live offspring. J Exp Zool 1988;246:180–186.

67. Wolf DP, VandeVoort CA, Meyer-Haas GR, Zelinski-Wooten MB, Hess DL, Baughman WL, Stouffer RL. In vitro fertilization and embryo transfer in the rhesus monkey. Biol Reprod 1989;41:335–346.

68. Hayashi S, Kobayashi K, Mizuno J, Saitoh K, Hirano S. Birth of piglets from frozen embryos. Vet Rec 1989;125:43–44.

69. Dixon TE, Hunter JW, Beatson NS. Pregnancies following the export of frozen red deer embryos from New Zealand to Australia. Theriogenology 1991;35:193 abstract.

70. Wenkoff MS, Bringans MJ, Embryo transfer in cervids. In: Renecker LA, Hudson RJ, eds. Wildlife Production: Conservation and Sustainable Development. AFES misc. pub. 91-6 University of Alaska, Fairbanks, AK, 1991, pp. 461–463.

71. Cranfield MR, Berger NG, Kempske S, Bavister BD, Boatman DE, Ialeggio DM. Macaque monkey birth following transfer of in vitro fertilized, frozen-thawed embryos to a surrogate mother. Therio-genology 1992;37:197.

72. Kasiraj R, Misra AK, Rao MM, Jaiswal RS, Rangareddi NS. Successful culmination of pregnancy and live birth following transfer of frozen-thawed buffalo embryos. Theriogenology 1993;39:1187–1192.

73. Morrow CJ, Asher GW, Berg DK, Tervit HR, Pugh PA, McMillan WH, et al. Embryo-transfer in fallow deer (dama-dama): superovulation, embryo recovery and laparoscopic transfer of fresh and cryopre-served embryos. Theriogenology 1994;42:579–590.

74. Lane M, Forest KT, Lyons EA, Bavister BD. Live births following vitrification of hamster embryos using a novel container-less technique. Theriogenology 1999;51:167, abstract.

75. Mochida K, Wakayama T, Takano K, Nogushi Y, Yamamoto Y, Suzuki O, et al. Successful cryopres-ervation of Mongolian gerbil embryos by vitrification. Theriogenology 1999;51:171, Abstract.

76. Watson PF. Recent developments and concepts in the cryopreservation of spermatozoa and the assess-ment of their post-thawing function. Reprod Fertil Dev 1995;7:871–891.

77. Holt WV. Alternative strategies for the long-term preservation of spermatozoa. Reprod Fertil Dev 1997;9:309–319.

78. Foote RH, Parks JE. Factors affecting preservation and fertility of bull sperm: a brief review. Reprod Fertil Dev 1993;5:665–673.

79. Graham JK. Cryopreservation of stallion spermatozoa. Vet Clin North Am Equine Pract 1996;12:131–147.

80. Farstad W. Semen cryopreservation in dogs and foxes. Anim Reprod Sci 1996;42:251–260.

81. Royere D, Barthelemy C, Hamamah S, Lansac J. Cryopreservation of spermatozoa: a 1996 review. Hum Reprod Update 1996;2:553–559.

82. Morrell JM, Hodges JK. Cryopreservation of non-human primate sperm: priorities for future research. Anim Reprod Sci 1998;53:43–63.

83. Duncan AE, Watson PF. Predictive water loss curves for ram spermatozoa during cryopreservation: Comparison with experimental observations. Cryobiology 1992;29:95–105

84. Curry MR, Millar JD, Watson PF. Calculated optimal cooling rates for ram and human sperm cryopreservation fail to conform with empirical observations. Biol Reprod 1994;51:1014–1021.

85. Henry MA, Noiles EE, Gao D, Mazur P, Critser JK. Cryopreservation of human spermatozoa. IV. The effects of cooling rate and warming rate on the maintenance of motility, plasma membrane integrity, and mitochondrial function. Fertil Steril 1993;60:911–918.

86. Karabinus DS, Evenson DP, Kaproth MT. Effects of egg yolk-citrate and milk extenders on chromatin structure and viability of cryopreserved bull sperm. J Dairy Sci 1991;74:3836–3848.

87. Thomas CA, Garner DL, DeJarnette JM, Marshall CE. Effect of cryopreservation on bovine sperm organelle function and viability as determined by flow cytometry. Biol Reprod 1998;58:786–793.

88. White IG. Lipids and calcium uptake of sperm in relation to cold shock and preservation: a review. Reprod Fertil Dev 1993;5:639–658.

89. de Leeuw FE, de Leeuw AM, den Daas JHG, Colenbrander B, Verkleij AJ. Effects of various cryoprotective agents and membrane-stabilizing compounds on bull and boar sperm plasma membrane integrity after cooling and freezing. Cryobiology 1993;30:32–44.

90. Wildt DE, Rall WF, Critser JK, Monfort SL, Seal US. Genome resource banks: living collections for biodiversity conservation. BioScience 1997;47:689–698.

91. Tucker MJ, Morton PC, Wright G, Sweitzer CL, Massey JB. Clinical application of human egg cryopreservation. Hum Reprod 1998;13:3156–3159.

92. Wolf DP, Meng L, Ouhibi N, Zelinski-Wooten M. Nuclear transfer in the rhesus monkey: practical and basic implications. Biol Reprod 1999;60:199–204.

93. Parks JE, Ruffing NA. Factors affecting low temperature survival of mammalian oocytes. Theriogenology 1992;37:59–73.

94. Van Blerkom J, Davis PW. Cytogenetic, cellular and developmental consequences of cryopreservation of immature and mature mouse and human oocytes. Microscop Res Tech 1994;27:165–193.

95. Carroll J, Wood MJ, Whittingham DG. Normal fertilization and development of frozen-thawed mouse oocytes: protective action of certain macromolecules. Biol Reprod 1993;48:606–612.

96. Bos-Mikich A, Wood MJ, Candy CJ, Whittingham DG. Cytogenetical analysis and developmental potential of vitrified mouse oocytes. Biol Reprod 1995;53:780–785.

97. Stachecki JJ, Cohen J, Willadsen S. Detrimental effects of sodium during mouse oocyte cryopreservation. Biol Reprod 1998;59:395–400.

98. Stachecki JJ, Cohen J, Willadsen S. Cryopreservation of unfertilized mouse oocytes: the effect of replacing sodium with choline in the freezing medium. Cryobiology 1998;37:346–354.

99. Fuku E, Kojima T, Shioya Y, Marcus GJ, Downey BR. In vitro fertilization and development of frozen-thawed bovine oocytes. Cryobiology 1992;29:485–492.

100. Zhang L, Barry DM, Denniston RS, Bunch TD, Godke RA. Birth of live calves after transfer of frozen-thawed bovine embryos fertilised in vitro. Vet Rec 1993;132:247–249.

101. Kubota C, Yang XZ, Dinnyes A, Todoroki J, Yamakuchi H, Mizoshita K, et al. In vitro and in vivo survival of frozen-thawed bovine oocytes after IVF, nuclear transfer, and parthenogenetic activation. Mol Reprod Dev 1998;51:281–286.

102. Chen C. Pregnancy after human oocyte cryopreservation. Lancet 1986;1(8486):884–886.

103. van Uem JF, Siebzehnrubl ER, Schuh B, Koch R, Trotnow S, Lang N. Birth after cryopreservation of unfertilized oocytes. Lancet 1987;1(8535):752–753.

104. Al-Hasani S, Diedrich K, van der Ven H, Reinecke A, Hartje M, Krebs D. Cryopreservation of human oocytes. Hum Reprod 1987;2:695–700.

105. Bernard A, Fuller BJ. Cryopreservation of human oocytes: a review of current problems and perspectives. Hum Reprod Update 1996;2:193–207.

106. Mandelbaum J, Belaisch-Allart J, Junca MA, Antoine JM, Plachot M, Alvarez S, et al. Cryopreservation in human assisted reproduction is now routine for embryos but remains a research procedure for oocytes. Hum Reprod 1998;13:161–174.

107. Kazem R, Thompson LA, Srikantharajah A, Laing MA, Hamilton MP, Templeton A. Cryopreservation of human oocytes and fertilization by two techniques: in-vitro fertilization and intracytoplasmic sperm injection. Hum Reprod 1995;10:2650–2654.

108. Porce E, Fabbri R, Seracchioli R, Ciotti PM, Magrini O, Flamigni C. Birth of healthy female after intracytoplasmic sperm injection of cryopreserved human oocytes. Fertil Steril 1997;68:724–726.

109. Frydman N, Selva J, Bergere M, Auroux M, Maro B. Cryopreserved immature mouse oocytes: a chromosomal and spindle study. J Assist Reprod Genet 1997;14:617–623.

110. Agca Y, Liu J, Peter AT, Critser ES, Critser JK. Effect of developmental stage on bovine oocyte plasma membrane water and cryoprotectant permeability characteristics. Mol Reprod Dev 1998;49:408–415.
111. Eppig JJ, O'Brien MJ. Development in vitro of mouse oocytes from primordial follicles. Biol Reprod 1996;54:197–207.
112. Candy CJ, Wood MJ, Whittingham DG, Merriman JA, Choudhury N. Cryopreservation of immature mouse oocytes. Hum Reprod 1994;9:1738–1742.
113. Eppig JJ, O'Brien MJ, Pendola FL, Watanabe S. Factors affecting the developmental competence of mouse oocytes grown in vitro: follicle-stimulating hormone and insulin. Biol Reprod 1998;59:1445–1453.
114. Suzuki T, Boediono A, Takagi M, Saha S, Sumantri C. Fertilization and development of frozen-thawed germinal vesicle bovine oocytes by a one-step dilution method in vitro. Cryobiology 1996;33:515–524.
115. Tucker MJ, Wright G, Morton PC, Massey JB. Birth after cryopreservation of immature oocytes with subsequent in vitro maturation. Fertil Steril 1998;70:578–579.
116. Wood CE, Shaw JM, Trounson AO. Cryopreservation of ovarian tissue: potential reproductive insurance for women at risk of early ovarian failure. Med J Australia 1997;166:366–369.
117. Oktay K, Newton H, Aubard Y, Salha O, Gosden RG. Cryopreservation of immature human oocytes and ovarian tissue: an emerging technology? Fertil Steril 1998;69:1–7.
118. Parrott DMV. The fertility of mice with orthotopic ovarian grafts derived from frozen tissue. J Reprod Fertil 1960;1:230–241.
119. Cox SL, Shaw J, Jenkin G. Transplantation of cryopreserved fetal ovarian tissue to adult recipients in mice. J Reprod Fertil 1996;107:315–322.
120. Candy CJ, Wood MJ, Whittingham DG. Effect of cryoprotectants on the survival of follicles in frozen mouse ovaries. J Reprod Fertil 1997;110:11–19.
121. Sztein JM, McGregor TE, Bedigian HJ, Mobraaten LE. Transgenic mouse strain rescued by frozen ovaries. Lab Anim Sci 1999;49:98–99.
122. Gosden RG, Baird DT, Wade JC, Webb R. Restoration of fertility to oophorectomized sheep by ovarian autografts stored at −196°C. Hum Reprod 1994;9:597–603.
123. Baird DT, Webb R, Campbell BK, Harkness LM, Gosden RG. Long-term ovarian function in sheep after ovariectomy and transplantation of autografts stored at −196°C. Endocrinology 1999;140:462–471.
124. Gosden RG, Boulton MI, Grant K, Webb R. Follicular development from ovarian xenografts in SCID mice. J Reprod Fertil 1994;101:619–623.
125. Candy CJ, Wood MJ, Whittingham DG. Follicular development in cryopreserved marmoset ovarian tissue after transplantation. Hum Reprod 1995;10:2334–2338.
126. Gunasena KT, Lakey JRT, Villines PM, Bush M, Raath C, Critser ES, McGann LE, Critser JK. Antral follicles develop in xenografted cryopreserved African elephant (Loxodonta africana) ovarian tissue. Anim Reprod Sci 1998;53:265–275.
127. Wood CE, Shaw JM, Trounson AO. Cryopreservation of ovarian tissue: potential reproductive insurance for women at risk of early ovarian failure. Med J Australia 1997;166:366–369.
128. Shaw JM, Bowles J, Koopman P, Wood EC, Trounson AO. Fresh and cryopreserved ovarian tissue samples from donors with lymphoma transmit the cancer to graft recipients. Hum Reprod 1996;11:1668–1673.

11 Satellite and Transport In Vitro Fertilization

Paul F. Kaplan, MD, Douglas J. Austin, MD, and Marsha J. Gorrill, MD

CONTENTS

INTRODUCTION
SATELLITE IN VITRO FERTILIZATION
TRANSPORT IN VITRO FERTILIZATION
CONCLUSIONS AND FUTURE CONSIDERATIONS
REFERENCES

INTRODUCTION

Celebrating 20 years of progressive advancement since the now-historic report of the first in vitro fertilization (IVF) birth by Steptoe and Edwards in 1978 *(1)*, IVF has become a standard therapy in the treatment of the infertile couple. Despite the remarkable progress in clinical IVF, many obstacles still remain in making this technology available to all couples who could benefit from its application. The high cost of IVF treatment and the relatively poor coverage of infertility services by health insurance in most of the US certainly head the list of these obstacles, but geographic limitations are an additional impediment for a large number of couples. The progressive complexity of the IVF laboratory with the inclusion of cryopreservation and micromanipulation equipment requires a high volume of cycles to justify the costs of both equipment and a highly skilled embryology staff *(2,3)*. All of these factors have created a need to make the IVF process more flexible in order to meet the requirements of a larger number of patients over a wider geographical area.

Successful IVF programs have found that the capacity of the embryology laboratory often exceeds that of the clinical program and have attempted to meet an expanded need for services by transporting either patients or gametes from distant sites *(4,5)*. Satellite IVF involves the stimulation and monitoring of patients according to a standard protocol at a site geographically distant from the IVF laboratory, with subsequent travel of the patient to the central program site for both oocyte retrieval and embryo transfer *(6)*. Transport IVF utilizes a similar model, but incorporates oocyte retrieval at the distant site with

From: *Contemporary Endocrinology: Assisted Fertilization and Nuclear Transfer in Mammals*
Edited by: D. P. Wolf and M. Zelinski-Wooten © Humana Press Inc., Totowa, NJ

the post-retrieval transportation of gametes to the centralized IVF laboratory for fertilization and later embryo transfer *(7)*. This review will summarize the benefits and challenges to patients, physicians, and IVF centers that utilize satellite and transport IVF programs.

SATELLITE IN VITRO FERTILIZATION

History and Development

The first report of satellite IVF in the US was Zarutskie *(8)* from the University of Washington program in 1988. Organizing nine sites in four states and Canada in the Northwest, this program utilized a rigid protocol including a 2-d on site training for participating physicians, standardized laboratory assays for endocrine testing, a specific algorithm for stimulation and cancellation, and travel of the patient to the IVF lab site for the final 1–4 d of monitoring in addition to oocyte retrieval and embryo transfer. Although pregnancy rates were not different between the central and satellite sites, a significantly greater percentage of satellite patients experienced canceled cycles (43 vs 22%) *(8)*.

Subsequent reports from the Mayo Clinic *(9)*, University of North Carolina, Chapel Hill *(10)*, Florida *(11)*, and Oregon *(6)* documented the use of more flexible stimulation protocols along with less rigid coordination of estradiol and ultrasound procedures. In addition, these programs demonstrated that monitoring of patients at the satellite site could be performed through human chorionic gonadotropin (hCG) administration without compromise in pregnancy rates. Our own experience in Oregon using a less rigid protocol has emphasized the satellite physician's understanding of his/her patient and has eliminated the difference in cancellation rates observed in other systems *(6)*. Satellite IVF has been reported from a limited number of programs in Europe and is also known as "travel IVF" *(5,12)*, European satellite IVF programs are organized similar to those in the U.S. Some programs even use a three-tiered approach with ovarian stimulation at a satellite site, oocyte retrieval at a different transport site, and fertilization and transfer at a third central site *(5)*.

Program Organization and Logistics

Successful satellite IVF requires both a coordinated set of protocols and a formal communication system between the satellite center and the central IVF laboratory site. Satellite physicians should have a working knowledge of advanced infertility treatments, gonadotropin stimulation, transvaginal ultrasound, and the management of complications including ovarian hyperstimulation syndrome. A commitment to a 7-d/wk laboratory and monitoring program is mandatory. Each satellite physician should have a minimum number of IVF cycles to maintain clinical competence. Regular meetings of all physicians and clinical staff at the central IVF site can greatly facilitate problem solving and communication.

An initial consultation for satellite patients is often performed at the main IVF campus for orientation, chart development, and trial embryo transfer *(6,9,10)*. Additional IVF screening, patient counseling, and informed consent, as well as stimulation and monitoring is performed at the satellite location under the standard protocol. Daily communication between the satellite site and central program during controlled ovarian stimulation is usually done by facsimile utilizing a standardized form with telephone consultation as needed. An IVF nurse coordinator at each satellite is in close contact with nursing personnel at the central facility as well as each IVF patient. After hCG administration (or sooner in some programs), couples travel to the central IVF program for the oocyte retrieval and additional treatment through embryo transfer. Follow-up care and all pregnancy management is then performed at the satellite center.

Benefits and Challenges of Satellite IVF

The benefits of satellite IVF to infertility couples are numerous. Patients can remain at home for the majority of their IVF cycle, significantly reducing the stress of IVF treatment. They can continue to work during stimulation and monitoring and minimize hotel and travel costs, reducing the expenses incurred during the cycle. In addition, the majority of their medical care continues in a familiar environment with their own personal physician. For many couples, these benefits may be the difference between taking advantage of IVF technology or foregoing further infertility treatment.

Benefits to physicians at satellite locations include greater participation in the assisted reproductive technologies (ART) and an expanded range of treatment options for their patients. Many satellite locations lack an adequate population base to support a full IVF laboratory. Without IVF available, couples may chose less effective treatment options such as surgery or repeated controlled ovarian hyperstimulation (COH)/intrauterine insemination (IUI) cycles. The laboratory requirements of a satellite IVF program generate the need for a complete endocrine testing system and a sophisticated andrology service. These features benefit other patients and improve the infertility care for the entire community.

The challenges of satellite IVF include patient convenience, communication, and cost. Although satellite IVF greatly reduces the inconvenience for patients, the process still requires potentially long distance auto or air travel, lodging away from home and family, and medical care with unfamiliar providers. As many programs move to blastocyst embryo transfer on d 5 or 6 after oocyte retrieval (*see* Chapters 8 and 9), patients will need to stay longer at the central location or make another trip for their transfer.

IVF patient communication is often difficult owing to the complexity of the process, and introducing new medical staff at the central site may compound this problem. Because of the geographical distances involved, even medical staff communication concerning ongoing changes in protocols between the central and satellite sites can be fraught with misunderstandings. Constant vigilance is necessary to minimize these communication problems and insure the best experience for each couple.

The cost of IVF will be greater for satellite patients owing to travel expenses, food and lodging away from home, and absence from employment. Our program has standardized medical costs for the actual IVF cycle at all sites, but additional nonmedical costs are inherent in the nature of the satellite concept. Every attempt needs to be made to minimize these expenses in order to allow the maximum number of infertile couples to take advantage of ART services.

Satellite IVF Results

Zarutskie et al. *(8)* at the University of Washington reported no difference in clinical pregnancy rates between satellite and central campus control cycles (Table 1). Although they found a significantly greater number of cycles completing oocyte retrieval among control vs satellite patients (78 vs 57%, respectively), there was no difference in the percentage of patients completing oocyte retrieval who proceeded to embryo transfer (95 vs 95%).

Milad et al. *(9)* at Mayo Clinic found no difference in cycle cancellation rate (13% satellite vs 23% central, respectively), mean number of oocytes per retrieval (7.0 vs 7.7),

Table 1
Satellite IVF Results

Author/ Reference	No. of satellite cycles	No. of central cycles	Satellite clinical pregnancies (%)	Central clinical pregnancies (%)	Significance
Zarutskie et al. (8)	72	175	20	20	NS
Milad et al. (9)	61	90	34	41	NS
Kaplan et al. (6)	54	222	33[b]	21[b]	NS
Talbert et al. (10)	500	394	15.6	15.0	NS
Roest et al. (5)	570	1637[a]	28.7	28.7	NS

NS, not significant
[a] Transport IVF cycles.
[b] Live births per retrieval.

or clinical pregnancies per retrieval (Table 1). Although they did observe a small difference in fertilization rate of oocytes between satellite and central clinics (74 vs 80%), they did not feel that this finding was clinically significant.

Kaplan et al. (6) at the Oregon Health Sciences University reported a 15% cancellation rate in both satellite and central cycle groups. There were no observed differences in mean number of oocytes per retrieval (16.4 satellite vs 15.3 central, respectively), mean peak estradiol level (3017 vs 2560 pg/mL), mean number of embryos achieved (9.8 vs 8.3), or number of live births per retrieval (Table 1).

Talbert et al. (10) at the University of North Carolina at Chapel Hill observed no difference in cycle cancellation rate (28% satellite vs 26% central, respectively) or clinical pregnancy rate per oocyte retrieval (Table 1). They also reported 62 satellite GIFT cycles compared to 35 central control cycles and again found no significant differences in cancellation or pregnancy rates.

A review of the current literature documents that transport IVF is more popular than the satellite approach in Europe. In one of only two publications on satellite IVF from Europe (5,12), Roest et al. (5) in Rotterdam, Netherlands demonstrated no difference in mean number of oocytes per retrieval (9.3 satellite vs 9.9 transport, respectively), fertilization rate (48.4 vs 51.5%), mean number of embryos per retrieval (4.5 vs 5.1), or clinical pregnancy rate (Table 1). The Rotterdam data are somewhat difficult to interpret as the satellite patients from other distant sites underwent oocyte retrieval at the transport clinic site rather than at a main campus, but still appear consistent with the U.S. experience in that no significant differences were noted among any groups. Bogdanskiene et al. (12) from Lithuania reported a 30.8% clinical pregnancy rate for patients selected for IVF and stimulated in Lithuania who then traveled to London with a Lithuanian physician for oocyte retrieval and transfer.

In summary, these results are consistent with the conclusion that satellite IVF does not compromise IVF success rates when compared to the central IVF laboratory program site. Although the use of a standardized protocol for all satellite sites is essential, patients may travel over long distances for oocyte retrieval, embryo culture, and transfer after satellite stimulation and monitoring with pregnancy rates equal to those achieved at a main campus program in a large population center.

TRANSPORT IN VITRO FERTILIZATION

History And Development

The concept of transport IVF developed in Europe and was first reported by Feichtinger et al. in Vienna in 1983 *(13)*. Whereas geographic and population density limitations in the United States generated the need for satellite IVF programs, European IVF centers found themselves instead with a different set of problems. High density urban populations within close proximity needed more clinical services than were available at traditional centers. Although IVF laboratory capacity was under utilized, limited clinical space for oocyte retrievals and related procedures resulted in unmet patient demands and long treatment delays. These needs generated systems for off-site oocyte retrieval with transport of the oocytes to a central IVF laboratory within 30–60 min. Successful transport IVF programs have now been reported from England *(14,15)*, Belgium *(16)*, Argentina *(17)*, The Netherlands *(5,18)*, Crete *(19)*, and Germany *(20)*, in addition to Austria *(13)*. Interestingly, transport IVF has not been an approach reported in the U.S. to date.

Variations on transport IVF include transport of only oocytes (in follicular fluid aspirates without examination or in culture media after isolation) or transport of both oocytes and sperm. Like satellite IVF, transport IVF programs still require travel from the clinic to the central IVF laboratory to transport the gametes and for subsequent embryo transfer.

Program Organization and Logistics

Transport IVF shares all of the requirements of satellite IVF including a successful central IVF program, standardized protocols, communication systems, equipment, and skilled infertility staff at the transport clinic site. Regular meetings, andrology laboratory services, and communications may actually be easier because the geographic distances are usually much shorter. Although many of the transport IVF reports do not refer specifically to an initial consultation visit at the central program, Kingsland et al. *(15)* in Liverpool note the requirement for counseling and maternal serum collection at the IVF laboratory before oocyte retrieval. Because embryo transfer is always performed at the central program, the logistics of trial embryo transfer and medical records may require this extra visit as in satellite IVF.

Controlled ovarian stimulation, monitoring, and hCG administration are again similar to satellite IVF. Oocyte retrieval is performed at the transport clinic and gametes are handled in a number of different ways. Some programs transport oocytes in follicular fluid without examination *(21)*, whereas others have an embryologist present at retrieval and transport isolated oocytes after transfer into culture medium *(16,21)*. Travel from the transport clinic to the central lab is required by either husband or an IVF team member for transportation of gametes. Temperature control of gametes is of utmost importance and has been attempted by husband transport (attached to male partner's chest) *(16)*, battery-powered heaters in insulated boxes *(16,17,21)*, car battery heaters in portable incubators *(14,15)*, and intravaginal capsules *(20,22)*. Elapsed time for oocyte transfer varied in reports from 30–185 minutes *(17,23)*. Sperm samples are most often obtained by the male partner at the central site when the oocytes are delivered but are sometimes transported separately *(17)*. All patients return to the central IVF laboratory program for embryo transfer, and subsequent follow-up and pregnancy care is performed at the transport clinic.

Table 2
Transport IVF Results

Author/ Reference	No. of transport cycles	No. of central cycles	Transport clinical pregnancies (%)	Central clinical pregnancies (%)	Significance
Roest et al. *(5)*	2207	3333	28.7	28.7	NS
Alfonsin et al. *(17)*	467	60	20.1	22.0	NS
Kingsland et al. *(15)*	26	26	42.3	30.7	NS

NS, not significant

Benefits and Challenges of Transport IVF

Transport IVF again shares many of the patient benefits of satellite IVF. Cost savings may not be quite as large because travel for gamete transport of more than 3 h may not be currently practical. Overall travel does not differ from satellite IVF since the gametes still must be delivered to the central IVF laboratory by either the male partner or another team member. In central IVF programs with limited clinical facilities, transport IVF may allow more patients to participate with a shorter waiting period for treatment.

The benefits of transport IVF for physicians and programs at the transport clinic sites may be even greater than with satellite IVF. Because the transport physicians perform the oocyte retrievals, they are more involved in the IVF process. As with satellite IVF, transport clinics benefit from expanded services to all patients and a smoother transition to IVF in the event of failure of conventional infertility treatment.

Current challenges for transport IVF include maximizing patient convenience, minimizing cost, and facilitating communication as for satellite IVF. The need for a skilled embryologist at the transport clinic for oocyte identification in some programs clearly adds to the cost of these services. Quality control is an even greater challenge in transport IVF. Pregnancy rates would be adversely affected if oocyte retrieval was less efficient under the care of physicians who had limited experience or volume of cases. Although results to date have been good, transport of gametes introduces another variable not found in the satellite IVF concept. Further research into the optimal methods for gamete transport and new technology for transport equipment will hopefully expand the horizons of this option.

Transport IVF Results

Roest et al. *(5)* compared transport IVF cycles with control cycles at the University Hospital of Rotterdam between 1989 and 1993 (Table 2). Oocytes were transported in follicular fluid aspirates without examination inside an insulated box and travel time ranged from 15–40 min. In this large series, they found no difference in mean number of oocytes retrieved (9.7 transport vs 9.3 central, respectively), fertilization rate (50.5 vs 48.4%), mean number of embryos per retrieval (4.9 vs 4.5), or clinical pregnancy rate.

Alfonsin et al. *(17)* in Argentina reported on the South American experience with transport IVF (Table 2). Oocytes were isolated and transported in culture media with the use of a battery-powered insulated box. Transport time varied from 45–185 min. They also observed no difference in mean number of oocytes retrieved (9.2 transport vs 7.4 central, respectively), fertilization rate (80.7 vs 78.0%), mean number of embryos per patient (3.8 vs 5.3), or clinical pregnancy rate per embryo transfer.

Kingsland et al. *(15)* in Liverpool compared transport IVF cycles with an equal number of controls from their conventional program (Table 2). Cycles were not randomized and oocytes were transported in follicular fluid without examination utilizing a car battery-powered transport incubator. Transport time was estimated at 40 min. They found a significantly lower mean number of oocytes retrieved from the transport site per patient (5.8 transport vs 8.0 central, respectively), but no difference between number of oocytes fertilized (70.8 vs 69.5%) or clinical pregnancy rate per cycle. In this small series, inexperience with oocyte retrieval may account for the lower number of oocytes obtained at the transport clinic and highlights one of the potential pitfalls in transport IVF.

In the only randomized clinical trial comparing satellite IVF with transport IVF, Coetsier et al. *(21)* from Gent, Belgium reported on 100 couples undergoing IVF with intracytoplasmic sperm injection (ICSI) in coordination with the Rotterdam group. Fifty patients were stimulated in Rotterdam and traveled to Gent for satellite IVF. A second group of 50 patients received oocyte retrieval in Rotterdam and oocytes were transported to Gent in follicular fluid aspirates without isolation. Transport time was estimated at 90–150 min. IVF with ICSI was then performed in Gent on the transported gametes. They found no difference in the mean number of fertilized oocytes (7.13 satellite vs 5.53 transport, respectively), the embryo implantation rate (17.7 vs 18.4%), or the clinical pregnancy rate per cycle (26 vs 36%). However, they observed a significantly different mean number of oocytes retrieved (10.8 vs 8.4), mean number of good quality embryos (4.6 vs 3.0), and mean number of embryos available for cryopreservation (2.7 vs 1.5). They conclude that IVF transport prior to ICSI does not affect oocyte fertilization and embryo implantation rates when compared to satellite IVF, but a negative effect on embryo quality cannot be excluded.

Sterzik et al. *(20)* from Munich reported on 72 couples completing 104 transport IVF with partial zona dissection (PZD) using intravaginal transport in plastic capsules. Oocytes were isolated, washed, and transferred to culture medium for transport with an estimated travel time of 90–120 min. The patient population consisted of a poor prognosis group who had all failed conventional IVF fertilization in the past. They observed a 20% fertilization rate with a total of 25 embryo transfers and 7 pregnancies (6.7% per cycle). Although intravaginal transport of gametes was successful, conclusions from this study are lacking due to absence of a control group for meaningful comparison to their very difficult patient population.

Transport IVF is an established, practical technique for gamete transport of 30–180 min. We could find no reports of transport IVF with travel time greater than 3 h. Pregnancy success rates are comparable to conventional and satellite IVF in several series *(4,15–17,21,24)*, including the large Rotterdam program *(5,25)*. Complications rates are low and comparable to conventional IVF with experience *(18)*. Although some reports have demonstrated a lower number of mean oocytes retrieved at the transport clinic as compared to the central program site *(15,21)*, this finding would be expected to decline in importance with adequate patient volume and continued transport physician experience with oocyte retrieval.

CONCLUSIONS AND FUTURE CONSIDERATIONS

Satellite and transport IVF are extensions of the assisted reproductive technologies that have a proven role in our field. They allow couples to take advantage of IVF treatment despite significant geographic barriers with a minimum of patient inconvenience and extra expense. They also allow the most efficient utilization of the highly sophisticated modern ART laboratory and can overcome the disproportionate capacities of clinical and laboratory services found in many European IVF programs. Whether satellite or transport IVF have distinct advantages over each other remains unclear at this time, and their indications clearly overlap in current reports. Satellite IVF remains the primary program option for couples who must travel more than 2–3 h by car with current limitations in gamete transport in studies to date.

The decision to use satellite or transport IVF as an alternative to establishing a separate IVF program will depend on a complex array of geographical, financial, and local considerations. The requirements for a highly skilled IVF team and a sophisticated, expensive IVF laboratory currently demand a minimum of 100 cycles annually for a separate IVF program to be cost-effective in the US. Physicians who are highly skilled in ovulation induction and transvaginal ultrasound follicle monitoring may participate in satellite or transport IVF with a much smaller volume of patients. Travel beyond 3 h from the decentralized site will favor satellite over transport IVF. As has been demonstrated in Europe, transport IVF will provide an excellent solution for shortages of clinical space for oocyte retrieval procedures at a central IVF laboratory site.

A new trend in this field in the U.S. has been the recent development of programs that offer satellite IVF laboratory networking. The concept of bringing the IVF program to the patient was first reported from Australia by Henessey et al. in 1989 (26). Although unreported in the literature to date, satellite IVF laboratory networking offers an adaptation of this concept with a mobile IVF lab, that comes to the satellite site on a periodic basis. Patients are scheduled in groups and the mobile IVF lab program brings all necessary laboratory personnel and equipment to the satellite clinic. Potential advantages include patient convenience, greater involvement of the satellite physicians in the IVF cycle, expert embryology staff with high-volume experience, and minimal financial outlay for the satellite center. Potential disadvantages include the reduced flexibility for patient scheduling with cycle grouping, high minimum patient volume requirements (e.g., 20 cycles at one time), limitations in physician oocyte retrieval and embryo-transfer experience at the satellite site, restrictions in scheduling frozen embryo-transfer cycles, and possible higher costs associated with moving IVF laboratory personnel and equipment. The overall feasibility of this new variation remains to be determined at this time.

The future of satellite and transport IVF programs is optimistic and developing rapidly. Managed care has made tremendous inroads in the U.S. and now frequently dictates the site of medical care. Patients are finding that their health insurance covers local services but not those considered "out-of-area." Satellite IVF allows some of the cost to be covered under these local restrictions and thus facilitates more couples to take advantage of this improving technology. Government regulation of IVF laboratories has already resulted in the development of many of the transport IVF systems in Europe (23,24). In the United Kingdom, each IVF clinic must be separately licensed by the Human Fertilisation and Embryology Authority with strict guidelines and a significant administrative workload. A satellite or transport IVF clinic can function under the umbrella of the central IVF laboratory and reduce the burden of these regulatory demands (24). In the U.S., the federal government has announced plans to further regulate IVF laboratories (see Chapter 12). Additional requirements for specifically credentialed personnel, laboratory certification, and administrative paperwork raise the very real possibility that many small programs may need to consolidate under satellite or transport IVF systems. The developing technology of in vitro maturation (IVM; see Chapter 4) of oocytes adds an additional incentive to the transport concept. If immature oocytes can routinely be harvested at the time of elective or incidental pelvic surgery or before cancer chemotherapy treatment for later use with IVM, the technology for transport of gametes will undoubtedly receive renewed attention around the world.

REFERENCES

1. Steptoe PC, Edwards RG. Birth after the replacement of a human embryo. Lancet 1978;2:336.
2. Gelety T, Surrey E. Cryopreservation of embryos and oocytes: an update. Current Opinion Obstet Gynecol 1993;5:606–614.
3. Paulson RJ. In vitro fertilization and other assisted reproductive techniques. J Reprod Med 1993;38:261–268.
4. Jansen CA, van Beek JJ, Verhoeff A, Alberda AT, Zeilmaker GH. In vitro fertilisation and embryo transfer with transport of oocytes. (Letter to the Editor.) Lancet 1986;8482:676.
5. Roest J, Verhoeff A, van Lant M, Huisman GJ, Zeilmaker GH. Results of decentralized in-vitro fertilization treatment with transport and satellite clinics. Hum Reprod 1995;10:563–567.
6. Kaplan PF, Gorrill MJ, Burry KA, Vos KL, Sherrill GM, Hollander JC. Satellite in vitro fertilization: the Oregon experience. Am J Obstet Gynecol 1995;172:1823–1827.
7. Plachot M, Mandelbaum J, Cohen J, Salat-Baroux J, Junca AM. Organization of human IVF centers on the basis of egg and embryo transportation. In: Feichtinger W, Kemeter P, eds. Recent Progress in Human In Vitro Fertilization. Cofese, Palermo, 1984, pp. 216–222.
8. Zarutskie PW, Kuzan FB, Moore DE, Soules MR, the University of Washington Satellite Physicians. An in vitro fertilization program using satellite physicians. Obstet Gynecol 1988;72:929–934.
9. Milad MP, Ball GD, Erickson LD, Ory SJ, Corfman RS. A successful assisted reproductive technology satellite program. Fertil Steril 1993;60:716–719.
10. Talbert LM, Hammond M, Bailey L, Wing R. A satellite system for assisted reproductive technologies: an evaluation. Fertil Steril 1991;55:555–558.
11. Williams RS, Drury K, Kipersztok S. Successful implementation of a regional in vitro fertilization program. J Florida Med Assoc 1994;81:106–108.
12. Bogdanskiene G, Masiliuniene J, Mehta J, Grudzinskas JG. Travel IVF: technology transfer to Lithuania. Hum Reprod 1994;4:135.
13. Feichtinger W, Kemeter P, Szalay S. The Vienna programme for in vitro fertilization and embryo transfer. A successful clinical treatment. Eur J Obstet Gynecol Reprod Biol 1983;15:63–70.
14. Aziz N, Taylor CT, Kingsland CR, Haddad N. First birth in a new transport in vitro fertilization program. J Vitro Fert Embryo Transfer 1991;8:362–363.
15. Kingsland CR, Aziz N, Taylor CT, Manasse PR, Haddad N, Richmond DH. Transport in vitro fertilization-a novel scheme for community-based treatment. Fertil Steril 1992;58:153–158.
16. De Sutter P, Dozortsev D, Verhoeff A, Coetsier T, Jansen CA, Van Os HC, Dhont M. Transport intracytoplasmic sperm injection (ICSI): a cost-effective alternative. J Assist Reprod Gen 1996;13:234–237.
17. Alfonsin AE, Amato AR, Arrighi A, Blaquier JA, Cogorno M, Feldman ES, et al. Transport in vitro fertilization and intracytoplasmic sperm injection: results of a collaborative trial. Fertil Steril 1998;69:466–470.
18. Roest J, Mous HV, Zeilmaker GH, Verhoeff A. The incidence of major clinical complications in a Dutch transport IVF programme. Hum Reprod Update 1996;2:345–353.
19. Fraidakis M, Mehta J, Gasparis P, Magarakis E, Anifanataki A, Grudzinskas JG. Transport IVF: a new concept. One year experience. Hum Reprod 1994;4:195.
20. Sterzik K, Rosenbusch B, Noss U. First pregnancies after intravaginal transport and partial zona dissection of human oocytes. Fertil Steril 1993;60:583–584.
21. Coetsier T, Verhoeff A, De Sutter P, Roest J, Dhont M. Transport-in-vitro fertilization/intracellular sperm injection: a prospective randomized study. Hum Reprod 1997;12:1654–1656.
22. Hewitt H. The intravaginal culture technique for supernumerary oocytes from gamete intrafallopian transfer. Hum Reprod 1991;6:76–78.
23. Balet R, Mehta J, Lower A, Wilson C, Grudzinskas JG. Transport in vitro fertilization: an old concept for the future. Assisted Reprod Reviews 1995;5:102–105.
24. Booker M. Transport in-vitro fertilization and embryo transfer. Br J Hosp Med 1993;50:369–370.
25. Verhoeff A, Huisman GJ, Leerentveld RA, Zeilmaker GH. Transport in vitro fertilization. (Letter to the Editor.) Fertil Steril 1993;60:187.
26. Henessey JF, Harrison KL, Fuller SM, Gutteridge BH, Wordsworth BA. Establishment of a visiting provincial in vitro fertilization (IVF) service. J Vitro Fert Embryo Transfer 1989;6:117–119.

12

The Assisted Reproductive Laboratory
Quality Control, Quality Assurance, and Continuous Quality Improvement in a Regulatory Environment

William Byrd, PHD

CONTENTS

INTRODUCTION

Since the birth of Louise Brown in 1978, over 300,000 children have been born worldwide because of in vitro fertilization (IVF) or assisted reproductive technology (ART) *(1)*. A conservative estimate suggests that if these successful live births represent about 1/5 of the total number of ART procedures, then approx 1.5 million ART cycles have been performed in the last 20 years. In the US, the most recent data from the Centers for Disease Control (CDC) for the year ending in 1997 reports a total of 24,582 babies born as a result of 71,826 ART cycles carried out using IVF, gamete intra gallopian transfer (GIFT), zygote intra fallopian transfer (ZIFT), frozen embryos, and donor oocytes *(2)*. Since the Society for Assisted Reproductive Technology (SART) first began data collection in 1985, there has been a dramatic increase in the number of ART cycles in the US and Canada and the percentage of cycles with a delivery has increased sixfold (Fig. 1) *(3–12)*. Examination of individual program success rates in the 1997 CDC data reveals a delivery rate that is highly variable from program to program. Possible reasons for these differences in delivery rates are numerous. Some programs may not follow the most effective follicular stimulation or treatment regimens. Patient selection varies from program to program. The skill levels and knowledge base of physicians and laboratorians are variable. Laboratories may not use the most efficacious insemination and culture techniques. Also, laboratories can lose embryos through mishaps or equipment failures. In addition to inherent errors, there have been numerous reports of mishandling of gametes

From: *Contemporary Endocrinology: Assisted Fertilization and Nuclear Transfer in Mammals*
Edited by: D. P. Wolf and M. Zelinski-Wooten © Humana Press Inc., Totowa, NJ

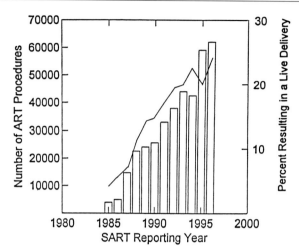

Fig. 1. Data complied from SART annual reports *(1–11)*. Bars represent the total number of ART procedures reported in a given year for the US and Canada. The line represents the percentage of these cycles that resulted in a live delivery.

or embryos, which have led to insemination of the wrong partner or implantation of embryos into the wrong patient *(13,14)*.

In the United States, there is no federal oversight on the laboratory practice of embryology (ART) because the Clinical Laboratory Improvement Amendment of 1988 (CLIA 88) did not include embryology as a high-complexity test. However, some high-complexity tests performed in ART laboratories, such as andrology and endocrine testing, are covered under CLIA 88. This means that there is some regulatory oversight of ART laboratories. Owing to concerns raised by both the public and by ART professionals, voluntary programs have been developed to address quality issues in ART. In response to the public need for information on the success of ART programs, the SART, a subsociety within the American Society for Reproductive Medicine (ASRM), developed a registry system in 1985. This registry system provided a mechanism for SART members to report and publish their results in a standardized fashion. The publication of this information on ART program success is now handled by the CDC. Because the ASRM is an educational body, it could not take on the responsibility of inspection and accreditation of ART laboratories. However, The College of American Pathologists (CAP) in cooperation with the ASRM developed a laboratory accreditation program for ART laboratories and began accrediting laboratories in 1992.

There has been considerable disagreement in the ART community as to whether or not embryology should be regulated by a mandatory government program *(15,16)*. The position of some members is that quality is not improved by either voluntary or government-mandated programs. Others argue that although negligence or human error cannot be eliminated in ART programs, mistakes can be examined, documented, and means to avoid them can be implemented. This latter group feels that mandatory standards are the best means to improve overall quality and service to the infertility community. Another issue is the ability of standards for practice to evolve rapidly enough to meet the onset of new technologies in the field. In this chapter, the role of quality assurance, quality control, and continuous quality improvement in the ART laboratory will be examined. In addition, the present and future regulatory environment and its effect on ART laboratories will be addressed.

Table 1
Internal QC of Sperm Morphology Using Kruger Strict Morphology[a]

	Slide 1	Slide 2	Slide 3	Slide 4	Slide 5
No. of cases	7	8	10	7	5
Minimum	8.000	0.000	2.000	4.000	19.000
Maximum	18.000	8.000	7.000	10.000	27.000
Range	10.000	8.000	5.000	6.000	8.000
Median	13.000	0.000	4.000	5.000	24.000
Mean	12.000	1.250	4.200	5.857	23.400
95% CI Upper	15.501	3.561	5.308	7.662	27.187
95% CI Lower	8.499	−1.061	3.092	4.052	19.613
Standard Error	1.431	0.977	0.490	0.738	1.364
Standard Deviation	3.786	2.765	1.549	1.952	3.050
Variance	14.333	7.643	2.400	3.810	9.300
C.V.[b]	0.315	2.212	0.369	0.333	0.130

[a] QC and ongoing training in the laboratory consists of determining the morphology of sperm using Kruger strict morphology. There is a set of 20 stained mounted slides that are kept specifically for this purpose. In this table are the multiple repeat readings of five of these slides by one technician. Data is analyzed for both intra- and inter-assay variation among all technicians. Morphology results are also traced for each technician and all technicians to determine if there are any trends in the data with time.

[b] Coefficient of variation (C.V.)

QUALITY CONTROL (QC), QUALITY ASSURANCE (QA), AND CONTINUOUS QUALITY IMPROVEMENT (CQI)

The goal of any ART program is to produce an environment in which patient care is optimized with the endpoint of a delivery of a healthy newborn after a cycle of treatment. The mechanism by which the laboratory reaches this goal is its overall QC, QA, and CQI program.

Quality Control (QC)

QC has been described by Diamond (18) as "a surveillance process in which the actions of people and performance of equipment and materials are observed in some systematic, periodic way which provides a record of consistency of performance and action taken when performance does not conform to standards which have been established in the laboratory." This surveillance mechanism requires that pre-existing standards or controls exist in the laboratory to serve as benchmarks and that records and documentation be kept of the surveillance. In the context of performing an assay, QC is a measure of precision of that laboratory. The ideal QC is to get the same result using the same analyte at different times and under different conditions. The goal of a QC program is to detect and correct deficiencies in any analytical process or procedure before that result is released.

QC can be divided into internal or external QC. Examples of internal QC could be control samples run with each endocrine assay, maintenance checks of machinery such as temperature and gas concentrations, determining sperm morphology using known slides, or calibration checks of equipment to ensure that they are running properly. An example of internal QC is seen in Table 1. In this case, there is a catalog of slides that have had their morphology determined by a skilled expert. Prior to analyzing patient specimens, technicians determine strict morphology on two blinded slides from the catalog.

Table 2
Results of Laboratories Participating in Strict Morphology Proficiency
Testing (PT) Offered by the American Association of Bioanalysts
(Second PT, 1988)[a]

Stain used	Number of labs	Mean percent normal	Standard deviation	Range
Diff quick	64	9.5	3.2	0–19
Papanicolau	15	15.8	5.3	0–32
Spermac	20	11.9	3.7	1–23
Wright giemsa	16	10.5	3.2	1–20

[a] The data presented here is taken from a PT test reported by the American Association of Bioanalysts from the second PT test in 1998. Only results for Kruger Strict Morphology are reported.

As long as their percent normal forms do not exceed two standard deviations of the known mean, they can then proceed with determining strict morphology on patient samples. On a monthly basis, all technicians are asked to read the same five blinded slides and these data are then recorded. Both daily QC and monthly review data are recorded and later analyzed for inter- and intra-technician variation. If kept for a long enough period, this data can be analyzed to determine if a particular technician or the entire laboratory has developed a drift or change in the way these reference slides are read.

External QC is a system by which unknown specimens are sent to the laboratory for evaluation. This external review is usually in the form of a proficiency test (PT). Alternatively laboratories can exchange specimens with each other to accomplish the same task. These tests, assays, or procedures must be run in the same manner as patient assays, if possible. PTs are a means of comparison between a laboratory's answer and the answer of all other laboratories performing the same assay with the same methodology. The ability of a laboratory to furnish an answer close to the group mean is a measure of accuracy. An example of PT is presented in Table 2. Because laboratories use different techniques, assays, and sometimes testing equipment, all PT is grouped by the technique used. In this case, only laboratories using strict morphology are grouped together. They are further divided into four different classes based on the type of stain used. Results are then submitted to and collated by the provider of the PT. If the analyte is graded, that is, you get a score of acceptable or unacceptable, then this information is provided to the laboratory and to the Health Care Finance Administration (HCFA) or its agent. If the answer is not graded, then based on the laboratory's procedure for evaluating PT, the laboratory director can determine if a successful result was obtained. If a PT is not acceptable, then there needs to be a determination of why the test was unsuccessful, and a plan of correction formulated. This review and itemization of any correction needs to be documented by the laboratory director or their designee.

QC in the ART laboratory is unique in that many of the procedures performed lack an immediate means of determining whether or not that process is in control. Some examples would be semen analysis and embryo culture. Previous studies have demonstrated that in andrology laboratories with trained personnel, there is a high degree of variation in the results of semen analysis performed in a single laboratory, and even more variability, between laboratories testing the same specimens (19–23). Reasons for this variation could be lack of standardization between laboratories, differences in training, and the absence of immediate controls. Fertilization, embryo culture, micromanipulation, and cryopreservation of gametes and embryos also lack immediate controls on the process. In addition, there are currently no recognized professional degree programs in this country that train individuals in human ART. This results in a loss of standardization.

There are several ways to address the absence of QC in a procedure. First, there must be commonly accepted laboratory standards and procedures in place. These standards and procedures provide a common point with which to develop an internal QC program. There also must be sufficient training of personnel and a mechanism to document this training. This training is usually the responsibility of a senior member of the lab who instructs the novice. For instance, in training the novice to count motile cells, the training period does not stop until the novice can count the same sample within an agreed upon difference (such as 95% confidence limits). Training a person to do intracytoplasmic sperm injection (ICSI) could consist of a series of steps that demonstrate that the novice can inject laboratory animal oocytes or nonviable human oocytes. Once they have reached a certain level of competency, they would be permitted to inject viable human oocytes. Training should not stop and it should be continued for all laboratory members on a regular and periodic basis. Although the ideal QC material should be processed or analyzed in the same fashion as patient samples, sometimes controls are less than ideal, e.g., daily QC for sperm counts with a known standard. Because samples (either immobilized sperm or small beads) are usually used for this control, they tend to be known, fixed amounts. This tends to put a bias in the system.

Quality Assurance (QA)

The concept of QA came after the development of QC and PT. QC and PT can be considered as the gold standards for controlling the analytical process and are an integral part of QA. The goal of QA was to expand beyond the analytical process to a consideration of all laboratory services involved in the delivery of patient care. As defined in CLIA 88 (17), QA is a program that is

"designed to monitor and evaluate the ongoing and overall quality of the total testing process (pre-analytic, analytic, post-analytic). The laboratory's quality assurance program must evaluate the effectiveness of its policies and procedures: identify and correct problems, assume the accurate, reliable and prompt report of test results and assure the adequacy and competency of staff. As necessary, the laboratory must revise policies and procedures based on the results of those evaluations. The laboratory must meet the standards as they apply to the services offered, the complexity of testing performed, and test results reported, and the unique practices of each testing entity. All quality assurance activities must be documented."

The development of QA came following the analysis of where error occurs in the testing of a sample. Surprisingly, only 7% of all laboratory errors occur in the analytical portion of the procedure (24). The other 93% of laboratory error occurs either in the pre-analytical or post-analytical portion of the process (Fig. 2). This suggests that the laboratory should focus not only on quality control of the process and proficiency testing, but also on development of a program that covers the pre- and post-analytical events. The pre-analytical portion includes a requisition of what is to be done with the specimen, patient instructions on proper specimen collection, the proper identification of the specimen

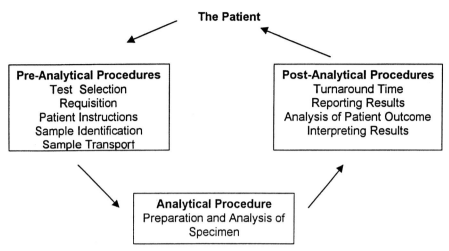

Fig. 2. Steps in the generation and application of a laboratory test.

with two unique forms of accompanying identification, the time of specimen collection and of receipt, and identification of who handles the specimen at all times. The analytical portion would include any analysis of the specimen and preparation for insemination. The post-analytical portion would include any action taken with the specimen, in this case, insemination. The turnaround time from receipt of the specimen until when the specimen is ready for insemination is analyzed on a routine basis to determine if patient needs are being met. The results have to be recorded, checked for errors, and reviewed by someone in the laboratory.

A good QA example is the chain of custody, processing, and preparation of a semen specimen that is to be used for insemination (Fig. 3).

Continuous Quality Improvement (CQI)

Following the development of QA, the next step by the laboratory industry was recognition that the laboratory is serving a customer and that customer care must be improved. Continuous Quality Improvement is composed of three areas:

1. Defining customers' expectations;
2. Describing and evaluating the laboratory processes; and
3. Continuously improving lab processes and outcome measures.

CQI can be defined as a continuous improvement process in the laboratory that is driven by customers' needs. The customer in this situation is not only the patient who benefits from the laboratory service, but also the physician who orders the test. Customers also include those organizations that may pay for any laboratory service such as managed care organizations and insurance companies. Once customer needs and expectations are known, then the laboratory processes can be streamlined and standardized. The next step is the reduction in error or variation in the process itself. Outcome data from the practice needs to be examined and appropriate action must take place to correct any problems. A goal or plan for the future must be initiated with specific objectives and timelines. These goals and how the organization meets them needs to be communicated throughout the ART practice. An ongoing part of the CQI program is creating in the laboratory a culture of customer service *(25)*.

Patient Test Management: Preparation of a Semen Sample for Intrauterine
Insemination

1. Patient receives written instructions regarding specimen collection prior to collection day. Written instructions are also posted in collection room.

2. Patients check into clinic on day of insemination
   Identities are verified and documented on requisition form
   Check schedule for procedure

3. Patient given label to fill out which is placed on specimen cup.

```
┌─────────────────────────────────────────┐
│    ANDROLOGY AND REPRODUCTIVE            │
│   ENDOCRINOLOGY LAB (214-648-2376)       │
│                                          │
│  NAME _____  │
│  SOC. SEC. #_____  │
│  TIME COLLECTED_____ DATE_____  │
│  PARTNER'S LAST NAME_____  │
│       IUI SPECIMEN CONTAINER             │
└─────────────────────────────────────────┘
```

4. Patient taken to collection room

5. Following collection, patient returns specimen in biohazard bag to a nurse who verifies ID and checks to see that specimen cup is labeled and that time of collection is noted.

6. Laboratory technician picks up specimen and requisition form from nurse

7. Requisition sheet is time/date stamped upon arrival in lab
   Patients name, date, time of collection, and time of receipt is put into specimen log. Entries reflect the technician who performs each step.

8. Specimen data is entered into Intrauterine Insemination sheet.
   Tubes for processing specimen are labeled with patient's identity and unique identifier number
   Specimen transferred to tube
   Label from specimen cup is transferred to Intrauterine Insemination sheet

9. Specimen is processed. Time of semen analysis and the time processing begins is entered into specimen log.

10. When specimen is prepared the Intrauterine Insemination sheet is date stamped.

11. Specimen is delivered to clinic, logged into Specimen Receipt Log (name, time, date, and technician), and placed in incubator. A copy of the

Fig. 3. Patient Test Management: Preparation of a semen sample for intrauterine insemination.

THE CURRENT REGULATORY ENVIRONMENT

United States (Federal Regulations and Laws)

As discussed earlier, existing lab QC, PT, QA, and CQI programs have evolved over the last 50 years. Currently then, why is there a need for government inspection and accreditation of laboratories? The simplest answer to this question is that only by external monitoring can we establish if standard operating procedures are being followed, if errors are being discovered and corrected, and if there is ongoing education in the laboratory.

Intrauterine Insemination sheet is left for the nurse or physician who will
perform the insemination.

12. The specimen is logged out by the person performing the insemination.

13. The patient is identified by the nurse or physician and it is documented on the
Intrauterine Insemination sheet. The tube with the prepared specimen and
the Intrauterine Insemination sheet with the patient's label are shown to the
patient for verification that the tube has the correct label and that the label on
the insemination sheet was made out by the partner.

14. The patient is inseminated

15. All data from the insemination is entered into the computer, which becomes a
permanent record.
A copy of the Intrauterine Insemination sheet is filed and saved for a minimum
of two years.

Fig. 3. (Continued)

The regulation of health industries, among others, is controlled in part by Federal
agencies such as the HCFA, Food and Drug Administration (FDA), and the CDC. These
agencies are sometimes referred to as the fourth branch of government. Proposed rules
or standards are published in the Federal Register. This is the first documentation of
potential laws. Once approved by congress and signed by the President, the final laws
become part of the Code of Federal Regulations (CFRs). These CFRs pertain to every
department of the federal government. Congressional and public concerns about the
quality of laboratory testing in the United States led to the development of two CFRs that
regulate the clinical laboratory (The Clinical Laboratory Improvement Act of 1967 and
the Clinical Laboratory Improvement Amendment of 1988 [CLIA 88]). The final rules
that implemented CLIA 67 were published on March 14, 1990. The final rules that implemented CLIA 88 were published on February 28, 1992. CLIA 88 expands federal oversight to almost all laboratories in the country that conduct testing on human specimens
for health assessment or the diagnosis, prevention, or treatment of disease. These final
rules can be further modified in the future by committee (CLIAC). The sets of rules, which
describe the laboratory requirements, are found in 42 CFR Part 493. There are five major
demands in CLIA 88.

PERSONNEL

These regulations cover the training, experience, and board certification required for
clinical laboratories. Staff performing high complexity or moderate complexity testing
must meet the personnel requirements for either the Director, Clinical Consultant, Technical Supervisor, General Supervisor, or testing personnel. Although qualified directors may
serve in all of these positions, they may delegate some portion of their duties and responsi-
bilities to others in the laboratory. The director is the person responsible for the laboratory
and has the overall responsibility for laboratory performance. The government has published, in CLIA 88, minimal educational standards for all positions, which implies that
more educated workers equal or result in higher quality laboratory performance.

QA/QC

There must be QC measures in place to ensure that the test results, answers, or procedures performed are accurate and precise. The laboratorian must establish that only

patient samples that fall within the reportable range of the test are reported. Controls need to be run with each shift (24 h) to ensure accuracy for quantitative tests. Qualitative tests require both a positive and a negative control. There has to be a comprehensive QA program in place that ensures there are procedure manuals with means of establishment and verification of method performance. Written procedures must be available. Procedures need to be approved, signed, and dated by the director; this documentation must be done on a regular basis. QA requires equipment maintenance and function checks. There must be a means to calibrate and verify calibration control procedure, remedial actions, and ensure adequate working facilities. The storage and disposal of materials used in the analyses must be defined. All lots of media or reagents must be labeled as to content, date of preparation or receipt by the lab, expiration date, and any other information necessary for use such as material safety data sheets (MSDS) labels. Documentation must exist on remedial action policies and procedures, and there has to documentation of any remedial actions taken. There must be mechanisms in place to detect errors. The laboratory must have a written QA plan, which provides for monitoring and evaluating the quality of the testing process.

PATIENT TEST MANAGEMENT

Each laboratory performing moderate- to high-complexity testing must maintain a system that provides for specimen preparation, collection, identification, preservation (if needed), transportation, processing, and finally analysis of the specimen. In addition, the laboratory must ensure that the test is appropriate for the patient. Tests may be performed only at the request of an authorized person. Oral requests must be accompanied by a written or electronic request within 30 d. Authorized persons are generally defined as individuals authorized under state laws to order tests. There must be oral or written instructions to patients on how to produce and transport specimens. Each laboratory must have written policies and procedures that cover all of these different steps. With such a series, the custody and identity of the specimen is critical, particularly when gametes are recovered, processed or manipulated in vitro, and then placed back into patients.

PROFICIENCY TESTING (PT)

CLIA 88 regulations stipulate that all labs must undergo successful PT testing to be considered qualified to perform testing. If PT testing is not available for a particular analyte, then each lab must develop its own and test at least twice a year. Failure to achieve a satisfactory score for two consecutive testing events or two out of three testing events is subject to sanction, which could include discontinuation of the assay until PT testing establishes the laboratory is in control. There are two HCFA approved providers of proficiency tests for reproductive laboratories; the American Association of Bioanalysts (AAB) offers PT tests for embryology and andrology, whereas the CAP offers PT tests for andrology.

REGISTRATION

Registration with HCFA is mandatory for clinical laboratories. Every lab must apply for or obtain either a certificate of waiver or a registration certificate, valid for a maximum of two years. Once the registration certificate is obtained, either the lab can receive a Certificate, if inspected by HCFA or its agents, or a Certificate of Accreditation by an accrediting agency with deemed status depending upon the type of testing offered. There are four major categories of testing. The regulations stratify the tests based on their technical complexity and the risk of harm in reporting an erroneous result. There are three categories of tests that are excluded from CLIA 88. These are 1) testing for forensic purposes, 2) research where patient-specific results are not generated, and 3) drug testing performed in laboratories that meet the National Institute of Drug Abuse guidelines and regulations.

The requirements for the four testing categories are listed in Table 3 and described in the following text.

WAIVED TESTS

The waiver allows a laboratory to perform waived tests. These tests are relatively simple assays that might be purchased over the counter such as urine dipsticks, blood glucose tests, pregnancy, and ovulation monitoring kits. Samples are not processed and are analyzed using a fully automated analyzer or self-contained system. The operator does not have to intervene or manipulate the assay. The waived tests are designed so that they yield no results if the test malfunctions or when the result is not in the reportable range of the test. The test requires little or no troubleshooting, and instructions must be written at a comprehension level no higher than seventh grade. These laboratories do not have to meet the CLIA requirements for moderate- to high-complexity and they are generally not inspected.

PROVIDER PERFORMED MICROSCOPY

These tests must be provided personally by a physician, dentist or midlevel practitioner, or physician assistant under the direct supervision of a physician during the patient's visit. The primary instrument for performing the test is the microscope. These specimens are usually labile, and a delay in performing the test could compromise accuracy. Control materials are used during the assay and little handling or processing is required. Examples of these tests are wet mount preparations, pinworm examinations, fern tests, urine sediment exams, and post-coital tests. These labs will have PT, patient test management, QA/QC, and are subject to random inspection.

MODERATE COMPLEXITY TESTING

All laboratories doing moderate-complexity testing must meet CLIA 88 standards, QC/QA, personnel requirements, and inspections. The testing methodology is generally an automated procedure that usually does not require reagent preparations. HCFA may conduct inspections at any time; however, these are usually announced and occur at 2-yr intervals. There can also be validation inspections. Sanctions may be imposed when laboratories are found not to comply with CLIA 88.

HIGH-COMPLEXITY TESTING

The same requirements apply as for moderate-complexity testing; however, the methodology of these tests is more complex and usually requires some sort of operator input into the test. An example of high-complexity testing would be semen analysis.

HCFA may impose sanctions against laboratories for failure to comply with the CLIA 88 requirements. These sanctions may be intermediate where there is a directed plan of correction with penalties of up to $10,000 per violation or per day of noncompliance. In addition, HCFA may suspend all or part of Medicare or Medicaid payment. HCFA may also impose a principal sanction of suspension, limitation, or revocation of a laboratory's certificate. In cases in which there is an immediate jeopardy to the public, HCFA may suspend the certificate before any hearing takes place.

Table 3
CLIA 88 Requirements for Obtaining HCFA Certification and Accreditation Based on Technical Complexity of Tests[a]

	Waived test	Provider performed microscopy	Moderate-complexity test	High-complexity test
Laboratory director	No stated requirement	Supervision by a physician required	MD, DO, or PhD BS or MS degree with training	MD, DO, or PhD
Complexity	Low	Low to moderate	Moderate	High
Personnel that can perform test without supervision	Staff with limited training	Physician, Dentist, midlevel prationer, or physician's assistant	Minimum high school degree with supervision	Minimum high school degree with supervision
Methodology	So simple and accurate as to render the likelihood of results negligible, or can do no harm if the test is erroneous	Primary instrument is the microscope. No control materials, specimen is sometimes labile	Varied, but generally assays do not require extensive intervention. Generally, kits and automated are employed	Requires operator intervention
Proficiency testing	Waived	As needed	Yes, for each analyte or test offered	Yes, for each test or analyte offered
Inspection	None	Subject to random inspection	Yes	Yes
Test examples	Dipstick, ovulation tests, urine pregnancy tests, blood glucose	Wet mounts, fern tests, post-coitals, urine sediments, qualitative semen analysis	Most endocrine tests	Semen analysis

[a] CLIA 88 requirements for obtaining HCFA certification or accreditation based on the technical complexity of tests.

Federal Action That May Result
in the Mandatory Inspection of ART Laboratories

In the late 1980s, Congressman Ron Wyden (Oregon) conducted public hearings regarding the conduct and possible oversight of ART programs. Owing to the concerns expressed by the public and Congress, Representative Wyden introduced the Fertility Clinic Success Rate and Certification Act of 1992. This bill became final on October 24, 1992 (Pub. L. 102-493, 42 U.S.C. 263a-1 et seq.), and requires that the Secretary of HSS, through the CDC, develop a registry of annual data on the pregnancy success rates of each ART program and on laboratory certification. This issue was addressed and published in a Federal Register notice (62 FR 45259, August 26, 1997). The second task for the Secretary was the development of a model program for certification of embryo labs. This model program has been developed and a proposal has been published (Federal Register, 63(215):60178-60189, 1998). Once the model program is in place, it would be distributed to the states for possible consideration and adoption. It is important to note that this is a voluntary program that may be adopted by the state; however, there is no way to force this program upon the state.

The Clinical Laboratory Improvement Advisory Committee (CLIAC) met with representatives from different professional societies regarding the classification of ART laboratories in 1998. Subsequently, the committee voted to recommend that embryology be classified as a high-complexity test, thereby imposing CLIA 88 requirements on embryology laboratories. This recommendation was then passed on to the Secretary of HHS for consideration, a decision that is pending in her office. In March of 1999, the AAB sued the Secretary of HHS. This suit asks the Secretary of HHS to follow the recommendation of CLIAC to classify embryology as a high complexity test.

Food and Drug Administration (FDA)

The FDA is developing regulations that would cover programs and/or people that procure or use reproductive tissue for reproductive purposes. If some of these proposed guidelines become regulations, it would mean that ART programs would have to register with the FDA and comply with a standard infectious disease control standard. These standards would be similar to those published as guidelines by the ASRM and the American Association of Tissue Banks.

State Regulation of ART Facilities

Several states have laws or codes in addition to Federal regulations. In California, there are laws for the prevention of sexually transmitted disease (Code 1644.5). California requires that all laboratory directors be licensed with the state. Unfortunately at this time, there is no mechanism to license PhDs who direct ART facilities. California requires that California-licensed Medical Technologists sign off on high complexity tests such as semen analysis. This puts an additional personnel burden on the laboratory if the director is not qualified.

Organizational Oversight of ART Facilities

ART laboratories that are part of larger institutions must also conform to organizational policy. Experimental procedures that may affect patient care must be approved by the local Institutional Review Board (IRB). These boards determine if the study is feasible and if it is of possible benefit to the patient. In most cases, a patient must sign a consent form if they are to be enrolled in an experimental program. What constitutes an experimental procedure? The Practice Committee of the ASRM has suggested that a procedure be considered experimental until at least two published manuscripts from two different laboratories prove that the procedure is useful in patient care. This Committee has been asked in the past to publish a Committee Opinion that declares that a particular procedure is no longer experimental. Often the push to rename an experimental procedure as a nonexperimental procedure is driven by insurance reimbursement. Generally, experimental procedures are not covered by insurance or are not reimbursed.

Organizations Involved in the Accreditation of ART Laboratories

An ART facility can be inspected and accredited in several ways. Because embryology is currently not classified under the complexity ruling of CLIA 88, ART lab inspection is voluntary. Because of this, there are only a few organizations that will inspect both embryology and andrology laboratories. There are several pathways for inspection and accreditation of a high-complexity laboratory.

First, the laboratory may be inspected and accredited by HCFA or one of its agents. In most states, the Department of Public Health has an accreditation/licensure department that can accredit a laboratory. An example would be the State of Texas in which the Public Health Department acts as agents for HCFA and performs all onsite inspections. A state can also decide that it wishes to run an accreditation program. To do so, the state must apply to HCFA and it may receive "deemed" status that permits the state to develop its own inspection/licensure program that must meet or exceed the requirements of CLIA 88. States with deemed status may allow organizations with deemed status to inspect laboratories in their state. The following states (with effective dates) have received deemed status: New York (1995), Oregon (1996), and Washington (1997). Some states, such as Georgia, have asked for a partial CLIA exemption that will only affect hospitals and independent laboratories, whereas others such as California and Florida have applied for deemed status.

The voluntary organizations that inspect and accredit laboratories are the CAP, the Joint Commission on Accreditation of Hospital Organizations (JCAHO), and the Commission on Laboratory Accreditation (COLA). The CAP was established in 1961 as a voluntary program for laboratory improvement through voluntary participation, peer review, education, and compliance with established performance standards. A peer-inspection program was developed specifically for andrology and embryology by the CAP in coordination with the ASRM. The Reproductive Biology Resource Committee, a committee of the CAP made up of CAP and ASRM members, used the practice guidelines developed for Andrology and Embryology Laboratories by the ASRM *(26,27)* as the basis for their program. These guidelines were developed into specific checklist questions to be used for inspection of ART facilities. The laboratory inspectors, deputy Commissioner, and Commissioner who run the program are members of the ASRM. The program is administered by the Laboratory Accreditation Program of the CAP. The Reproductive Laboratory Accreditation Program inspected its first ART laboratory in 1992. Since that time, over 220 ART laboratories have signed up for inspection and accreditation. COLA does not have a specific program at this time for the inspection of embryology. However, COLA will inspect smaller andrology laboratories. JCAHO is developing an inspection program for embryology laboratories.

FUTURE PROSPECTS

The development of embryonic and adult somatic cell cloning, cytoplasmic and nuclear transfers, stem cell isolation and culture, and pre-implantation genetic diagnosis, to mention a few areas, have raised both ethical and moral arguments. Typically, when the first successful use of a technique is published there is a great deal of attention. In the absence of any regulatory body, most universities, hospitals, and other organizations require laboratories to submit their proposed research for IRB approval. Practice guidelines to cover these new techniques can be developed by professional societies, but the development and publication of these documents can take years. In the absence of any federal regulation of ART laboratories and funding by the National Institutes of Health, there is, unfortunately, no federal oversight of new controversial areas. In this regulatory vacuum, the thought that some of these techniques, such as cloning, might be used on humans has stimulated the proliferation of many state-supported bills. Specifically, California has outlawed cloning, whereas Connecticut (HB 5042), New York (S 1179), South Carolina (HB 3036), Massachusetts (S 1399 and S 1394), New Jersey (A 329), and Virginia (HB752) all have pending legislation on cloning of humans.

SUMMARY/CONCLUSION

This chapter has reviewed some of the means by which ART facilities are regulated, or in some cases, not regulated, by state and federal government agencies. Although some aspects of ART remain unregulated, it is still important for the laboratorian to understand the concepts of QC, QA, and CQI. Once these concepts have been applied to the laboratory, they should make for a better laboratory environment and improve patient care. It is still possible at this time for a patient to undergo treatment involving ART in a laboratory that is not accredited, and in which there is little or no oversight over embryology. Although the mandatory regulation of embryology labs is not anticipated in the near future, approximately two-thirds of all ART laboratories have opted for voluntary accreditation. There are two options available to the patient; one is to choose a laboratory that has been accredited. If a lab is accredited, this does not necessarily guarantee success, but it suggests that at least a minimum review of the program has taken place. If the accreditation is from the CAP, then the inspection was done by a volunteer who was a peer and is familiar with ART. Alternately, the patient can choose a nonaccredited laboratory. Statistical data on IVF success rates in laboratories, although available, is usually two or more years out of date, and such rates for individual laboratories are not directly comparable for a number of reasons. Therefore, relying on past performance is not always a good indication of the potential quality of the laboratory. However, although patients cannot inspect the quality of a laboratory, inspection and accreditation offer the patient consumer the best treatment option because, if nothing else, the effort put into voluntary accreditation reflects a commitment to quality.

REFERENCES

1. ISLAT Working Group. ART into Science: regulation of fertility techniques. Science 1998;281:651–652.
2. 1996 Assisted Reproductive Technology Success Rates, National Summary and Fertility Clinic Reports, Center for Disease Control, Atlanta Georgia, http://www.cdc.gov/nccdphp/drh/art97.htm. 1999.
3. Medical Research International, The American Fertility Society Special Interest Group: In vitro fertilization/embryo transfer in the United States: 1985 and 1986 results from the National IVF-ET Registry. Fertil Steril 1988;49:212.

 4. Medical Research International, The American Fertility Society Special Interest Group: In vitro fertilization/embryo transfer in the United States: 1987 results from the National IVF-ET Registry. Fertil Steril 1989;51:13–20.
 5. Medical Research International, The Society for Assisted Reproductive Technology. In vitro fertilization/embryo transfer in the United States: 1988 results from the IVF-ET Registry. Fertil Steril 1990;53:13–20.
 6. Medical Research International, The Society for Assisted Reproductive Technology. In vitro fertilization/embryo transfer in the United States: 1989 results from the IVF-ET Registry. Fertil Steril 1991;55:14–23.
 7. Medical Research International, Society for Assisted Reproductive Technology (SART), The American Fertility Society. In vitro fertilization-embryo transfer in the United States: 1990 results from the IVF-ET Registry. Fertil Steril 1992;57:15–24.
 8. Society for Assisted Reproductive Technology, The American Fertility Society. Assisted reproductive technology in the United States and Canada: 1991 results from the Society for Assisted Reproductive Technology generated from the American Fertility Society Registry. Fertil Steril 1993;59:956–962.
 9. Society for Assisted Reproductive Technology, The American Fertility Society. Assisted reproductive technology in the United States and Canada: 1992 results generated from The American Fertility Society/Society for Assisted Reproductive Technology Registry. Fertil Steril 1994;62:1121–1127.
10. Assisted Reproductive Technology in the United States and Canada: 1993 results generated from the American Society for Reproductive Medicine/Society for Assisted Reproductive Technology Registry, Birmingham, AL. Fertil Steril 1995;64:13–21.
11. Assisted Reproductive Technology in the United States and Canada: 1994 results generated from the American Society for Reproductive Medicine/Society for Assisted Reproductive Technology Registry. Society for Assisted Reproductive Technology and the American Society for Reproductive Medicine, Birmingham, AL. Fertil Steril 1996;66:697–705.
12. Assisted Reproductive Technology in the United States and Canada: 1995 results generated from the American Society for Reproductive Medicine/Society for Assisted Reproductive Technology Registry. Fertil Steril 1998;69:389–398.
13. Robertson JA, The case of the switched embryos. Hastings Center Report, G1-7, Nov–Dec. 1995.
14. Van Kooij RJ, Peeters MF, te Velde ER. Quality control and quality assurance in IVF. Twins of mixed races: consequences for Dutch IVF laboratories. Hum Reprod 1997;12:2585–2593.
15. Keel BA. The assisted reproductive technology laboratories and regulatory agencies. Infertility Reprod Med Clinics North Am 1998;9(2):311–330.
16. Pool TB. Practices contributing to quality performance in the embryo lab and the status of laboratory regulation in the US. Hum Reprod 1997;12:2591–2594.
17. 42 Code of Federal Regulations, Ch. IV (10-1-96 Edition) Part 493.1701.
18. Diamond I. Quality control revisited. Pathologist 1980;34(7):333–336.
19. Dunphy BC, Kay R, Barratt CLR, Cooke, ID. Quality control during the conventional analysis of semen: an essential exercise. J Androl 1989;10:378–385.
20. Mortimer D, Shu MA, Tan R. Standardization and quality control of sperm concentration and motility counts in semen analysis. Hum Reprod 1986;1:299–303.
21. Freund M, Carol B. Factors affecting haemocytometer counts of sperm concentration in human semen. J Reprod Fertil 1964;8:149–155.
22. Clements S, Cooke ID, Barratt CLR. Implementing comprehensive quality control in the andrology laboratory. Hum Reprod 1995;10:2096–2106.
23. Matson PL. External quality assessment for semen analysis and sperm antibody detection: results of a pilot scheme. Hum Reprod 1995;10:620–625.
24. Sainato D. Proficiency testing: friend or foe? Clin Lab News 1997;24:1–5.
25. Corriveau B. Customer service in the clinical laboratory. Clin Lab Manage Rev 1993;7:49–55.

II   NUCLEAR TRANSFER

13 Somatic Cell Nuclear Transplantation in Cattle

James M. Robl, PhD

CONTENTS

INTRODUCTION

One of the primary goals of research in mammalian nuclear transplantation has been to develop a method of propagating valuable genotypes in species with agricultural value. This is of particular importance in cattle since generation interval and reproductive rate influence genetic progress. Cattle are a challenge in both areas because the generation interval is long, about two years, and reproductive rate is low, one calf per cow per year. Regardless, cattle are one of the most important agricultural species, economically, both in the United States and in the world.

A second important reason for developing procedures for nuclear transplantation in cattle is to use this method for genetic modification of cattle. Genetic modification would be important for improving the efficiency of meat and milk production for agriculture, and could be applied to the development of strains of cattle used to produce unique products, in large volume, for human health. Production of novel pharmaceutical proteins in milk is one well-known example *(1–3)*. Another is the production of proteins, such as human antibodies, in the blood of cattle. Furthermore, work is being done on the use of bovine cells for human therapeutics.

Development of a system for nuclear transplantation, that would allow genetic modification and large-scale propagation of cattle genotypes, involves several aspects. The first aspect is the development of and refinement in micromanipulation technologies. The second is an analysis of the cell biology of nuclear transplantation, including the

From: *Contemporary Endocrinology: Assisted Fertilization and Nuclear Transfer in Mammals*
Edited by: D. P. Wolf and M. Zelinski-Wooten © Humana Press Inc., Totowa, NJ

development of an understanding of nuclear reprogramming and an investigation of the consequences of combining two different cells into one. The third aspect is finding a source of donor nuclei that could be obtained in large supply and could support development of nuclear-transplant embryos to term. Finally, the cells used in nuclear transplantation should be capable of being genetically manipulated, particularly, of having DNA sequences inserted into selected sites in the genome.

TECHNICAL REFINEMENTS
IN NUCLEAR-TRANSFER TECHNOLOGY

Research on nuclear-transplantation technology in agricultural mammals was initiated in 1983 following a report in the mouse of a highly efficient, noninvasive method of pronuclear transfer (4). The method involved treating the embryos with cytoskeletal inhibitors and removing the pronuclei in a membrane-enclosed pocket of cytoplasm. Pronuclei, from another embryo, could be inserted into a recipient cytoplast using viral-mediated cell fusion. The technique was nearly 100% efficient and stimulated interest in the application of nuclear transfer for cloning in the larger domestic mammals. Several key modifications were made in the procedure and, soon thereafter, success was reported with a method that could be used to clone mammals of several different species (5–7).

The key modifications that were made consisted of using a mature oocyte as a recipient cell and the development of methods for enucleating the oocyte, use of electrically induced cell fusion, and activation of the oocyte to induce development of the nuclear-transplant embryo. These modifications, in addition to species differences, required extensive development and refinement of procedures and considerable effort at investigating the control of events during the first cell cycle of the embryo, which is critical for the success of nuclear transplantation.

Enucleation of the mature oocyte involved removal of the metaphase plate of the second meiotic division. Willadsen (5) chose a method that involved cutting the ovine oocyte in half and fusing a donor cell to each half. Only the enucleated half would develop properly and form blastocysts. In addition to fusing enucleated hemi-oocytes with donor cells in the bovine, Prather et al. (6) also used a technique in which the chromosomes were located by their proximity to the first polar body and were removed in a small cytoplast. Stice and Robl (7) were able to locate the chromosomes in the rabbit oocyte beneath the first polar body. Subsequently, Collas and Robl (8) verified enucleation of the rabbit oocyte by observing the chromosomes in the enucleation pipet. The most common method used currently is location of the chromosomes and confirmation of enucleation by labeling the DNA with a fluorescent dye (9). Other methods of enucleation have also been developed (10).

Sendai virus fusion methods that worked so successfully with the mouse were not effective for transplantation of nuclei to bovine or porcine oocytes (11,12). Electrically induced fusion has been highly successful with all species attempted. The mechanisms of electrically induced cell fusion and variables that affect the efficiency of cell fusion have been studied extensively (for review, see refs. 13 and 14). Overall, the primary factor that limits fusion, assuming that the voltage parameters are correct and the two cells are in contact, is alignment of the membranes to be fused. These should be parallel to the electrodes so that the current passes directly through the membranes. This is particularly difficult with current procedures that use very small somatic cells.

Activation of the oocyte is a process normally induced by the sperm. In nuclear transplantation this process must be done by an artificial stimulus. Although essentially nothing was known about activation in bovine oocytes when nuclear transplantation techniques were first developed, some information was available for mouse and hamster oocytes *(15,16)*. In these laboratory species, oocyte activation was mediated by a series of elevations in free intracellular calcium concentration. Many studies have been done in the past 10 years verifying that the sperm does induce oscillations in calcium in bovine ooctyes *(17)*, and that these oscillations are responsible for suppressing the elevated levels of H1 kinase activity in the oocyte *(18)*. This presumably results in a dephosphorylation of many different proteins and pronuclear formation. Electrical pulses were effective for inducing activation of the oocyte following nuclear transfer *(19,20)*. Electrical pulses induce pore formation in the oocyte membrane, allowing free extracellular calcium flow into the oocyte, causing increases in free intracellular levels of calcium *(19)*. The importance of multiple elevations in calcium as necessary for suppressing the levels of H1 kinase activity over a period of several hours during the first cell cycle were demonstrated in the rabbit oocyte. Further work on investigating the mechanisms of sperm-induced oocyte activation resulted in the development of chemical activation procedures that have been very successful in the cow *(21)*. The chemical methods act by inducing an elevation in free intracellular calcium concentration followed by the maintenance of low H1 kinase activity by the use of a phosphorylation inhibitor. Several methods of artificially activating oocytes are now available and appear to be quite successful. However, effort continues on developing methods that better duplicate the action of the sperm *(22)*.

The evolution of current techniques of nuclear transplantation, along with improved methods for oocyte maturation and embryo culture, allowed the development of large-scale cloning systems and improvements in the efficiency of cloning cattle. These improvements facilitated the production of large numbers of cloned cattle *(23)* but limitations, particularly that of using embryonic blastomeres, still restricted the numbers of animals that could be produced in a clonal line.

CELL BIOLOGY OF NUCLEAR TRANSFER

Czolowska and coworkers *(24)* and Stice and Robl *(7)* reported remodeling of the donor nucleus following nuclear transplantation in mammalian oocytes (*see* Chapter 14). Nuclear remodeling consisted primarily of nuclear swelling, but also a change in the morphology of the nucleolus, so that both the size and morphology of the nucleus resembled that of a pronucleus. Reprogramming of the developmental schedule was also reported in the rabbit *(7)*, wherein nuclear transplant embryos developed on a schedule similar to that of a pronuclear embryo and not on the schedule of the donor blastomere. The mechanism of nuclear reprogramming was hypothesized to involve an exchange of donor nuclear proteins with cytoplasmic nuclear proteins present in the metaphase oocyte (Fig. 1). This hypothesis was supported by data from Prather et al. *(25)*, who observed the exchange of nuclear lamin proteins in the pig. Likewise, Bordignon et al. *(26)* documented exchange of histone H1 variants in the cow, and Pinto-Correia et al. *(27)* demonstrated the loss of nucleolar fibrillarin in the rabbit.

The mechanism for remodeling of the donor nucleus has been investigated and involves, first, nuclear-envelope breakdown and premature chromosome condensation (PCC) in the donor nucleus, followed by chromatin decondensation and swelling of the

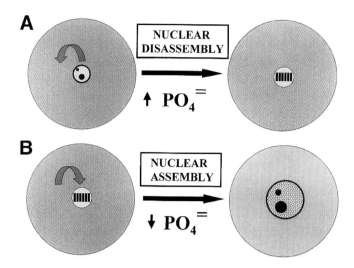

Fig. 1. Hypothetical mechanism of nuclear reprogramming. Nuclear reprogramming involves disassembly of the transplanted nucleus followed by reassembly of the transplanted nucleus into a pronucleus. (**A**) The process of nuclear disassembly involves phosphorylation of specific nuclear proteins by an M-phase kinase. (**B**) Reassembly of the nucleus occurs following activation of the oocyte and a decrease in phosphorylation owing to a decrease in an M-phase kinase and the action of phosphatases. Disassembly and reassembly involves a dilution and replacement of regulatory proteins from the transplanted nucleus by oocyte regulatory proteins.

nucleus upon activation of the oocyte *(28)*. Presumably, nuclear proteins are released at PCC with subsequent incorporation of oocyte nuclear proteins upon reformation of the nucleus.

PCC has been extensively described in somatic-cell fusion studies *(29,30)* that found that G1 and G2 nuclei display elongated, but essentially normal chromosomes when fused with mitotic cells. In contrast, induction of PCC in the S phase leads to incomplete condensation with both dispersed and condensed regions. These studies indicate that only nonreplicating chromatin can condense when placed in metaphase cytoplasm.

In light of the induction of PCC as a component of nuclear reprogramming, it was necessary to investigate the effect of the donor cell cycle on the response of the nucleus following transplantation into an oocyte. Would transplantation of an S-phase donor nucleus into a metaphase recipient cell oocyte cause irreparable damage to the chromatin, thus reducing developmental potential?

The influence of the donor cell-cycle stage on chromatin and spindle morphology has been investigated in the rabbit (Fig. 2) *(31)*. Within 2 h after fusion with the donor cell, the recipient oocyte cytoplasm was able to induce formation of a metaphase plate associated with spindle microtubules. Metaphase chromosomes and spindle microtubules were intact and normal, in most cases, in G1 transplants. However, these structures displayed minor abnormalities in early S-phase transplants and gross abnormalities in late S-phase transplants, such as incomplete chromosome condensation and incomplete or abnormal spindle microtubules. From observations of the metaphase chromosomes in embryos resulting from these nuclear transplants, G1-derived embryos displayed normal chromosomes; some abnormalities were observed in early S-phase transplants, and late S-phase, nuclear- transplant embryos displayed frequent chromosome abnormalities. Fur-

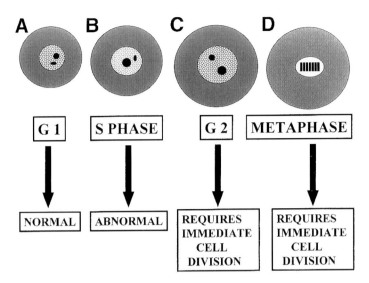

Fig. 2. States of the donor nucleus cell cycle and interaction with the recipient oocyte cytoplasm. (**A**) Following nuclear transplantation, G1 nuclei are able to undergo nuclear disassembly and chromatin condensation and form a normal embryonic nucleus. (**B**) Donor nuclei in S phase of the cell cycle cannot undergo normal chromatin condensation and form abnormal embryonic nuclei, resulting in decreased embryo viability. (**C**) and (**D**) Donor nuclei in G2 and M phase are likely to form normal condensed chromatin following nuclear transfer, but the oocyte must extrude half the DNA or the cell will be tetraploid.

thermore, induction of PCC in S-phase nuclei results in re-replication of DNA following decondensation of the chromatin and nuclear-envelope formation *(32)*. These results indicated that transplanting an S-phase nucleus into an unactivated oocyte is likely to result in chromosomal defects and impede development of the resulting embryos.

We investigated this hypothesis in the rabbit by transplanting G1, early S-, and late S-phase donor cells into oocytes and observing the rate of development to the blastocyst stage *(31,33)*. For G1/early S-phase donor blastomeres, 59% developed to the blastocyst stage; for mid S-phase blastomeres, 32% developed to the blastocyst stage; and for late S-phase blastomeres, only 3% developed to the blastocyst stage. These results confirmed our belief that the cell cycle of the donor nucleus is important for development of nuclear-transfer embryos. Unfortunately, the results also indicated that nuclear transfer with embryonic blastomeres would be of limited success because the cell cycle of early embryos consists mostly of S-phase, with G1 being only 15–30 min in length *(33)*.

SOURCES OF DONOR NUCLEI
FOR NUCLEAR TRANSPLANTATION

Development of a method for producing large clonal lines of cattle required an alternative source of donor cells. The ideal characteristics of these cells include that they 1) be relatively undifferentiated, 2) could be obtained in large numbers, and 3) had an inherently long G1 phase. The first choice was embryonic stem (ES) cells. ES cells are typically derived from the inner-cell mass of an embryo and are grown in a culture system that inhibits significant further differentiation. Because embryos and offspring had been produced from inner-cell mass cells *(34,35)* the expectation was that they could also be produced from ES cells. Furthermore, ES cells have been very useful in generating genetic modifications, both random insertions and targeted integrations, in the mouse (for review, *see* ref. *36*). This would also be a tremendous benefit for using ES cells in the cow.

Cells have been produced from bovine blastocyst inner-cell masses plated on top of mouse fetal fibroblasts. The characteristics of the cells were first described by Saito et al. *(37)*. A subsequent report demonstrated that inner-cell mass-derived cell lines could support development through organogenesis following nuclear transplantation *(38)*. More recently, Cibelli et al. *(39)* derived "ES-like" cells that were used to form chimeric cattle. Cells were cultured on mouse-fibroblast feeder layers and could be passaged indefinately without changing morphology. Unfortunately, the cells could not be clonally propagated nor efficiently transfected. Transgenic colonies were made by microinjection of individual cells and selection of colonies using G418. Use of these cells as nuclear donors resulted in a low rate of development to the blastocyst stage compared to fibroblast controls. Because of these limitations, other types of cells were investigated.

Somatic cells had been used for nuclear transplantation in previous studies. Collas and Barnes *(34)* injected granulosa cell nuclei into bovine oocytes and obtained blastocyst development, but not survival beyond 40 d of gestation. Furthermore, Campbell et al. *(40)* showed that cells derived from cultured embryonic cells, and displaying a somatic-cell phenotype, supported development of sheep nuclear-transplant embryos to term. Experiments in the cow indicated that fibroblasts supported development of nuclear-transplant embryos to the blastocyst stage. Furthermore, the blastocysts could be used to derive ES-like cells, which could contribute to many different tissues in the body *(41)*. Also, embryos derived from fibroblasts could support development of morphologically normal fetuses to d 45 of gestation *(42)*. Fibroblasts appeared to fit the aforementioned criteria of a cell type that might be ideal for nuclear-transplantation and development of cloned calves. Development of nuclear-transplant embryos, derived from both fetal and adult somatic cells, to term was first demonstrated by Wilmut et al. *(43)* in the sheep. Cibelli et al. *(39)* confirmed that fetal fibroblasts could support development to term in the cow. Several other studies have recently confirmed that somatic cells, of a variety of different types, from adult cows can support development to term *(44–46)*.

Offspring have been produced from different types of somatic cells in cattle. Cibelli et al. *(39)* used fetal fibroblasts, Kato et al. *(44)* used both cumulus cells and oviductal cells from an adult cow, Vignon et al. *(45)* used skin fibroblasts, and Wells et al. *(46)* used oviductal cells. Although the results of Kato et al. *(44)* indicate that cumulus cells may support a higher rate of development to term than oviductal cells, further work is necessary to make any definite conclusions about the characteristics of a cell type that allows them to support development following nuclear transfer. These recent results indicate that current methods, however inefficient, are sufficient for the production of clonal lines of cattle.

NUCLEAR TRANSPLANTATION
AS A METHOD FOR GENETIC MODIFICATION OF CATTLE

Several methods have been used to randomly insert genes into cattle. Genetically modified cattle have been produced in many laboratories using direct microinjection of pronuclei *(3)*. This approach, although feasible, is highly inefficient, therefore, it cannot be used to genetically modify high-value genotypes. A second method that has been attempted is based on the widely used ES cell system in the mouse. ES-like cells, produced from bovine embryos, have been genetically modified and chimeric calves with cells containing the transgene have been produced *(39)*. Two limitations of this method were observed. First, the ES cells were difficult to grow and passage, therefore, the genetic modifications were made by microinjection of the cells. This is only a modest advantage over pronuclear injection methods. This limitation was overcome by genetically modifying fibroblasts, using the fibroblasts in nuclear transfer and producing ES-like cells from the resulting nuclear-transfer embryos. A second limitation was that contribution of the ES-like cells to the germline, regardless of how they were derived, was not confirmed, so the modifications would not likely be passed on to offspring. Subsequent work demonstrated that fibroblasts could be used in nuclear transfer to produce offspring with a randomly inserted gene. Nuclear transfer was shown to be much more efficient than either pronuclear microinjection or use of ES-like cells and the technique could be used to insert a gene into a high-value genotype.

However, for applications in agriculture, random gene insertion has several drawbacks *(47)*. The site of insertion affects expression levels and, consequently, several transgenic lines must be produced to obtain one line with appropriate levels of expression to be useful. Because integration is random, it is advantageous that a line of transgenic animals be started from one founder animal and, with the inefficient microinjection approach, that animal is unlikely to be of specified genetics. The use of a single founder would avoid difficulties in monitoring zygosity and potential difficulties that might occur with interactions among multiple insertion sites *(48)*. However, if inbreeding is to be avoided, starting a transgenic line from one hemizygous animal with a random insert would require breeding several generations and significant time for introgression of the transgene into the population before breeding and testing homozygotes *(48)*. Even without concern for inbreeding, it would take 6.5 yr before reproduction could be tested in homozygous animals *(49)*. Finally, the quality of the genetics of a homozygous transgenic line would lag behind that of the general population because of the reduced population within which to select future generations of transgenic animals and the difficulty of bringing new genetics into a population in which the transgene is fixed.

An ideal system for producing transgenic animals for agricultural applications would, preferably, be insertion of the gene into a predetermined site. The specified site could confer high expression and not affect general viability or productivity of the animal. Furthermore, the identification of a locus for insertion would allow multiple lines to be produced and crossed to produce homozygotes. The ability to insert genes into a specified site would allow the integration of new genetics into the transgenic line at any time. Therefore, the development of methods for homologous recombination in cell lines from cattle that could subsequently be used in cloning would be of great benefit for both agricultural and biomedical uses of cattle.

Targeted insertion of DNA sequences by homologous recombination has been successful in rat and human primary fibroblasts *(50,51)*. Furthermore, elevated selection antibiotic was successfully used to produce homozygous insertions. However, for cattle the task of inserting DNA sequences by homologous recombination may prove more difficult. Fibroblasts collected from 40-d-old fetuses only have a life span of 30–35 population doublings *(39)*, and cells obtained from adult animals have a reduced life span of about 20–25 population doublings (unpublished observations). This has been sufficient for random insertion of a transgene in fetal-derived cells and selection of a clonal line of cells for nuclear transplantation and production of calves *(39)*. Although it was possible to produce clonal lines of transgenic cells from adult animals, no calves were obtained from over 500 nuclear-transfer embryos in one experiment. Although many factors could have been responsible for this result, the effect of cell senescence may have been involved. Because propagation of a cell line from a single, cloned, genetically modified cell requires 20 population doublings to produce 500,000 cells, two sequential rounds of selection would be a challenge.

CONCLUSION

Tremendous progress has been made in the development of procedures for the propagation of specific genotypes in cattle. With the use of somatic cell cloning it is now possible to produce large clonal lines of cattle. Furthermore, production of cattle with transgenes randomly inserted into the genome is now relatively efficient; opening up many possibilities for the production of novel products for human health care. One of the remaining challenges is the development of procedures for the targeting of DNA sequences into selected sites in the genome by homologous recombination.

REFERENCES

1. Ziomek CA. Commercialization of proteins produced in the mammary gland. Theriogenology 1998;49: 139–144.
2. Bremel RD. Potential role of transgenesis in dairy production and related areas. Theriogenology 1996;45: 51–56.
3. Wall RJ. Transgenic livestock: progress and prospects for the future. Theriogenology 1996;45:57–68.
4. McGrath J, Solter D. Nuclear transplantation in the mouse embryo by microsurgery and cell fusion. Science 1983;220:1300–1302.
5. Willadsen SM. Nuclear transplantation in sheep embryos. Nature 1986;320:63–65.
6. Prather RS, Barnes FL, Sims ML, Robl JM, Eyestone WH, First NL. Nuclear transplantation in the bovine embryo: assessment of donor nuclei and recipient oocyte. Biol Reprod 1987;37:859–866.
7. Stice S, Robl J. Nuclear reprogramming in nuclear transplant rabbit embryos. Biol Reprod 1988;39: 657–664.
8. Collas P, Robl JM. Factors affecting the efficiency of nuclear transplantation in the rabbit embryo. Biol Reprod 1990;43:877–884.
9. Westhusin ME, Pryer JH, Bondioli KR. Nuclear transfer in the bovine embryo: a comparison of 5-day, 6-day, frozen thawed and nuclear transfer donor embryos. Mol Reprod Dev 1991;28:119–123.
10. Bordignon V, Smith LC. Telophase enucleation: an improved method to prepare recipient cytoplasts for use in bovine nuclear transfer. Mol Reprod Dev 1998;49:29–36.
11. Robl JM, Prather R, Barnes F, Eyestone W, Northey D, Gilligan B, First NJ. Nuclear transplantation in the bovine embryo. J Anim Sci 1987;64:642–647.
12. Robl JM, First NL. Manipulation of gametes and embryos in the pig. J Reprod Fert Suppl 1985;33: 101–114.
13. Robl JM, Collas P, Fissore R, Dobrinsky JR. Electrically induced fusion and activation in nuclear transplant embryos. In: Chang D, Chassy BM, Saunders JA, Sowers AE, ed. Guide to Electroporation and Electrofusion. Academic, San Diego, CA, 1992, pp. 535–551.
14. Collas P, Fissore R, Robl JM. Preparation of nuclear transplant embryos by electroporation. Anal Biochem 1993;208:1–9.
15. Cuthbertson KSR, Whittingham DG, Cobbold PH. Free Ca^{2+} increases in exponential phases during mouse oocyte activation. Nature 1981;294:754–757.
16. Miyazaki S, Igusa Y. Fertilization potential in golden hamster eggs consists of recurrent hyperpolarizations. Nature 1981;290:702–704.
17. Fissore RA, Dobrinsky JR, Duby RT, Robl JM. Patterns of intracellular calcium concentrations in fertilized bovine eggs. Biol Reprod 1992;47:960–969.

18. Collas P, Sullivan EJ, Barnes FL. Histone H1 kinase activity in bovine oocytes following calcium stimulation. Mol Reprod Dev 1993;34:224–231.

19. Fissore RA, Robl JM. Intracellular Ca^{2+} response of rabbit oocytes to electrical stimulation. Mol Reprod Dev 1992;32:9–16.

20. Collas P, Fissore R, Robl JM, Sullivan EJ, Barnes FL. Electrically induced calcium elevation, activation and parthenogenetic development of bovine oocytes. Mol Reprod Dev 1993;34:212–223.

21. Susko-Parrish JL, Leibfried-Rutledge ML, Northey DL, Shutzkus V, First NL. Inhibition of protein kinases after an induced calcium transient causes transition of bovine oocytes to embryonic cycles without meiotic completion. Dev Biol 1995;169:729–739.

22. Fissore RA, Gordo AC, Wu H. Activation of development in mammals: is there a role for a sperm cytosolic factor? Theriogenology 1998;49:43–52.

23. Bondioli KR, Westhusin ME, Looney CR. Production of identical bovine offspring by nuclear transfer. Theriogenology 1990;33:165–174.

24. Czolowska R, Modlinski JA, Tarkowski AK. Behavior of thymocyte nuclei in nonactivated and activated mouse oocytes. J Cell Sci 1984;69:19–34.

25. Prather R, Sims MM, First NL. Nuclear transplantation in the pig embryo: nuclear swelling. J Exp Zool 1990;255:355–358.

26. Bordignon V, Clarke HJ, Smith LC. Effect of cytoplast cell cycle stage on the reprogramming of somatic histone H1 in reconstructed bovine embryos. Theriogenology 1998;49:178.

27. Pinto-Correia C, Long CR, Chang T, Robl JM. Factors involved in nuclear reprogramming during early development in the rabbit. Mol Reprod Dev 1995;40:292–304.

28. Collas P, Robl JM. Relationship between nuclear remodeling and development in nuclear transplant rabbit embryos. Biol Reprod 1991;5:455–465.

29. Johnson RT, Rao PN. Mammalian cell fusion: induction of premature chromosome condensation interphase nuclei. Nature 1970;76:151–158.

30. Rao PN, Johnson RT. Mammalian cell fusion: studies on the regulation of DNA synthesis and mitosis. Nature 1970;225:159–164.

31. Collas P, Pinto-Correia C, Ponce de Leon FA, Robl JM. Effect of donor cell cycle stage on chromatin and spindle morphology in nuclear transplant rabbit embryos. Biol Reprod 1992;46:501–511.

32. Campbell KHS, Ritchie WA, Wilmut I. Nuclear-cytoplasmic interactions during the first cell cycle of nuclear transfer reconstructed bovine embryos: implications for deoxyribonucleic acid replication and development. Biol Reprod 1993;49:933–942.

33. Collas P, Robl JM. Influence of the cell cycle stage of the donor nucleus on development of nuclear transplant rabbit embryos. Biol Reprod 1992;46:492–500.

34. Collas P, Barnes FL. Nuclear transplantation by microinjection of inner cell mass and granulosa cell nuclei. Mol Reprod Dev 1994;38:264–267.

35. Sims M, First NL. Production of calves by transfer of nuclei from cultured inner cell mass cells. Proc Natl Acad Sci USA 1994;91:6143–6147.

36. Doetschman T. Gene transfer in embryonic stem cells. In: Pinkert CA, ed. Transgenic Animal Technology. Academic, New York, NY, 1994, pp. 115–146.

37. Saito S, Strelchenko N, Niemann H. Bovine embryonic stem cell- like cell lines cultured over several passages. Roux's Arch Dev Biol 1992;201:134–141.

38. Stice SL, Strelchenko NJ, Keefer CS, Matthews L. Pluripotent bovine embryonic cell lines direct embryonic development following nuclear transfer. Biol Reprod 1996;54:100–110.

39. Cibelli JB, Stice SL, Golueke PJ, Kane JJ, Jerry J, Blackwell C, et al. Cloned transgenic calves produced from nonquiescent fetal fibroblasts. Science 1998;280:1256–1258.

40. Campbell KHS, Ritchie WA, Wilmut I. Nuclear-cytoplasmic interactions during the first cell cycle of nuclear transfer reconstructed bovine embryos: implications for deoxyribonucleic acid replication and development. Biol Reprod 1996;49:933–942.

41. Cibelli JB, Stice SL, Golueke PJ, Kane JJ, Jerry J, Blackwell C, et al. Transgenic bovine chimeric offspring produced from somatic cell-derived stem-like cells. Nature Biotechnol 1998b;16:642–646.

42. Zwada MW, Cibelli JB, Choi PK, Clarkson ED, Golueke PJ, Witta SE, et al. Somatic cell cloning-produced transgenic bovine neurons for transplantation in Parkinsonian rats. Nature Med 1998;4:569–574.

43. Wilmut I, Schnieke AE, McWhir J, Kind AJ, Campbell KHS. Viable offspring derived from fetal and adult mammalian cells. Nature 1997;385:810–813.

44. Kato Y, Tani T, Sotomaru Y, Kurokawa K, Kato J, Doguchi H, et al. Eight calves cloned from somatic cells of a single adult. Science 1998;282:2095–2098.

45. Vignon X, LeBourhis D, Chesne P, Marchal J, Heyman Y, Renard JP. Development of bovine nuclear transfer embryos reconstructed with quiescent and proliferative skin fibroblasts. Theriogenology 1999; 51:216.

46. Wells DN, Misca PM, Forsyth JT, Berg MC, Lange JM, Tervit HR, Vivenco WH. The use of adult somatic cell nuclear transfer to preserve the last surviving cow of the Enderby Island cattle breed. Theriogenology 1999;51:217.

47. Robl JM, Cibelli JB, Golueke PG, Kane JJ, Blackwell C, Jerry J, et al. ES cell chimeras and somatic cell nuclear transplantation for production of transgenic cattle. In: Murray JD, et al., ed. Transgenic Animals Agriculture. CAB International, Wallingford, UK, 1998.

48. Cundiff LV, Bishop MD, Johnson RK. Challenges and opportunities for integrating genetically modified animals into traditional animal breeding plans. J Anim Sci 1993;71(Suppl 3):20–25.

49. Seidel GE Jr. Resource requirements for transgenic livestock research. J Anim Sci 1993;71(Suppl 3): 26–33.

50. Mateyak MK, Obaya AJ, Adachi S, Sedivy JM. Phenotype of c-Myc-deficient rat fibroblasts isolated by targeted homologous recombination. Cell Growth Differentiat 1997;8:1039–1048.

51. Brown JP, Wei W, Sedivy JM. Bypass of senescence after disruption of p21 CIP1/WAF1 gene in normal diploid human fibroblasts. Science 1997;277:831–834.

14

Nuclear Modifications and Reprogramming After Nuclear Transfer

Randall S. Prather, BS, MS, PHD

INTRODUCTION

The birth of Dolly *(1)*, the first mammal cloned from an adult cell, has focused much attention, both scientific and public, on early embryo development, molecular biology, and genetic manipulations. Many scientific meetings over the past year have had, and in the next year will have, sessions devoted to cloning technology or to the ethics of cloning. This review is written with a focus on the normal course of nuclear modifications that occur during development and the changes that occur when a nucleus is transferred to the cytoplasm of an oocyte, as in the cloning process. This is written with a focus on nuclear transfer in domestic animals. Data from other species will be included where appropriate (*see* Chapter 6).

A few definitions early in this review will prove useful for the discussion later. Complete nuclear remodeling is defined as a complete change in the morphology of the nucleus, such that it appears to be a pronucleus in a zygote. Nuclear size, antibody reactivity, or a change in the appearance as visualized by TEM may measure these changes in morphology. Nuclear reprogramming, on the other hand, will be defined as a change in RNA synthesis such that the developmental sequence of differential RNA production (or lack thereof) is reset to the zygote stage. However, it should be kept in mind that complete remodeling or reprogramming during the first cell cycle might not be necessary for term development. This apparent dilemma will be discussed later in this review. A brief discussion of the normal course of nuclear transformations during early development will be followed by a description of the changes in nuclear structure and function that have

From: *Contemporary Endocrinology: Assisted Fertilization and Nuclear Transfer in Mammals*
Edited by: D. P. Wolf and M. Zelinski-Wooten © Humana Press Inc., Totowa, NJ

been observed after nuclear transfer. This will be followed by a review of the degree of development of nuclear transfer embryos, and finally a look to the future with questions that need to be answered regarding nuclear modifications.

CHROMATIN CHANGES
AT FERTILIZATION AND DURING DIFFERENTIATION

Fertilization-Induced Changes in Chromatin

The mammalian egg is arrested at metaphase II of meiosis. The maternal chromosomes are in a condensed state similar to what occurs during a normal mitosis. In contrast, during spermatogenesis the sperm are packaged with protamines rather than histones. Upon sperm entry into the cytoplasm, the protamines are released and oocyte-derived histones are assembled on the sperm chromatin. The maternal chromosomes separate as in mitosis, releasing the second polar body. Both sets of chromosomes are transformed into pronuclei and they migrate to the center of the oocyte. The pronuclei come into direct contact, pronuclear envelopes interdigitating. The compartments stay separated until the first mitotic division, when the pronuclear envelopes breakdown, and the paternal- and maternal-derived chromosomes intermix (syngamy) and then segregate to the two daughter cells.

Changes in Chromatin Function and Structure During Differentiation

In general, mammalian embryos produce little, if any, RNA during the first few cleavage divisions. The major onset of RNA synthesis occurs at a species-specific cell stage. RNA synthesis can readily be detected either directly or indirectly by the 2-cell stage in mice, 4-cell stage in pigs and humans, and the 8–16-cell stage in sheep and cattle *(2)*. In fact, prior to this stage there appears to be an active repression of transcription *(3)*. However, it is not clear which factor(s) are responsible for the transcription permissive stage *(4)*. There are many changes that occur in the structure of the chromatin that are temporally correlated with this change in transcription. Some of these include changes in the presence or absence of both peripheral and internal nuclear-matrix antigens that are associated with transcription *(5)*. Some specific proteins that have been identified that appear or dissappear during this time period include nuclear lamins *(6)*, small nuclear ribonuclear proteins (snRNPs) *(7)*, and somatic-type histones *(8)*. Some of the internal nuclear-matrix antigens, nuclear lamins, and snRNPs will be discussed later. To follow we present a detailed discussion of the structure and function of histones. This detailed discussion is included, in part, because very little is known about the changes in histone composition and structure during early development, and in part to stimulate more research in this area.

Histones are a group of water and dilute acid-soluble basic proteins found associated with DNA in chromosomes. They have high levels of the amino acids lysine and arginine. Histones can be acetylated, methylated, or phosphorylated. The model for chromatin packaging is a 200-bp segment coiled on the outside of a histone unit composed of $(H3)_2$ $(H4)_2$ tetramer and two each of H2a and H2b. This octomer (nucleosome) is linked to other octomers via histone H1. Histone H1 is phosphorylated during mitosis.

Nucleosomes can repress transcription and replication. Each strand of DNA in a nucleosome is inaccessible along most of its length in every helical turn *(9)*. Because most genes are longer than a single nucleosome, a mechanism must be in place to pass the transcription complex through the nucleosome. However, if a nucleosome covers a promoter, the transcription complex can not bind and initiate RNA synthesis *(10)*. Once transcription is initiated, then the position of the nucleosome complex can be altered, or removed; resulting in DNA that is more or less available to the transcription complex or even not packaged *(11,12)*. The result is dependent on the concentration of DNA relative to histones, and the rate of transcription.

Histone acetylation has been implicated in transcriptional regulation, cell-cycle progression, and chromatin assembly after DNA replication *(13)*. Acetylation of lysine residues near the NH2-terminus of histones is thought to regulate the accessibility of transcription factors to their enhancer and promoter sequences. Histone H4 is acetylated in the order lysine 16, then lysine 8 or 12, followed by lysine 5 *(14)* in somatic and embryonic stem cells *(15)*. These N-terminal tail regions of histones H3 and H4 play a critical role in the quartenary structure of chromatin *(16)*. Hyper-acetylation is correlated with transcriptional activity, because increased histone acetylation can facilitate the binding of some transcription factors, such as TFIIIA, to chromatin templates *(17,18)*. In contrast to the active X chromosome in female cells the inactive X chromosome is composed of less acetylated histone H4 *(19)*.

In early mouse and cow embryos, histone content and acetylation is correlated with gene expression. The first paper to suggest this was Clarke et al. *(8)*. In this study they affinity-purified antibodies with rat thymus histone H1 and found that this preparation did not recognize histones in 1- or 2-cell stage mouse embryos. It was not until the embryos reached the 4-cell stage that the antibodies cross-reacted with the nuclei. However, microinjection of somatic H1 did not alter early development *(20)*. Overall, mice contain at least seven nonallelic subtypes of H1, including the somatic variants H1a through H1e, the testis-specific variant H1t, and the replacement linker histone H1(o).

Adenot et al. *(21)* found that histone H4 was not hyeracetylated in sperm or meiotic metaphase II-arrested oocytes. However, immediately following fertilization, paternal, but not maternal, pronuclei had hyperacetylated histone H4. This is in contrast to parthenogenetically activated oocytes where the maternal pronucleus contained hyperacetylated histone H4. Further studies found that histone H4 is transiently acetylated (at lysine 5, 8, and 12) during the 2-cell stage of mouse embryogenesis *(22)* as is H3 (at lysine 9 or 18), and H2A (at lysine 5) at the nuclear periphery *(23)*. In contrast, H3 (lysine 14 or 23) and H2B, like H3 (lysine 16), remain distributed throughout the nucleoplasm. A transgene expressed in mouse 1-cell stage embryos was found to be positively correlated with histone H4 acetylated at lysine 5 *(24)*. In addition, inhibition of histone deacetylases with trapoxin increases endogenous gene expression in 2-cell stage mouse embryos *(25)*. Treatments that result in hyper-acetylation result in higher levels of gene expression in 1-cell stage mouse embryos *(21,26,27)* and reduce the requirement of enhancers for reporter gene expression *(28,29)*.

Similar to the mouse, immunoreactive somatic H1 in bovine embryos became detectable during the third or fourth cell cycle (4- to 8-cell stage) and this appearance was blocked by alpha-amanitin *(30)*. Levels of Histone H3 mRNA decrease from the 1-cell to the 8-cell stage in early bovine embryos, and then begin to increase twofold at the blastocyst stage *(31)*. However, the absolute level of histone H3 mRNA at the blastocyst stage is still less (~55%) than that of the unfertilized egg. In the mouse, the amount of histone H3 mRNA at the blastocyst stage was about the same as in the unfertilized egg *(32)*.

Histone changes during early development are not unique to mammals, because switching of histone H1 subtypes occurs in early embryos of sea urchins, sea worms, mud snails *(33)*, *Drosophila (34)*, and *Xenopus (35)*.

It is anticipated that this discussion will illustrate how little is really known about the structure of the nucleus as the embryo begins development. Clearly, further research is needed to elucidate the structural and functional changes that occur during even this short period of development.

CHROMATIN CHANGES
AND GENE EXPRESSION AFTER TRANSFER TO AN OOCYTE

The structure of the chromatin can be dramatically altered when exposed to the cytoplasm of an oocyte. This change in structure will be termed "nuclear remodeling." This is not to be considered synonymous with term development of the nuclear-transfer embryo. This change in structure is dependent on the levels of various kinases within the cytoplasm of the oocyte. The level of the kinase activity is generally dependent on whether the oocyte has been activated or is still arrested at metaphase II of meiosis. Later, we will discuss the consequences of changes in chromatin structure of using oocytes or pre-activated oocytes as recipients for nuclear transfer. A section will follow this on DNA synthesis and the benefits of serial nuclear transfer. Finally, these effects will be discussed in terms of specific gene expression.

Pre-Activated vs Metaphase II Oocytes

In many cases, nuclear transfer is performed by using a pre-activated or aged oocyte as a recipient cell. As will be discussed later, this is a good strategy when using donor cells in S phase or G2 phase of the cell cycle, but does not result in a complete remodeling of the transferred nucleus. A few examples will illustrate the point. The first example is that of the nuclear lamins. The nuclear lamins are a set of intermediate filament-type proteins that reside on the inner surface of the nuclear envelope and aid in anchoring the DNA to the nuclear envelope. In mammals there are three main types of lamins and they have been designated A, B, and C. They differ in molecular weight. Lamins A and C are identical except for an 82 amino-acid tail on lamin A. Lamin B has a distinct protein sequence. Nuclear lamins polymerize and depolymerize with the cell cycle. In metaphase they are distributed throughout the cytoplasm. Many studies have evaluated nuclear lamins using immunocytochemistry and the antibodies generally used do not discriminate between lamins A or C; thus they will be referred to as A/C. Lamins A/C are present in interphase nuclei in mice, pigs, and cows before the respective species makes the major transition from maternal control of development to the stage at which the embryo begins producing large amounts of RNA and begins to direct its own development (2-cell, 4-cell, and 8-cell stage, respectively *(6,36)*. If a nucleus beyond this stage of development, i.e., lamin A/C negative, is transferred to a pre-activated oocyte, then the transferred nucleus does not acquire the cytoplasmic lamins from the oocyte. This is in contrast to a nucleus transferred to an oocyte at metaphase II. Here the nuclear envelope is broken down (if only transiently) and the nucleus assembled using lamins from the cytoplasm of the oocyte *(6,37,38)*.

The second example is that of the nucleoli. The nucleoli are the sites of rRNA synthesis. Under transmission electron microscopy (TEM), the morphology of the nucleus can readily be determined and correlated with rRNA synthesis. A compact agranular, non-reticulated morphology is correlated with the absence of rRNA synthesis. In contrast a granular, reticulated morphology is correleated with active rRNA synthesis. This transition in morphology occurs during the 2-cell stage in the mouse, 4-cell stage in the pig, and the 8-cell stage in cattle. Nuclear transfer to a pre-activated or aged oocyte results in a change in the structure of the nucleoli, but not a complete transformation back to the agranular, nonreticulated morphology of the 1-cell stage embryo (39,40,41). This is in contrast to nuclear transfer to an oocyte in metaphase II of meiosis followed by egg activation where the nucleoli make a complete transformation (42–45).

The final example is that of nuclear swelling. Upon transfer of a nucleus to a metaphase II oocyte and activation, the transferred nuclei swell in diameter. In most cases the nuclei swell to a diameter that is similar to that of a zygotic pronucleus (46,47). However, when nuclei are transferred to an aged or pre-activated oocyte, the nuclei do not swell in diameter (47), unless sequentially treated with ionomycin and 6-DMAP (41). Presumably swelling is owing to the exchange of protein between the cytoplasm of the oocyte and the nucleus that serve to remodel the chromatin to be similar to the pronucleus of a zygote. Interestingly, if this swelling does not occur during the first cell cycle, it will not occur in subsequent cell cycles (48). The swelling appears to be correlated with levels of maturation promoting factor (MPF). When male pronuclear growth is evaluated in species that fertilize at the germinal vesicle (GV) stage, metaphase II, or the pronuclear stage, this relationship is clearly seen. In the surf clam, fertilization occurs at the GV stage. MPF levels oscillate with the condensed state of the chromosomes, i.e., at fertilization the male pronucleus does not grow until germinal vesicle breakdown (GVB) begins. During meiosis I and II, when the chromosomes are maximally condensed and (MPF) levels are the highest, the male pronucleus begins to shrink. After extrusion of the second polar body, both the male and female pronuclei resume growth (49). A similar pattern, although abbreviated, exists with fertilization at different stages of meiosis (50,51).

Overall, these changes in chromatin structure, depicted in Fig. 1, are dependent on the stage of the recipient cell. There appears to be a window of opportunity shortly before to shortly after activation of the oocyte in which these changes in chromatin structure are maximal (52,53).

Effects on DNA Synthesis

The cell cycle is composed of four broad phases, G1, S, G2, and M. G0 is another phase that is generally considered a subset of G1. G1 is the period after mitosis, but before DNA synthesis has been initiated. There is a restriction point in G1 at which cells will go into G0 if nutrients are limiting. DNA synthesis phase (S) follows G1. G1, G0, S, and G2 comprise interphase. Mitosis follows G2 and the cells divide to form two daughter cells. The total length of the cell cycle would be 16–24 h in rapidly dividing cell lines.

When the nuclear transfer is conducted at the same time as oocyte activation, there is a transient nuclear envelope breakdown owing to the high cytoplasmic levels of MPF. According to Blow and Laskey (54), this short period of nuclear instability would allow licensing factors to enter the nucleus, thus licensing the DNA to undergo replication (conversely, the nuclear instability could allow for certain factors to be released). This occurs regardless of the stage of the cell cycle. Thus after nuclear transfer, nuclei that were in G1 will undergo one complete round of replication, whereas nuclei that were in G2 also will undergo another complete round of DNA synthesis (55). This is not a problem for the

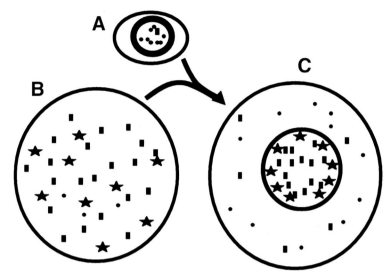

Fig. 1. Exchange of proteins during nuclear transfer. (**A**) Cell containing the donor nucleus. (**B**) Enucleated recipient oocyte. (**C**) Nuclear-transfer embryo after nuclear envelope breakdown and subsequent oocyte activation. Star, Nuclear lamins A/C; Dot, B core protein of the snRNP; Rectangle, Transcription repressing factors. After nuclear transfer and formation of the new "pronucleus" the nucleus acquires nuclear lamins releases transcript splicing machinery (snRNPs) acquires transcription repressors and assumes a transcriptionally repressed state.

nuclei transferred in G1, but the nuclei transferred in S or G2 become polyploid. The licensing factors do not, however, enter if the oocyte is pre-activated and MPF levels are low, likely because the nuclear envelope does not breakdown. In the nuclear-transfer embryos, resulting from oocytes with low levels of MPF, DNA content remains correct *(56–60)*, but remodeling is often incomplete (for example, *see* refs. *40,51,52*). Thus for complete remodeling a nucleus must be used that has not begun DNA synthesis (or entered S phase). A few studies do show better development after using nuclei in G1 vs S or G2 *(61,62)*. This is part of the basis for the claim by Wilmut et al. *(1)*; that a nucleus must be in G0 for the best development after nuclear transfer. However, Cibelli et al. *(63)* show that much effort toward cell-cycle synchronization may not be necessary.

Serial Nuclear Transfer

Many have shown that improved development results from some sort of serial nuclear transfer *(64–67)*. This serial nuclear transfer involves transferring a nucleus to an enucleated oocyte, followed by some period of development (hours to days). A nucleus from the developing nuclear-transfer embryo is then transferred to another enucleated recipient oocyte or zygote. Peura and Trounson *(68)* would classify some of these nuclear transfers as serial nuclear transfer and some as recycling. With sequential exposure to cytoplasm of either oocytes or zygotes, the resulting development appears to be improved. An indirect indicator of a more complete reprogramming is also provided by the expression of some of the TEC antigens (TEC-2, -4) *(69)*.

Nuclear Reprogramming and Gene Expression

Owing to the basic lack of information on the developmental expression of genes in domestic animals, there is a general lack of good information regarding the pattern of gene expression after nuclear transfer. One of the best studies evaluating the pattern of gene expression in nuclear-transfer embryos was by Schultz et al. *(70)*. Here they showed marked differences in mRNA content of IGF-1, IGF-2, and IGF-1R between normal and nuclear-transfer embryos. Some examples of indirect indicators of changes in gene expression are provided in this section, but first two examples from nuclear transfer in Xenopus will set the stage for the mammalian studies.

XENOPUS

Some excellent work was performed a number of years ago in frogs. Here I will list two examples of the specificity of the reprogramming that can occur after nuclear transfer. In frogs, genes for muscle-specific actin are turned on to begin RNA synthesis at a specific stage in the development of the myotome cells, but these genes can be turned off (RNA synthesis stops) after nuclear transfer. These genes are not only turned on again when the nuclear-transfer embryo reaches the correct stage of development, but they are turned on only in the developing myotome cells *(71)*. A similar regulatory control is seen with the $5S^{ooc}$ gene. The $5S^{ooc}$ gene is transcribed for only a short period during the late blastula stage, never to be seen again in development. Nuclei from neurulae-stage embryos (beyond the blastula stage) can express this gene again at the correct time if the nuclei are transferred to an oocyte and the resulting embryo develops to the blastula stage *(72)*. These results illustrate the regulatory control of cytoplasm of the oocyte on gene expression.

INDIRECT INDICATORS OF NUCLEAR REPROGRAMMING

Without direct measurement of the entire repertoire of mRNA synthesis at all developmental stages during normal development, as well as after nuclear transfer, complete reprogramming of the developmental program cannot be confirmed. Thus to follow are some indirect indicators of the reprogramming of the nucleus.

DEVELOPMENTAL OBSERVATIONS

One of the best indirect evidences of genomic reprogramming is a gross morphological recapitulation of development. One example from studies of early cattle embryos illustrates this point. The nuclei from a normally developing embryo at the 32-cell stage will, after 24 h, direct the development of the blastocoele cavity and formation of a blastocyst. If nuclear transfer does not reprogram the donor nuclei to recapitulate development, then 24 h after the nuclear transfer, these nuclei will attempt to direct the development of a blastocoele cavity while the nuclear transfer-embryo is only at the 2-cell stage. If this were to happen, the resulting embryo would likely form just the trophectoderm and not the inner cell mass, i.e., just a placenta without a fetus. On the other hand, if the nucleus is reprogrammed, then 24 h after nuclear transfer the nucleus should produce very little RNA and participate in cleavage to the 2-cell stage. After retraversing the early cleavage divisions, followed by compaction and blastocoele formation a few days later, the nuclear-transfer embryo would then be at the blastocyst stage and be suitable for transfer to the uterus of a cow 5–7 d after the onset of estrus. This example of the recapitulation of development, although the timing is not exact, is what occurs after nuclear transfer *(73)*.

CHANGES IN NUCLEAR ANTIGENS

Owing to the limited amount of material available, often the only way to evaluate nuclear reprogramming on early embryos is to indirectly evaluate changes in antigenicity of specific structures. A few examples will be provided here. The first deal with nuclear structure. The change in nuclear structure is illustrated by the change in antibody binding after nuclear transfer. Monoclonal antibodies (MAbs) I1 and Y12 bind to internal nuclear matrix antigens and a core protein (B) of the snRNPs, respectively. Both become detectable in the pig during the 4-cell stage and the appearance of Y12 is alpha- amanitin sensitive. After nuclear transfer using 8-cell nuclei, or beyond, the presence of each antigen is altered. For example, both I1 and Y12 disappear during the first cell cycle. This illustrates a change in structure, that can be interpreted as a change in function, i.e., there is no RNA processing because the snRNPs are no longer present (5,74).

Similarly, because there is a change in the composition of histone H1 during early development, it was tested in the bovine if a nucleus with somatic-type H1 would be modified after nuclear transfer to an oocyte. Bordignon et al. (75) showed that the somatic-type H1 disappeared after nuclear transfer, and that the rate of disappearance was dependent on the phase of the cell cycle of the oocyte. The fastest disappearance was in nuclei transferred to nonactivated oocytes. In addition, localization of fibrillarin to nuclei that are undergoing active transcription revealed that, for the most part, nuclear-transfer embryos recapitulate the normal pattern of localization (76).

The final indirect indicator of nuclear reprogramming is the appearance of the TEC antigens during bovine embryogenesis. Van Stekelenburg-Hamers et al. (77) show the stage-specific appearance of the TEC-3 antigen, and how the presence of the antigen during development after nuclear transfer is recapitulated. Trounson et al. (69) further show that serial nuclear transfer is necessary for complete recapitulation of the expression patterns of TEC-2 and -4.

Epigenetic Modifications

Little will be discussed in this section, because little is known. The reason for including this section is to not overlook other factors that may affect development of the nuclear-transfer embryos. These epigenetic factors include protein sources in culture media, mitochondria, histone acetylation (as discussed earlier), and DNA methylation. DNA methylation is perhaps one of the most interesting. However, it appears that nuclear transfer may actually result in few changes in DNA methylation (78). The methylation patterns appear to be established during gametogenesis and nuclear transfer may not change them. However, Dean et al. (79) present evidence that in vitro conditions may affect the methylation pattern. Thus further research is sorely needed in these areas.

SUMMARY AND FUTURE DIRECTIONS

The main concern for understanding the nuclear remodeling and nuclear reprogramming that occurs after nuclear transfer is the inconsistency between full remodeling during the first cell cycle after nuclear transfer and term development. Although some factors appear to be fully understood (nuclear lamins), other factors that we know little about (histone acetylation and DNA methylation) may have a profound influence on gene expression. In addition, there are likely unknown and therefore undescribed factors that are affecting the remodeling and reprogramming observed after nuclear transfer. The large calf/lamb syndrome, first associated with nuclear transfer embryos, but now thought to be a result of culture conditions (80), illustrates some of the problems with studies like these. Here, a condition present during the first week of development has profound implications for birth weight and gestation length almost 9 mo later.

Although some nuclear transfer techniques remove the cytoplasm associated with the nuclear donor cell *(81,82)*, it is known that cytoplasmic RNAs are transferred with the cell-fusion method of nuclear transfer *(83)*. A better understanding of the ramifications of cytoplasmic transfer on subsequent development of the embryo is needed.

ACKNOWLEDGMENTS

I would like to thank the many people in my and B.N. Day's laboratories that have contributed to the nuclear-transfer experiments: L.R. Abeydeera, J.E. Anderson, A. Bonk, A. Boquest, R.A. Cabot, T.C. Cantley, H.-J. Do, J.-H. Kim, Z. Machaty, C.N. Murphy, B. Nichols, A.L. Petersen, A. Rieke, N.T. Ruddock, Tao Tao, and W.-H. Wang. This manuscript was prepared while supported by BioTransplant, Inc. (Charlestown, MA), the National Center for Research Resources, NIH (RR13438), the Cooperative State Research, Education and Extension Service, U.S. Department of Agriculture under agreement #95-37203-2073, and Food for the 21st Century. This manuscript is a contribution from the Missouri Agricultural Experiment Station, Journal Series No. 12,818.

REFERENCES

1. Wilmut I, Schnieke AE, McWhir J, Kind AG, Campbell KHS. Viable offspring derived from fetal an adult mammalian cells. Nature 1997;385:810–813.
2. Prather RS. Nuclear control of early embryonic development in domestic pigs. J Reprod Fertil Suppl 1993;48:1–29.
3. Martinez-Salas E, Linney E, Hassell J, DePamphilis ML. The need for enhancers in gene expression first appears during mouse development with formation of the zygotic nucleus. Genes Dev 1989;3:1493–1506.
4. Latham KE, Soltor D, Schultz RM. Acquisition of a transcriptionally permissive state during the 1-cell stage of mouse embryogenesis. Dev Biol 1992;149:457–462.
5. Prather RS, Schatten G. Construction of the nuclear matrix at the transition from maternal to zygotic control of development in the mouse: an immunocytochemical study. Mol Reprod Dev 1992;32:203–208.
6. Prather RS, Sims MM, Maul GG, First NL, Schatten G. Nuclear lamin antigens are developmentally regulated during porcine and bovine embryogenesis. Biol Reprod 1989;41:123–132.
7. Prather RS, Rickords LF. Developmental regulation of a snRNP core protein epitope during pig embryogenesis and after nuclear transfer for cloning. Mol Reprod Dev 1992;33:119–123.
8. Clarke HJ, Obelin C, Bustin M. Developmental regulation of chromatin composition during mouse embryogenesis: somatic histone H1 is first detectable at the 4-cell stage. Development 1992;115:791–799.
9. Luger K, Mader AW, Richmond RK, Sargent DF, Richmond TJ. Crystal structure of the nucleosome core protein at 2.8 A resolution. Nature 1997;389:251–260.
10. Kornberg RD, Lorch Y. Interplay between chromatin structure and transcription. Curr Opin Cel Biol 1995;7:371–375.
11. O'Donohue M, Duband-Goulet I, Hamiche A, Prunell A. Octamer displacement and redistribution in transcription of single nucleosomes. Nucleic Acids Res 1994;22:937–945.
12. Studitsky VM, Clark DJ, Felsenfeld G. A histone octamer can step around a transcribing polymerase without leaving the template. Cell 1994;76:371–382
13. Turner BM. Histone acetylation and control of gene expression. J Cell Sci 1991;99:13–20.
14. Turner BM, Fellows G. Specific antibodies reveal ordered and cell-cycle-related use of histone H4 acetylation sites in mammalian cells. Eur J Biochem 1989;179:131–139.
15. Keohane AM, O'Neill LP, Belyaev ND, Lavender JS, Turner BM. X-inactivation and histone H4 acetylation in embryonic stem cells. Dev Biol 1996;180:618–630.
16. Moor SC, Ausio J. Major role of the histones H3-H4 in the folding of the chromatin fiber. Biochem Biophys Res Commun. 1997;230:136–139.
17. Lee DY, Hayes JJ, Pruss D, Wolffe AP. A positive role for histone acetylation in transcription factor access to nucleosomal DNA. Cell 1993;72:73–84.
18. Vettese-Dadey M, Grant PA, Hebbes TR, Crane-Robinson C, Allis CD, Workman JL. Acetylation of histone H4 plays a primary role in enhancing transcription factor binding to nucleosomal DNA in vitro. EMBO J 1996;15:2508–2518.

19. Jeppesen P, Turner BM. The inactive X chromosome in female mammals is distinguished by a lack of histone H4 acetylation a cytogenetic marker for gene expression. Cell 1993;74:281–289.

20. Lin P, Clarke HJ. Somatic histone H1 microinjected into fertilized mouse eggs is transported into the pronuclei but does not disrupt subsequent preimplantation development. Mol Reprod Dev 1996;44:185–192.

21. Adenot PG, Mercier Y, Renard J-P, Thompson EM. Differential H4 acetylation of paternal and maternal chromatin precedes DNA replication and differential transcriptional activity in pronuclei of 1-cell mouse embryos. Development 1997;124:4615–4625.

22. Worrad DM, Turner BM, Schultz RM. Temporally restricted spatial localization of acetylated isoforms of histone H4 and RNA polymerase II in the 2-cell mouse embryo. Development 1995;121:2949–2959.

23. Stein P, Worrad DM, Belyaev ND, Turner BM, Schultz RM. Stage-dependent redistributions of acetylated histones in nuclei of the early preimplantation mouse embryo. Mol Reprod Dev 1997;47:421–429.

24. Thompson EM, Legouy E, Christians E, Renard J-P. Progressive maturation of chromatin structure regulated HSP70.1 gene expression in the preimplantation mouse embryo. Development 1995;121:3425–3437.

25. Aoki F, Worrad DM, Schultz RM. Regulation of transcriptional activity during the first and second cell cycles in the preimplantation mouse embryo. Dev Biol 1997;181:296–307.

26. Wiekowski M, Miranda M, DePamphilis ML. Requirements for promoter activity in mouse oocytes and embryos distinguish paternal pronuclei from maternal and zygotic nuclei. Dev Biol 1993;159:366–378.

27. Davis W Jr, DeSousa PD, Schultz RM. Transient expression of translation initiation factor eIF-4c during the 2-cell stage of the preimplantation mouse embryo: identification by mRNA differential display and the role of DNA replication. Dev Biol 1996;174:190–201.

28. Wiekowski M, Miranda M, DePamphilis M. Regulation of gene expression in preimplantation mouse embryos: effects of the zygotic clock and the first mitosis on promoter and enhancer activities. Dev Biol 1991;147:403–414.

29. Henery CC, Miranda M, Wiekowski M, Wilmut I, DePamphilis ML. Repression of gene expression at the beginning of mouse development. Dev Biol 1995;169:448–460.

30. Smith LC, Meirelles FV, Bustin M, Clarke HJ. Assembly of somatic histone H1 onto chromatin during bovine early embryogenesis. J Exp Zool 1995;73:317–326.

31. Bilodeau-Goeseels S, Schultz GA. Changes in the relative abundance of various housekeeping gene transcripts in in vitro-produced early bovine embryos. Mol Reprod Dev 1997;47:413–420.

32. Graves RA, Marzluff WF, Giebelhaus DH, Schultz GA. Quantitative and qualitative changes in histone gene expression during early mouse embryo development. Proc Natl Acad Sci USA 1985;82:5685–5689.

33. Poccia D. Remodeling of nucleoproteins during gametogenesis fertilization and early development. Int Rev Cytol 1986;105:1–65.

34. Ner SS, Travers AA. HMG-D Drosophila melanogaster homologue of HMG 1 protein is associated with early embryonic chromatin in the absence of histone H1. EMBO J 1994;13:1817–1822.

35. Bouvet P, Dimitrov S, Wolffe AP. Specific regulation of Xenopus chromosomal 5S rRNA gene transcription in vivo by histone H1. Genes Dev 1994;8:1147–1159.

36. Schatten G, Maul GG, Schatten H, Chaly N, Simerly C, Balczon R, Brown DL. Nuclear lamins and periperal nuclear antigens during fertilization and embryogenesis in mice and sea urchins. Proc Natl Acad Sci USA 1985;82:4727–4731.

37. Prather RS, Kubiak J, Maul GG, First NL, Schatten G. The association of nuclear lamins A and C is regulated by the developmental stage of the mouse oocyte or embryonic cytoplasm. J Exp Zool 1991;257:110–114.

38. Kubiak JZ, Prather RS, Maul GG, Schatten G. Cytoplasmic modification of the nuclear lamina during pronuclear-like transformation of mouse blastomere nuclei. Mech Dev 1991;35:103–111.

39. King WA, Shepherd DL, Plante L, Lavoir MC, Looney CR, Barnes FL. Nucleolar and mitochondrial morphology in bovine embryos reconstructed by nuclear transfer. Mol Reprod Dev 1996;44:499–506.

40. Lavoir M.-C, Kelk D, Rumph N, Barnes F, Betteridge KJ, King WA. Transcription and translation in bovine nuclear transfer embryos. Biol Reprod 1997;57:204–213.

41. Loi P, Ledda S, Fulka J Jr, Cappai P, Moor RM. Development of parthenogenetic and cloned ovine embryos: effect of activation protocols. Biol Reprod 1998;58:1177–1187.

42. Kanka J, Fulka J Jr, Fulka J, Petr J. Nuclear transplantation in bovine embryo: fine structural and autoradiographic studies. Mol Reprod Dev 1991;29:110–116.

43. Mayes MA, Stogsdill PL, Parry TW, Kinden DA, Prather RS. Reprogramming of nucleoli after nuclear transfer of pig blastomeres into enucleated oocytes. Dev Biol 1994;163:542.

44. An M, Liu L, Sun T, Chen Y. Nuclear transplantation in rabbit embryos: ultrastructural studies. Theriogenology 1994;41:156 (Abstract).
45. Ouhibi N, Kanka J, Horska M, Moor MR, Fulka J Jr. Nuclear transplantation in pigs: M-phase to M-phase cytoplast fusion. Reprod Fertil Dev 1996;36:661–666.
46. Prather RS, Sims MM, First NL. Nuclear transplantation in the pig embryo: nuclear swelling. J Exp Zool 1990;255:355–358.
47. Liu L, Moor RM, Laurie S, Notarianni E. Nuclear remodeling and early development in cryopreserved porcine primordial germ cells following nuclear transfer into in vitro-matured oocytes. Intl J Dev Biol 1995;39:639–644.
48. Collas P, Robl JM. Relationship between nuclear remodeling and development in nuclear transplant rabbit embryos. Biol Reprod 1991;45:455–465.
49. Luttmer SJ, Longo FJ. Sperm nuclear transformations consist of enlargement and condensation coordinate with stages of meiotic maturation in fertilized spisula solidissima oocytes. Dev Biol 1988;128:89–96.
50. Luttmer SJ, Longo FJ. Rates of male pronuclear enlargement in sea urchin zygotes. J Exp Zool 1987;243:289–298.
51. Wright SJ, Longo FJ. Sperm nuclear enlargement in fertilized hamster eggs is related to meiotic maturation of the maternal chromatin. J Exp Zool 1988;247:155–165.
52. Czolowska R, Modliniski JA, Tarkowski AK. Behavior of thymocyte nuclei in nonactivated and activated mouse oocytes. J Cell Sci 1984;69:19–34.
53. Szollosi D, Czolowsska R, Szollosi MS, Tarkowski AK. Remodeling of mouse thymocyte nuclei depends on the time of their transfer into activated homologous oocytes. J Cell Sci 1988;91:603–613.
54. Blow JJ, Laskey RA. A role for the nuclear envelope in controlling DNA replication within the cell cycle. Nature 1988;32:546–547.
55. Thommes P, Blow JJ. The DNA replication licensing system. Cancer Surveys 1997;29:75–90.
56. Stumpf TT, Schoenbeck RA, Prather RS. DNA synthesis during the porcine embryo two-cell stage. Biol Reprod Suppl 1992;46:71.
57. Campbell KHS, Ritchie WA, Wilmut I. Nuclear-cytoplasmic interactions during the first cell cycle of nuclear transfer reconstructed bovine embryos: implications for DNA replication and development. Biol Reprod 1993;49:933–942.
58. Campbell KHS, Loi P, Cappai P, Wilmut I. Improved development to blastocyst of ovine nuclear transfer embryos reconstructed during the presumptive S-phase of the enucleated activated oocyte. Biol Reprod 1994;50:1385–1393.
59. Stice SL, Keefer CL, Matthews L. Bovine nuclear transfer embryos: oocyte activation prior to blastomere fusion. Mol Reprod Dev 1994;38:61–68.
60. Liu L, Dai YF, Moor RM. Nuclear transfer in sheep embryos- the effect of cell cycle coordination between nucleus and cytoplasm and the use of in vitro matured oocytes. Mol Reprod Dev 1997;47:255–264.
61. Collas P, Pinto-Correia C, Ponce de Leon FA, Robl JM. Effect of donor cell cycle stage on chromatin and spindle morphology in nuclear transplant rabbit embryos. Biol Reprod 1992;46:501–511.
62. Collas P, Balise JJ, Robl JM. Influence of cell cycle stage of the donor nucleus on development of nuclear transplant rabbit embryos. Biol Reprod 1992b;46:492–500.
63. Cibelli JB, Stice SL, Golueke PJ, Kane JJ, Jerry J, Blackwell C, et al. Cloned transgenic calves produced from nonquiescent fetal fibroblasts. Science 1998;280:1256–1258.
64. Gurdon JB, Laskey RA. Methods of transplanting nuclei from single cultured cells to unfertilized frogs' eggs. J Embryol Exp Morph 1970;24:227–248.
65. DiBerardino MA, Hoffner NJ. Origin of chromosomal abnormalities in nuclear transplants- a reevaluation of nuclear differentiation and nuclear equivalence in amphibians. Dev Biol 1983;23:185–209.
66. Tsunoda Y, Kato Y. Full-term development after transfer of nuclei from 4-cell and compacted morula stage embryos to enucleated oocytes in the mouse. J Exp Zool 1997;278:250–254.
67. Kwon OY, Kono T. Production of identical sextuplet mice by transferring metaphase nuclei from four-cell embryos. Proc Natl Acad Sci USA 1996;93:13,010–13,013.
68. Peura TT, Trounson AO. Recycling bovine embryos for nuclear transfer. Reprod Fertil Dev 1998;10:627–632.
69. Trounson A, Lacham-Kaplan O, Diamente M, Gougoulidis T. Somatic cell reprogramming. Reprod Fertil Dev 1998;10:645–650.
70. Schultz GA, Harvey MB, Watson AJ, Arcellana-Panlilio MY, Jones K, Westhusin ME. Regulation of early embryonic development by growth factors: growth factor gene expression in cloned bovine embryos. J Anim Sci 1996;74(Suppl 3):50–57.

71. Gurdon JB, Brennan S, Fairman S, Mohun TJ. Transcription of muscle specific actin genes in early Xenopus development: nuclear transplantation and cell dissociation. Cell 1984;38:691–700.

72. Wakefiled L, Gurdon JB. Cytoplasmic regulation of 5S RNA genes in nuclear-transplant embryos. EMBO J 1984;2:1613–1619.

73. Prather RS, Barnes FL, Sims MM, Robl JM, Eyestone WH, First NL. Nuclear transplantation in the bovine embryo: assessment of donor nuclei and recipient oocyte. Biol Reprod 1987;37:859–866.

74. Prather RS, Stumpf TT, Rickords LF. Reprogramming the nucleus and synchronizing it with the cytoplasm. International Symposium on: Cloning Mammals by Nuclear Transplantation, Fort Collins CO, 1992, pp. 26–27.

75. Bordignon V, Clarke HJ, Smith LC. Effect of cytoplast cell cycle stage on the reprogramming of somatic histone H1 reconstructed bovine embryos. Theriogenology 1998;49:178 (Abstract).

76. Pinto-Correia C, Long CR, Chang T, Robl JM. Factors involved in nuclear reprogramming during early development in the rabbit. Mol Reprod Dev 1995;40:292–304.

77. Van Stekelenburg-Hamers AEP, Rebel HG, Van Inzen WG, DeLoos FAM, Drost M, Mummery CL, et al. Stage-specific appearance of the mouse antigen TEC3 in normal and nuclear transfer bovine embryos: re-expression after nuclear transfer. Mol Reprod Dev 1994;37:27–33.

78. Obata Y, Kaneko-Ishino T, Koide T, Takai Y, Ueda T, Domeki I, et al. Disruption of primary imprinting during oocyte growth leads to the modified expression of imprinted genes during embryogenesis. Development 1998;125:1553–1560.

79. Dean W, Bowden L, Aitchison A, Klose J, Moore T, Meneses JJ, et al. Altered imprinted gene methylation and expression in completely ES cell-derived mouse fetuses: association with aberrant phenotypes. Development 1989;125:2273–2282.

80. Holm P, Walker SK, Seamark RF. Embryo viability duration of gestation and birth weight in sheep after transfer of in vitro matured and in vitro fertilized zygotes cultured in vitro or in vivo. J Reprod Fert 1996; 107:175–181.

81. Collas P, Barnes FL. Nuclear transplantation by microinjection of inner cell mas and granulosa cell nuclei. Mol Reprod Dev 1994;38:264–267.

82. Wakayama T, Perry ACF, Zuccotti M, Johnson KR, Yanagimachi R. Full-term development of mice from enucleated oocytes injected with cumulus cell nuclei. Nature 1998;394:369–371.

83. Parry TW, Prather RS. Protein reprogramming after nuclear transfer? Reprod Nut Dev 1995;35:313–318.

15

Application of ARTs and Nuclear Transfer in Exotic or Endangered Species

Kenneth L. White, PHD,
Thomas D. Bunch, PHD,
Shoukhrat Mitalipov, PHD,
and William A. Reed, PHD

Contents

INTRODUCTION

With the production of Dolly, the first somatic cell cloned sheep *(1)*, the potential impact of cloning became apparent with respect to the ability to produce live offspring, which are genetically identical to adult animals. Other recent reports confirm this potential. Wakayama et al. *(2)* reported the birth of several offspring produced from the nuclear transfer of terminally differentiated, adult, cumulus cells of mice. Scientists in New Zealand *(3,4)* used cumulus cells to successfully clone a rare cow, the last of the herd that had died in isolation on Enderby Island, a barren, sub-Antarctic piece of the Auckland Islands. Applications of the use of adult cells as donor nuclei in cloning can range from duplication of valuable animals or animals with unique characteristics, to species that survive in limited numbers.

Species extinction has occurred since life began on earth, but human activities are causing the loss of biological diversity at an unprecedented rate. During the last 100 years, the rate of extinction is considered by some scientists to have reached crisis proportions. The United States Department of the Interior, Fish and Wildlife Service (USFW), list 310 mammalian species as threatened or endangered (59 US and 251 foreign; Endangered Species Bulletin, April 30, 1998), with the number of other threatened or endangered life forms far exceeding that number. Recovering endangered species is an enormous challenge that requires cooperation from all sectors of society and may have profound ecological, economic, and social consequences.

From: *Contemporary Endocrinology: Assisted Fertilization and Nuclear Transfer in Mammals*
Edited by: D. P. Wolf and M. Zelinski-Wooten © Humana Press Inc., Totowa, NJ

Although habit restoration is the single most important factor in safeguarding threatened or endangered species, the use of technological advances in reproduction, specifically cloning, is a method that now potentially can be used to safeguard some species against extinction. Somatic cells or embryos from endangered or threatened species can be cryopreserved and maintained in what has been referred to as the "frozen zoo" and then later used as nuclear donors for cloning purposes. All samples from aged or infirm animals could be saved and used to produce a new "generation" thereby preserving their genetic diversity. Distant populations could benefit from the introduction of a clone of an isolated animal carrying rare alleles.

If cloning is to become a viable option in any animal recovery program, at least two areas must be considered: are embryo-transfer procedures established for the species of concern or a closely related species (e.g., wild or domestic); and is there an available, closely related recipient/surrogate species (e.g., wild or domestic) that will carry cloned embryos to term? A candidate endangered species that fits these requirements and will be further discussed in this chapter is the Argaliform wild sheep (*Ovis ammon*) of central Asia.

The argalis comprise a cluster of closely related subspecies, representing one of the six major taxons of wild sheep: *O. orientalis, O. vignei, O. ammon, O. nivicola, O. dalli, and O. canadensis. (5).* There are eight subspecies of argalis: the Kara Tau sheep (*O. a. nigrimontana*), Severtzov sheep (*O. a. severtzovi*), Marco Polo's sheep (O. *a. polii*), Tibetan *sheep (O. a. hodgsoni = dalai-lamae)*, Tien Shan sheep (*O. a. karelini*), Mongolian or Gobi *sheep (O. a. darwini)*, Shansi sheep (*O. a. jubata*), and Altai sheep (*O. a. ammon*) *(6)*. The U.S. Fish and Wildlife Service has listed *O. ammon* as an endangered or threatened species with historic ranges occurring in Afghanistan, China, India, Kazakhstan, Kyrgyzstan, Mongolia, Nepal, Pakistan, Russia, Tajikistan, and Uzbekistan (USFW, 2000) *(6a)*. The Convention on International Trade in Endangered Species list *O. a. darwini, O. a. jubata*, and *O. a. nigrimontana* as endangered and *O. a. ammon, O. a. collium, O. a. hodgsoni, O.a. karelini*, and *O. a. polii* as vulnerable (CITES, 2000) *(6b)*.

Herein, we describe the background of current efforts to recover exotic or endangered species using emerging technologies within the broad category of assisted reproduction. Further, we discuss the potential application of nuclear-transfer technology and results of early experimental efforts using nuclear transfer in a specific endangered specie.

ASSISTED REPRODUCTION

There are several examples of the application of assisted reproductive technologies (ART) in exotic or endangered species. Often, when programs are restricted to only a few pairs of breeding animals, no genetic selection of any kind is possible *(7)*. In many cases the limiting factor in recovery of a species is the number of suitable female animals available for reproduction. This low number of animals results in a failure of the birth rate to maintain pace with the mortality rate of the species. The net result is the ultimate loss of the species. Although not all, many of the approaches used to facilitate recovery of species focus on maximizing the number of female resources available. Many of these efforts have used either intra- or interspecies embryo transfer as a tool for recovery of suitable species.

Intraspecies Embryo Transfers

Intraspecies embryo transfers have been used and suggested as an important tool for species preservation *(8)*. Most of the development of these technologies has occurred in domestic animals with attempts to apply the resultant protocols to exotic species. The application of in vitro fertilization (IVF) to exotics, in conjunction with embryo transfer, has been proposed as a way to advance wildlife conservation efforts. This has already resulted in important impacts on recovery of gametes from the gonads of wildlife after death *(8)*.

Interspecies Embryo Transfers

Interspecies embryo transfers provide unique challenges because success depends on the ability to select an appropriately suitable recipient animal. There are several examples of successful interspecies embryo transfers involving rare or endangered species. Some examples are bongo embryos transferred into elands *(9)*, Przewalski's horse embryos into domestic horses *(10)*, gaur and banteng embryos into domestic cattle *(11,12)*, and Indian desert cats into domestic cats *(13)* as well as nonendangered species, e.g., cyno-molgus monkey embryos into rhesus macaque *(14)*.

One of the fundamental considerations when identifying a potential recipient species is the similarity in basic reproductive characteristics such as length of gestation, type of placentation, mechanism of maternal recognition, pregnancy maintenance, and estrous menstrual cycle with the donor specie. Clearly, if the two species have the ability to hybridize, it is believed they would also have a high probability for successful interspecies embryo transfer. Some of the problems that have been associated with both successful and failed interspecies embryo transfer are poor placentome formation *(11,15)* and maternal immunological rejection *(16,15)*. These would presumably be some of the same considerations when attempting to identify a suitable combination of donor nucleus–recipient oocyte in nuclear-transfer combination.

Hybrid Embryos

Several attempts have been made to produce and evaluate the developmental potential of hybrid embryos. Slavik et al. *(17)* reported the development of ovine-bovine hybrid embryos. These embryos, as defined by the presence of two well-developed pronuclei, were produced by the insemination of in vitro-matured bovine oocytes with ovine spermatozoa. Sixty-seven percent of bovine oocytes were fertilized by ovine spermatozoa as compared to 83% of control bovine oocytes inseminated with bovine spermatozoa. Fourteen percent of hybrid embryos developed to the 2-cell stage and subsequently 19% of these 2-cell embryos developed to the 8-cell stage, which was comparable to control embryos (16% 2-cell and 24% 8-cell). Experiments were also carried out to evaluate the relative uptake of ^{3}H-uridine at the 8-cell stage (maternal to embryonic transition) using these hybrid embryos and comparing them to control in vitro-fertilized bovine embryos. These results indicated a slightly lower uptake of radiolabel. These data may indicate a decrease in the developmental compatibility of the hybrid nuclei produced from the fertilization of a bovine oocyte by an ovine sperm. In addition, the data further support the hypothesis that developmental barriers may be in place to protect the integrity of mammalian species, at least in the case of specific hybridizations (*see* ref. *18* for review).

In efforts at conservation of the endangered lion-tailed macaque (LTM, Macaca silenus), scientists at the Baltimore Zoo created hybrid pig-tailed macaque (PTM, Macaca nemestrina) × LTM embryos by IVF of PTM oocytes with LTM sperm *(19)*. Frozen/thawed 4-cell stage hybrid embryos were transferred into the fallopian tubes of a PTM recipient. A morphologically normal hybrid male was born after 162 d gestation who has shown normal development during the first 2 yr of observation.

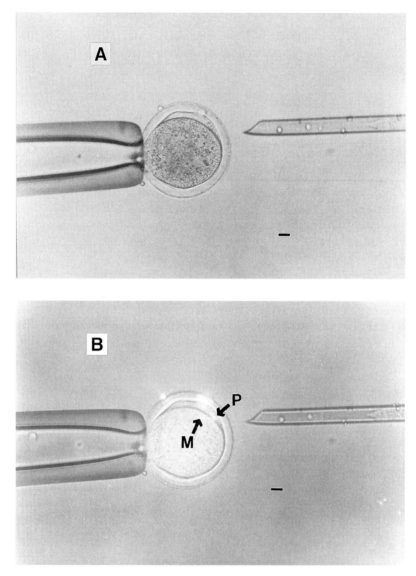

Fig. 1. Demonstration of an enucleation of a sheep oocyte after staining with Hoechst 33342. (**A**) Before enucleation viewed under visible light, 200×. (**B**) Before enucleation viewed with combined visible and UV illumination. Arrows indicate the first polar body (P) and the metaphase II plate (M).

NUCLEAR TRANSFER

In the majority of current nuclear-transfer reports involving somatic cells, fibroblasts (or other somatic cell types) are synchronized in the G_0–G_1 phase of the cell cycle by culture under conditions that either maintain or induce a large proportion of cells to enter into this phase of the cell cycle *(1,20–22)*. Typically, in vitro-matured, MII oocytes are transferred into drops of manipulation medium (i.e., HECM/HEPES), *(23)* containing 7.5 µg/ml cytochalasin B and subsequently enucleated to create recipient cytoplast. The first polar body and the metaphase plate of an oocyte are removed using a 25–28-µm ID enucleation pipet. Confirmation of complete removal of nuclear components is often

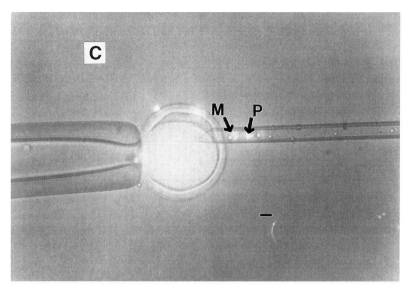

Fig. 1. (Continued) (**C**) The same oocyte after enucleation viewed as in (**B**). Polar body and metaphase II plate have been drawn into the enucleation pipet. In actual production of nuclear-transfer embryos the oocyte is not exposed to UV light. The polar body and a portion of cytoplasm proximal to the polar body is removed under visible light, the oocyte is moved out of the field of illumination, and the enucleation pipet illluminated with UV light to check for the presence of both the polar body and metaphase plate in the pipet to confirm complete enucleation. Bar, 19 μm.

accomplished by visualization of metaphase plate and polar body in the pipet under UV light (*see* Fig. 1). The same enucleation pipet is then used to create a fusion couple by aspirating a disaggregated donor cell and placing it into the perivitelline space of the cytoplast. Fusion is induced by two DC pulses after individual couples are appropriately oriented in a fusion chamber. Fused nuclear-transfer embryos are activated, within 2–6 h of fusion, by exposure to calcium ionophore or other agents that induce intracellular calcium release *(24)*. A delay in activation after fusion of a somatic nucleus with an enucleated MII oocyte appears beneficial in most, but not all situations. Exposure of the transferred nucleus to various factors present in the cytoplasm of a nonactivated, metaphase-arrested oocyte may facilitate prerequisite nuclear remodeling and reprogramming. Such a delay, for 4–6 h before activation significantly increased development of bovine nuclear transfer (NT) embryos to blastocyst *(21,25,26)* and resulted in viable cloned calves using fetal fibroblasts *(21)* and adult mural granulosa cells *(26)* as a source of donor nuclei. Similarly in the mouse, embryo and fetal development were both improved following exposure of cumulus cell nuclei to MII cytoplasm for 1–6 h *(2)*. Finally, nuclear-transfer embryos are cultured to a suitable stage of development and transferred to a synchronized recipient animal to be carried to term.

Hybrid Nuclear-Transfer Embryos

The success of nuclear-transfer strategies using somatic cell lines provides new opportunities that were not previously envisioned. One of these applications is as a tool for species preservation, because the potential exists to recover tissue samples from dead, dying, or incapacitated animals that could serve as a source of genetic material for nuclear transfer. This approach would provide an endless supply of donor cells, which could be used to generate nuclear-transfer embryos for transfer to suitable recipient animals in efforts to establish term pregnancies. Under these circumstances, the limiting factor would be the number of available oocytes that could be enucleated and subsequently receive donor nuclear material. The ability to use closely related animals for production of recipient oocytes (cytoplasts) would further augment the potential impact of this technology. In addition, the ability to produce developmentally competent "hybrid" nuclear-transfer embryos and use them in conjunction with interspecies embryo transfer could have an important impact on species preservation. The subsequent sections will describe early efforts to assess the feasibility of applying nuclear transfer in such a manner.

Xenogenic Nuclear Transfer

Xenogenic nuclear transfer will be used here to define the use of interspecific (animal of one species or genus into one of another) karyoplasts and cytoplasts to produce resultant nuclear-transfer embryos. One of the earliest studies examining the developmental capacity of nuclear-transfer embryos produced with nuclei from genetically diverse and widely separated species was reported in 1990 *(27)*. In vivo-produced blastomeres from bovine 4.5–5.5-d embryos were used as a source of nuclear donors, while enucleated ova from American bison, Spanish goats, Syrian hamsters, and domestic cows served as recipient cytoplasts. During the interim, fused nuclear-transfer embryos were cultured in the oviducts of, recipient ewes for 6 d, after which time embryos were recovered and evaluated. No cleavage was observed when hamster ova served as the recipient cytoplast, however, cleaved embryos and blastocysts were found among bovine-bison (1.9%), bovine-goat (1.2%) and bovine-bovine (19.4%) nuclear-transfer embryos. This was the first evidence suggesting that mammalian nuclei may be capable of interacting with cytoplasm from another mammalian species and direct early development after nuclear transfer. More recently, the bovine oocyte has been used as a type of "universal" cytoplast for nuclear transplantation. Mitalipova et al. *(28)* and Dominko et al. *(29)* reported in vitro development of nuclear-transfer embryos produced following the transfer of nuclear-donor cells from cattle, sheep, pigs, monkeys, and rats into enucleated bovine, MII cytoplasts. Evaluations in these experiments were based on development to the morula and blastocyst stages. Donor-cell lines with fibroblast-like morphology were established from skin biopsies of adult animals. Development to the morula and blastocyst stages in these sheep-bovine, pig-bovine, monkey-bovine, and rat-bovine nuclear-transfer embryos was comparable to control (bovine-bovine) nuclear-transfer embryos. Timing of the first cleavage division and rate of development was dictated by donor nuclei and corresponded to that described for embryos of the nuclear donor species *(28)*. Furthermore, ICM cells of control bovine-bovine nuclear-transfer blastocyst were positive for oocyte-specific proteins, i.e., c-Kit receptor staining and the receptor for stem-cell factor, when compared to nuclear donor fibroblasts that showed no c-Kit staining *(28)*.

Additional reports by White et al. *(20,30)* using a cell line from a wild sheep (argali) as the nuclear donor source and enucleated bovine cytoplast support the conclusion of Mitalipova et al. *(28)* and Dominko et al. *(29)* that these "hybrid" nuclear-transfer embryos can develop in vitro to the blastocyst stage. Specifically, from a total of 166 argali-bovine nuclear-transfer couples, 128 (77%) successfully fused, 100 (78% of fused) of which developed to the 8- to 16-cell stage and 2 (1.6%) to the blastocyst stage. The presence of argali nuclei in 8- to 16-cell stage, argali-bovine, nuclear-transfer embryo clones was confirmed on Hoechst 33342 stained embryos under UV light. Chromosome analysis of metaphase spreads from blastomeres revealed the presence of the argali karyotype.

Results of these "hybrid" (XX-bovine) nuclear transfers indicate that the bovine oocyte provides adequate factors to support at least limited development to the blastocyst stage following xenonuclear transplantation. Bovine oocytes may also be useful in generating embryonic cell lines from species where obtaining or using embryos for this purpose is either impractical or not feasible. However, no data exist that evaluate the effects of this hybridization of cytoplasmic and nuclear elements on subsequent development or on the cell biology of the resulting cell type.

Another potential example of the use of xenonuclear transplantation derives from two independent announcements in 1998 *(31,32)* that human embryonic stem (ES) cells had been isolated in the first case from ICM cells of IVF-produced blastocysts (*31; see* Chapter 16) and in the second, from primordial germ cells of gonadal ridges and mesenteries of 5–9-wk-old fetuses *(32)*. The most useful and important property of these cells is their totipotency and the ability to differentiate in vivo and in vitro into ectodermal, endodermal, and mesodermal derivatives or into a wide variety of cell types in culture. Such cells would be invaluable for studies of human embryogenesis and for the development of transplantation therapies. Many diseases, for example Parkinson's or juvenile-onset diabetes mellitus, result from the death or dysfunction of just one or a few cell types, replacement of which could offer an effective lifelong treatment. However, based on moral status of the early human embryo, the Congress of the United States established a moratorium on federal funding for experimentation on human embryos and fetal tissue (*see* Chapter 17). Xenonuclear transplantation of donor human cells into suitable nonhuman recipient cytoplasts to create ES cells would be one possible avenue of escape from the moral enigmas of this research. In fact, Advanced Cell Technologies, a biotech company, claims it has already established stem cells from human-bovine nuclear-transfer embryos *(33)*. If this approach becomes routine, human stem cell lines derived from adult cells would not only resolve problems with the use of human embryonic tissue and the availability of a suitable donor oocyte source, but may also have superior therapeutic properties because problems of secondary immune rejection may be minimized.

A potential problem in the use of xenonuclear transplantation derives from the fact that two different mitochondrial DNAs (mtDNA) would be present in the newly constructed embryo. Although mitochondrial transfers could be considered, some information is available on the consequences of creating xenomitochondrial hybrids. Nuclear-transfer techniques were used intensively to create heteroplasmic mouse embryos and live offspring carrying two different mtDNA genotypes in studies of mechanisms controlling mtDNA segregation and inheritance in mammals *(34–36)*. These studies have shown that the ratio of donor:host mtDNA genotypes increases at the 8-cell to blastocyst stage of embryogenesis, suggesting that the nucleus is either preferentially replicating its own mtDNA or selectively destroying the host mtDNA. The nuclear and mitochondrial genomes co-evolve to optimize approx 100 different interactions necessary for an efficient ATP-generating system. This co-evolution led to a species-specific compatibility between these genomes. Introduced by nuclear transfer, mtDNA from common chimpanzee, pygmy chimpanzee, and gorilla into mtDNA-less human cells were able to restore oxidative phosphorylation in the context of a human nuclear background *(37)*. Xenomitochondrial cybrids produced by transfer of mtDNA from orangutan and species representative of

Old-World monkeys, New-World monkeys, and lemurs into human cells failed to replace functionally human mtDNA, suggesting the presence of one or a few mutations affecting critical nuclear-mitochondrial genome interactions between these species. This finding suggests that nuclear-transfer embryos resulting from distant species may not fully develop owing to, at least, nuclear-mitochondrial incompatibilities. However, this may not be a universal problem in all species. Successful development may depend on the compatibility between the nuclear and cytoplast donors *(20)*.

Allogenic Nuclear Transfer

Allogenic nuclear transfer will be used here to define the use of karyoplasts and cytoplasts from different species within the same genus to produce resultant nuclear-transfer embryos. Results of experiments using wild-sheep (argali) cell lines as nuclear donor cells and enucleated domestic-sheep oocytes as cytoplasts (argali-sheep) and domestic-sheep as recipient animals have been reported *(20; see* Fig. 2). In these studies, nuclear-transfer embryos were allowed to develop to the early morula stage and disaggregated blastomeres were used again as nuclear donors in combination with domestic-sheep cytoplasts to generate new or second-generation nuclear-transfer embryos. Following a 72-h culture period, the resultant second-generation nuclear-transfer embryos were transferred to synchronized domestic sheep recipients *(see* Fig. 3). A control group of nuclear-transfer embryos (sheep-sheep), was also generated using the same protocols and adult domestic-sheep fibroblast cell lines as nuclear donor cells. In these experiments, a total of 28 argali-sheep and 21 sheep-sheep nuclear-transfer embryos were separately transferred into 10 recipient animals. At 49 d of putative gestation, all recipient animals were evaluated for pregnancy using ultrasound. Two animals had increased fluid in their uterine horns but were not pregnant. Two additional recipients were determined to be pregnant, one carrying sheep-sheep and the other argali-sheep nuclear-transfer embryos. The sheep-sheep recipient was carrying >1 fetus and the other recipient appeared to be carrying a single fetus *(20)*. In addition, the sheep-sheep pregnancy resulted from the transfer of first-generation nuclear-transfer embryos, whereas, the argali-sheep pregnancy resulted from second-generation clones. Recipients pregnant at d 49 were again evaluated at 59 d gestation using ultrasonography; both displayed increased fluid within the uterine horns relative to that seen at 49 d, but neither carried a viable fetus. These results *(20)* provide the first report of a >49-d pregnancy resulting from the transfer of a "hybrid" nuclear-transfer embryo. In these experiments, several reasons for the reported failure of both the sheep-sheep and argali-sheep pregnancies prior to 59 d gestation can be considered.

Primary losses of ongoing nuclear-transfer pregnancies between 40–60 d gestation have been noted by others *(1,25,38)*. It appears that the failure of normal placentation is a problem frequently observed with cloned embryos and also with a proportion of in vitro-produced (IVP) embryos. Approximately 25% of early embryo mortality with IVP embryos appears to be owing to an unsuccessful transition from yolk sac to allantoic nutrition, whereby the growth of the allantois is severely retarded, or even nonexistent, and characterized by a lack of vascularization *(26)*. It is likely that cloned embryos will have a similar deficiency during this stage of development. All of these reports are concerned with intraspecies nuclear transfers rather than interspecies transfers, which further support the idea that failure may not be the result of complications introduced by interspecies interactions. This gestational time is obviously a stage in development that requires sig-

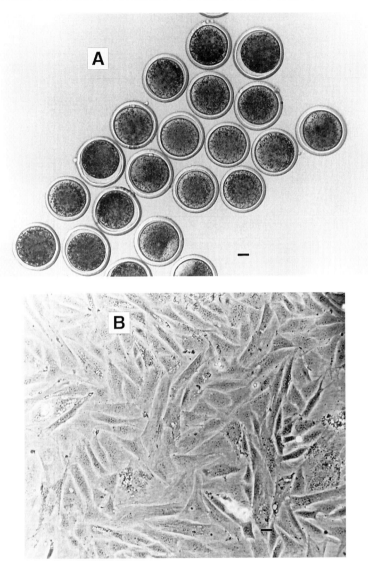

Fig. 2. (A) Domestic sheep (*O. aries*) oocytes used as cytoplasts (bar, 19 µm) and **(B)** passage 5 argali (*O. ammon*) dermal fibroblasts before dispersion in trypsin used as karyoplasts (bar, 38 µm) in constructing argali-sheep nuclear transfer em bryos.

nificant interaction between the fetal unit and the maternal environment *(39)*, such that any developmental failure in the fetal unit could adversely affect the maintenance of pregnancy. The transfer of additional numbers of nuclear-transfer embryos could lead to the establishment of pregnancies that develop to term in these interspecies transfers.

An additional reason for failure of the argali pregnancy could be owing to problems associated with the chromosomal composition of the cell line used as the nuclear donor source. These researchers reported normal argali karyotype on early passages of the cell line, which was subsequently used as nuclear donor. However, re-evaluation of later passages that were used to generate the transferred nuclear-transfer embryos indicated a high percentage of chromosomal abnormalities. Use of either a polyploid or aneuploid

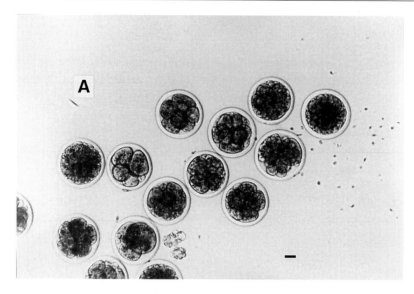

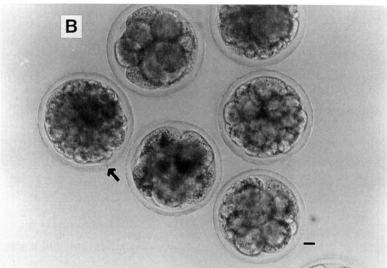

Fig. 3. Argali-sheep nuclear-transfer embryos after 72 h in culture just before transfer to recipient domestic ewes (*O. aries*) viewed with 100× (**A**) bar, 19 μm and 200× (**B**) bar, 38 μm magnification. Arrow in (**B**) points to the small hole in the zona pellucida of one of the embryos made during the nuclear-transfer procedure.

nucleus as the nuclear donor would result in a high probability of premature termination of pregnancy *(40)*. Although it is not clear at which stage of gestation failure would occur under these circumstances, it cannot be ruled out as a possible factor for termination between 40 and 60 d.

Finally, potential developmental incompatibility of the karyoplast-cytoplast (argali-sheep) union, which resulted in the subsequent nuclear-transfer embryo, cannot be eliminated as a cause of pregnancy failure. There are differences in the number of chromosomes found in *O. aries (54)* as compared to *O. ammon (56)*, which could potentially contribute to developmental incompatibilities between the cytoplasm of one strain and the nucleus of another. The developmental consequences of the interaction of "foreign" cytoplasmic factors, such as mitochondria, with nuclear elements has not yet been elucidated, although hybrid animals resulting from the breeding of argali animals with domestic sheep have been reported *(41)*. It is certainly possible that incompatibilities at a molecular level could result in developmental failure, because it is clear there are several milestones in development, each of which is pivotal to the next.

CONCLUSION

The encouraging interspecies nuclear-transfer results discussed herein should provide the impetus to continue exploratory efforts on the use of nuclear transfer involving oocytes from plentiful, closely related species to help preserve endangered, threatened, or even extinct species. With regard to the latter, efforts have been described to resurrect the woolly mammoth *(42)*. Japanese scientists are looking for a viable sperm or other cells with intact DNA from mammoth remnants found in Russian Siberia; fossils on Wrangel Island are the youngest that have ever been found at only 3,800 years old. Although most findings include only bones, in a few cases the Siberian permafrost has preserved skin and muscle as well. Most of the cells in these tissue samples are degraded, although in the past decade a few proteins and fragmented genes have been rescued from such samples. If viable mammoth sperm or other cells are found, it would provide the opportunity to fertilize an elephant female for cloning using elephant eggs as cytoplasts and elephant females as recipients.

The successful production of viable young using this approach would provide a tremendous impact on the ability to re-generate animal numbers in these species and to expand the number of resident populations. Given the absence of habitat limitations, the realization of the utility of cryobanking cells for genomic preservation would be possible. Great efforts could then be applied to the production and storage of suitable cell lines with normal chromosomal composition for future use in conjunction with nuclear-transfer technologies to facilitate the rescue of endangered species.

REFERENCES

1. Wilmut I, Schnieke AE, McWhir J, Kind AJ, Campbell KHS. Viable offspring derived from fetal and adult mammalian cells. Nature 1997;385:810–813.
2. Wakayama T, Perry ACF, Zuccotti M, Johnson KR, Yanagimachi R. Full-term development of mice from enucleated oocytes injected with cumulus cell nuclei. Nature 1998;394:369–374.
3. Wells DN, Misika PM, Forsyth JT, Berg MC, Lange JM, Tervit HR, Vivanco WH. The use of adult somatic cell nuclear transfer to preserve the last surviving cow of the Enderby Island cattle breed. Theriogenology 1999;51:217.
4. Weiss R. Scientists clone last of a rare cow breed. The Oregonian, August 20, 1998;A20.
5. Geist V. On the taxonomy of giant sheep (Ovis ammon Linnaeus, 1766). Can J Zool 1991;69:706–723.
6. Bunch TD, Vorontsov NN, Lyapunova EA, Hoffmann RS. Confirmation of diploid chromosome number in Severtzov's sheep (Ovis ammon severtzovi Nasonov 1914): G-band karyotype comparisons within Ovis. J Hered 1998;89:267–269.
6a. U.S. Fish and Wildlife Service. Threatened and Endangered Species System (TESS). 2000.http://ecos.fws.gov/servlet/lTESSSpeciesReport/generate.
6b. Convention on International Trade in Endangered Species of Wild Fauna and Flora. 200.http://environment.about.com/newissues/environment/gi/dynamic/offsite.htm? sit e=http%3A%2F%2Fwww.cites.org
7. Lasley BL, Loskutoff NM, Anderson GB. The limitation of conventional breeding programs and the need and promise of assisted reproduction in nondomestic species. Theriogenology 1994:41:119–132.

8. Loskutoff NM, Bartels P, Meintjes M, Godke RA, Schiewe MC. Assisted reproductive technology in nondomestic ungulates: a model approach to preserving and managing genetic diversity. Theriogenology 1995;43:3–12.

9. Dresser BL, Kramer L, Dalhausen RD. Successful transcontinental and interspecies embryo transfer from bongo antelope (Tragelaphus euryceros) at the Los Angeles Zoo to eland antelope (Taurotragus oryx) and bongo at the Cincinnati Zoo. Proc Amer Assoc Zool Parks Aquariums, 1984, pp. 166–168.

10. Summers PM, Shephard AM, Hodges JK, Kydd J, Boyle MS, Allen WS. Successful transfer of the embryo of Przewalski's horse (Equus przewalskii) and grant's zebra (E. burchelli) to domestic mares (E. caballus). J Reprod Fert 1987;80:13–20.

11. Stover J, Evans J, Dolensek EP. Interspecies embryo transfer from the gaur to the domestic holstein. Proc Amer Zoo Vet 1981:122–124.

12. Wiesner H, Lampeter WW, Rietschel W. Erfahrungen beim unblutigen embryotransfer vom banteng auf hausrinder. Verhandlungen 26. Int Symp Erkrankungen Zootiere Brno Czech 1984:99–102.

13. Pope CE, Gelwicks EJ, Wachs KB, Keller GL, Maruska EJ, Dresser BL. Successful interspecies transfer of embryos from the indian desert cat (Felis silvestris ornata) to the domestic cat (Felis catus). Biol Reprod 1989;40:61.

14. Balmaceda JP, Pool TB, Arana JB, Heitman TS, Asch RH. Successful in vitro fertilization and embryo transfer in cynomolgus monkeys. Fertil Steril 1984;42(5):791–795

15. MacLaren LA, Anderson GB, BonDurant RH, Edmondson AJ, Bernoco D. Maternal serum reactivity to species-specific antigens in sheep-goat interspecific pregnancy. Biol Reprod 1992;46:1–9.

16. Dent J, McGovern PT, Hancock JL. Immunological implications of ultrastructural studies of goat x sheep hybrid placentae. Nature 1971;231:116–117.

17. Slavik T, Kopecny V, Fulka J. Developmental failure of hybrid embryos originated after fertilization of bovine oocytes with ram spermatozoa. Mol Reprod Dev 1997;48:344–349.

18. McGovern PT. The barriers to interspecific hybridization in domestic and laboratory mammals. Br Vet J 1975;131:691–706.

19. Cranfield MR, Bavister BD, Boatman DE, Berger NG, Schaffer N, Kempske SE, et al. Assisted reproduction in the propagation management of the endangered lion-tailed macaque (Macaca silenus). In: Wolf DP, Stouffer RL, Brenner RM, eds. In Vitro Fertilization and Embryo Transfer in Primates. Springer-Verlag, 1993, pp. 331–348.

20. White K L, Bunch TD, Mitalipov S, Reed WA. Establishment of pregnancy after the transfer of nuclear-transfer embryos produced from the fusion of Argali (Ovis ammon) nuclei into domestic sheep (Ovis aries) enucleated oocytes. Cloning 1999;1:47–54.

21. Cibelli J, Stice S, Golueke P, Kane J, Jerry J, Blackwell C, Ponce de Leon FA, Robl J. Cloned transgenic calves produced From nonquiescent fetal fibroblasts. Science 1998;280:1256–1258.

22. Campbell KHS, McWhir J, Ritchie WA, Wilmut, I. Sheep cloned by nuclear transfer from a cultured cell line. Nature 1996;380:64–66.

23. Seshagiri PB, Bavister BD. Phosphate is required for inhibition by glucose of development of hamster 8-cell embryos in vitro. Biol Reprod 1989;40:607–614.

24. Mitalipov SM, Farrar VR, Reed WA, White KL. Parthenogenic development of bovine oocytes following activation by inositol 1,4,5-trisphosphate (IP3) and ryanodine (RYR). Mol Biol Cell 1996;7(S):1789.

25. Stice SL, Strelchenko NS, Keefer CL, Matthews L. Pluripotent bovine embryonic cell lines direct embryonic development following nuclear transfer. Biol Reprod 1996;54:100–110.

26. Wells DN, Misika PM, Tervit HR. Production of cloned calves following nuclear transfer with cultured adult mural granulosa cells. Biol Reprod 1999;60:996–1005.

27. Wolfe BA, Westhusin ME, Levanduski MJ Bondioli KR, Kraemer DC. Preimplantation development of embryos produced by intergeneric nuclear transplantation. Theriogenology 1990;33(1):350.

28. Mitalipova M, Dominko T, Haley B, Beyhan Z, Memili E, First N. Bovine cytoplasm reprograms somatic cell nuclei from various mammalian species. Theriogenology 1998;49(1):389.

29. Dominko T, Mitalipova M, Haley B, Beyhan Z, Memili E, First N. Bovine oocyte as a universal recipient cytoplasm in mammalian nuclear transfer. Theriogenology 1998;49:385.

30. White KL, Mitalipov SM, Reed WA, Farrar VR, Bunch TD. Embryo clones derived from Tibetan argali (Ovis ammon) nuclear-donor fibroblast cells and enucleated bovine oocytes. Theriogenology 1998;49(1):396.

31. Thomson JA, Itskovitz-Eldor J, Shapiro SS, Waknitz MA, Swiergiel JJ, Marshall VS, Jones JM. Embryonic stem cell lines derived from human blastocysts. Science 1998;282:1145–1147.

32. Shamblott MJ, Axelman J, Wang S, Bugg EM, Littlefield JW, Donovan PJ, et al. Derivation of pluripotent stem cells from cultured human primordial germ cells. Proc Natl Acad Sci USA 1998;95:13,726–13,731.
33. Easterbook G. Medical evolution: will Homo sapiens become obsolete? The New Republic. March 1999;1:20–25.
34. Jenuth JP, Peterson AC, Shoubridge EA. Tissue-specific selection for different mtDNA genotypes in heteroplasmic mice. Nature Genet 1997;16:93–95.
35. Meirelles FV, Smith LC. Mitochondrial genotype segregation in a mouse lineage produced by embryonic karyoplast transplantation. Genetics 1997;145:445–451.
36. Meirelles FV, Smith LC. Mitochondrial genotype segregation during preimplantation development in mouse heteroplasmic embryos. Genetics 1998;148:877–883.
37. Kenyon L, Moraes C. Expanding the functional human mitochondrial DNA database by the establishment of primate xenomitochondrial cybrids. Proc Natl Acad Sci USA 1997;94:9131–9135.
38. Wells DN, Misica PM, Day TAM, Tervit HR. Production of cloned lambs from an established embryonic cell line: a comparison between in vivo- and in vitro-matured cytoplasts. Biol Reprod 1997;57:385–393.
39. Anderson GB. Interspecific pregnancy: barriers and prospects. Biol Reprod 1988;38:1–15.
40. Hare WCD, Singh EL. Cytogenetics in Animal Reproduction. Commonwealth agricultural bureaux, England 1979;96.
41. Gray AP. Mammalian hybrids: A check list with bibliography. C.A.B. England 1954;76–144.
42. Stone R. Mammoth: cloning the woolly. Discover 1999;April:56–63.

16 Assisted Fertilization and Nuclear Transfer in Nonhuman Primates

Nadia Ouhibi, PHD, Mary B. Zelinski-Wooten, PHD, James A. Thomson, VMD, PHD, and Don P. Wolf, PHD

CONTENTS

INTRODUCTION

Progress over the last decade has firmly established the feasibility and success of the nonhuman primate as a model for basic studies concerning many aspects of the assisted reproductive technologies (ARTs) including folliculogenesis, oocyte maturation, fertilization, embryonic development and implantation. Ethical and practical reasons preclude investigation of many of these processes, including nuclear transfer, in women. Similarities between the reproductive processes of female nonhuman primates and women make them ideal animal models for the investigation of clinically relevant therapies for alleviating infertility. Evolution of the nonhuman primate model to its current status has encompassed many exciting "firsts" in macaques, e.g., live births of nonfrozen *(1)* and frozen-thawed *(2)* in vitro fertilization (IVF)-derived embryos, an infant from ultrasound-guided transabdominal intrauterine insemination with cryopreserved sperm *(3)*, blastocysts produced from in vitro matured (IVM)/IVF embryos *(4)*, infants from intracytoplasmic sperm injection (ICSI; 5), and individuals derived from nuclear transfer *(6)*. Using information gathered from women and macaques, the ARTs have been applied

From: *Contemporary Endocrinology: Assisted Fertilization and Nuclear Transfer in Mammals*
Edited by: D. P. Wolf and M. Zelinski-Wooten © Humana Press Inc., Totowa, NJ

in zoo programs to enhance the propagation of endangered primates leading to, for example, the first IVF- and ICSI-derived embryos from the lion tailed macaque at the Baltimore Zoo *(7)* and an IVF-derived female gorilla born at the Cincinnati Zoo *(8)*. Although the number of live-born offspring worldwide are orders of magnitude less than the current population of humans derived from the ARTs (discussed below), their very existence lends credibility to the utility of nonhuman primates as models for clinical reproductive therapies and the propagation of endangered species. In fact, the production of thousands of macaque oocytes and embryos annually is now a reality, and concerted efforts are currently underway to utilize this precious resource in basic and applied research, not only in the area of infertility, but in the study of other human diseases. This chapter summarizes recent developments and applications of the ARTs in nonhuman primates, focusing primarily on the rhesus monkey.

FOLLICULAR STIMULATION

The application of ARTs requires a large consistent supply of oocytes, harvested in the immature germinal vesicle (GV)-intact stage for IVM/IVF research, or mature, i.e. metaphase II (MII) stage for IVF, ICSI or nuclear transfer experimentation. Oocytes have been recovered in vivo from unstimulated primates such as marmosets, chimpanzees, rhesus and pig-tailed macaques during spontaneous menstrual cycles *(9)*. Oocyte collection from nonstimulated animals is tedious and of low yield, but may provide important comparisons relative to oocytes obtained from stimulated cycles. Early methods for stimulating the growth and maturation of multiple preovulatory follicles and their enclosed oocytes in nonhuman primates have been extensively reviewed *(9,10)*. Typically these methods*(1,2,9–20)* involve:

1. Urinary (u)-derived human (h) gonadotropins, follicle stimulating hormone (FSH) and luteinizing hormone (LH) with the inclusion of human chorionic gonadotropin (hCG) to induce oocyte maturation, luteinization and/or follicle rupture (i.e., superovulation); and, to a lesser extent,
2. Clomiphene citrate which elevates endogenous gonadotropin levels,
3. Pregnant mare's serum gonadotropin (PMSG), typically used in nonprimate species,
4. Relatively impure pituitary preparations of FSH and LH.

VandeVoort and colleagues *(20)* established a "standardized" protocol in rhesus monkeys of urinary human gonadotropins used clinically in women; beginning at menses, 6 d of FSH (30 IU, bid, im; Metrodin, Serono Laboratories, Norwell, MA) followed by 3 d of FSH + LH (1:1, 30 IU each, bid, im; Pergonal, Serono) with hCG (1000 IU, sid, im; Profasi, Serono) as the ovulatory stimulus. This sequential regimen consistently stimulated the growth of multiple follicles capable of ovulation in rhesus monkeys, and was used for many years by our laboratories in various experimental paradigms, e.g., titration of the dose and duration of the ovulatory stimulus, oocyte maturation and luteinization, evaluation of the role of steroids in folliculogenesis and, oocyte harvest for in vitro embryo culture experimentation *(9,10,21–23)*. We subsequently determined that this regimen could be "individualized" for optimal development of multiple follicles and mature oocytes by varying the exposure to FSH + LH from 1–3 d *(14)*. Transabdominal ultrasonography is routinely performed on anesthetized animals on the 7th day of follicular stimulation to assess the numbers and diameters of ovarian follicles. In previous studies, follicles were visualized using a 7.5 MHz sector scanner with an Ultramark 4

(Advanced Technologies Laboratory [ATL], Bothell, WA) system; currently we use a C-8 curved array scanhead with an HDI 1000 system (ATL). When three follicles ≥4 mm diameter are observed on each ovary, hCG is administered the following day *(14)*.

Although successful with respect to recovery of fertilizable oocytes, the sequential regimen of follicular stimulation with urinary human gonadotropins had two major disadvantages: the occurrence of spontaneous LH surges in some individuals that compromised oocyte number and quality *(9)*, and the production of neutralizing antibodies. The latter results in ovarian refractoriness to further gonadotropin therapy restricting follicular stimulation to a single protocol per animal, a feature noted in both rhesus monkeys *(10,24)* and olive baboons *(17)*. Fortunately, the presence of circulating anti-human gonadotropin antibodies that result from follicular stimulation regimens do not interfere with subsequent conception and maintenance of pregnancy in rhesus monkeys *(25)*. Furthermore, existing antibody titers do not increase during gestation or pregnancy. Continued fertility and normal gestations in antibody positive females are apparently due to failure of these antibodies to cross-react appreciably with endogenous macaque (m) FSH/LH and mCG *(25)*. Based on these results, it is possible that maximal oocyte recovery following gonadotropin stimulation in a limited number of endangered primate species would not compromise future breeding potential in such females; however, testing in each species is required.

Based on its effectiveness and reversibility in macaques (for review, *see* ref. *26*) administration of a gonadotropin releasing hormone (GnRH) antagonist, Antide (0.5–1.0 mg/kg body weight of a solution of 10 mg/mL [w/v] in propylene glycol:water [1:1, v/v], sid, sc; Laboratories Serono SA, Aubonne, Switzerland) was used throughout follicular stimulation with sequential human gonadotropins which eliminated endogenous LH surges in >95% of rhesus monkeys. Initiation of Antide treatment in the midluteal phase, prior to gonadotropin administration at menses, did not confer any advantage with respect to follicular development and oocyte maturation/fertilization *(27)*. Short intervals of Antide treatment initiated during the middle of gonadotropin stimulation protocols also suppressed endogenous LH surges in macaques *(28)*.

Ideally, the use of nonhuman primate gonadotropins would overcome the problem of antibody production in response to human gonadotropins; however, ample supplies of macaque hormones for follicular stimulation are not currently available. With the recent advent of recombinant (r) DNA technology, highly purified human gonadotropins, e.g. FSH devoid of LH activity and vice versa, became available for use in macaques. Initial trials in Antide-treated rhesus monkeys demonstrated the effectiveness of r-hFSH (Gonal F ™, Laboratories Serono SA) alone or in combination with r-hLH (Lahdi; Laboratories Serono SA) for follicular stimulation, oocyte maturation, fertilization and subsequent embryonic development *(26,27)*. Additional studies showed that 1000 IU r-hCG as well as 2500 IU r-hFSH were equivalent to the standard 1000 IU u-hCG for induction of periovulatory events (oocyte nuclear maturation, luteinization) in rhesus monkeys *(29,30)*. Controlled experiments investigating the repeated use of rhesus monkeys subjected to follicular stimulation with r-hFSH/LH and r-hCG as the ovulatory stimulus *(31)* found that circulating antibodies were absent following one stimulation cycle. However, at the start of the third stimulation cycle, 1 of 10 and 3 of 10 animals were FSH and hCG antibody-positive, respectively. At the end of the third cycle, modest levels of antibodies to FSH were noted in 6 of 10 animals, and anti-hCG antibodies were observed in 7 of 10 animals. Nonetheless, 5 antibody-positive animals yielded mature oocytes from the third cycle that fertilized in vitro. Oocyte maturation and fertilization rates were similar between the first and third stimulation cycles, although the total number of animals yielding fertilizable oocytes declined with repeated gonadotropin stimulation. Thus, three follicular stimulation cycles per macaque can be achieved using recombinant human gonadotropins without major impact on oocyte maturation at collection or fertilization in vitro *(31)*.

Our current follicular stimulation regimen in use for rhesus monkeys begins at menses with co-administration of Antide (1.0 mg/kg bw, sid, sc as described previously) with 6 d of r-hFSH (30 IU bid, im), followed by 1–3 d of r-hFSH + r-hLH (30 IU each, bid, im) depending on the number and size of follicles observed on ultrasound on d 7 of stimulation as described earlier. The following morning, or in the evening of the final day of FSH/LH treatment, animals receive a single injection of 1000 IU r-hCG (im), and oocytes are collected 27 h or 32–34 h later, respectively. During 1997–1998 *(32)*, 45 females underwent follicular stimulation, with recovery of 668 oocytes from 36 animals for an average of 17 oocytes/aspiration. Oocyte yield from the initial stimulation cycle was greater (520 oocytes from 27 aspirations, average of 19/retrieval) than from repeat stimulation cycles (148 oocytes from 12 aspirations, average of 12/retrieval). Although the optimal time from hCG injection to oocyte retrieval led us to routinely use a 27 h interval, oocytes are collected 32–34 hours for nuclear transfer studies which allows earlier retrievals during the working day and a higher yield of mature oocytes at collection *(33)*.

Follicular Stimulation in Prepubertal Monkeys

The immature, gonadotropin-treated female mouse currently reigns as the rodent model most widely used for studies involving the ARTs (*see* Chapters 1 and 2). Prepubertal calves can also be stimulated with FSH for oocyte harvest and embryo production (*see* Chapter 1). However, it is not known whether a similar primate model could produce large follicles as well as mature oocytes capable of IVF in response to gonadotropins. Therefore, four prepubertal female rhesus monkeys with no history of menstrual cyclicity each underwent two follicular stimulation protocols. Table 1 displays the outcome of gonadotropin treatment and IVF in prepubertal macaques. First, females at 13–14 months of age were treated with Antide (as described earlier) simultaneously with a sequential regimen of 9 d of r-hFSH followed by 1–2 d of r-hFSH + r-hLH to stimulate the growth of multiple preovulatory follicles, followed by r-hCG as the ovulatory stimulus. In 2 of 4 animals (Protocol 1, Table 1), follicles ≥4 mm diameter were observed on ultrasound and mature oocytes were collected that yielded a 75% fertilization rate and a 44% cleavage rate to the 2- to 4-cell stage. The remaining 2 females did not respond to the gonadotropin treatment. In the second protocol, the 2 responders in the first protocol, now at 15–17 mo of age, received Antide with 10 d of r-hFSH alone followed by r-hCG. Although the percentage of follicles ≥4 mm diameter and total number of oocytes retrieved tended to be lower than in the first protocol, the inseminated oocytes had high fertilization and cleavage rates (2- to 4-cell; Table 1). In contrast, the 2 females who did not respond to the first protocol did elicit growth of multiple follicles with a second protocol of 6 d of u-hFSH (Metrodin, Serono) followed by 4 d of u-hFSH + u-hLH (Pergonal, Serono) with u-hCG (Profasi, Serono) as the ovulatory stimulus. Although mature oocytes were retrieved, fertilization and cleavage rates were low (Table 1). Thus, mature oocytes capable of fertilization in vitro and early cleavage can be obtained from gonadotropin-treated prepubertal rhesus monkeys. In addition, two gonadotropin protocols were successful in some of the animals, while nonresponders were capable of yielding fertilizable oocytes after

Table 1
Follicular Stimulation and IVF in Prepubertal Rhesus Monkeys

Protocol	No. responders	Total no. follicles	% Follicle ≥ 4 mm	Total no. oocytes	Proportion of Total Oocytes				No. fert./ no. insem.	Fertilization %	Cleavage %
					%MII	%MI	%GV	%Atretic			
1 r-hFSH/LH	2	32	22	43	21	44	25	10	21/28	75	44
2 r-hFSH	2	44	14	19	11	79	0	10	16/17	94	88
2 u-hFSH/LH	2*	35	11	34	9	47	23	21	7/19	37	nd

* These 2 females did not respond to protocol 1 (r-hFSH/LH).
nd = not determined

a second, altered, stimulation protocol. It is not known whether embryos derived from gonadotropin-stimulated immature primates would lead to live young comparable to IVF-produced embryos from mature macaques.

IN VITRO MATURATION

The success or failure of in vitro maturation (IVM) is determined by the quality and maturational status of the gametes. Simple (TALP) or complex culture media (CMRL) supplemented with serum, exogenous gonadotropins (FSH, LH, hCG) or granulosa cells have been employed for the nuclear and cytoplasmic maturation of GV-intact oocytes, morphologically normal (spherical, medium to lightly pigmented and no vacuoles present in the cytoplasm) and enclosed by at least two to three layers of tightly condensed cumulus cells *(34)*. The production of live young from in vitro matured GV-intact oocytes would allow the rescue of genetic material from important females who died before reproducing or from endangered species, circumvent the need for ovarian stimulation, provide a larger potential source of oocytes, and lead to knowledge that may improve human IVM/IVF success. The ability to support nuclear and cytoplasmic maturation of immature primate oocytes collected during non-stimulated cycles has important implications for women going through IVF (*see* Chapter 4).

Ovary and Oocyte Recovery

Ovaries can be recovered at necropsy or ovariectomy from anesthetized rhesus monkeys by paramedian pelvic laparotomy as described by Alak and Wolf *(35)*. Excised ovaries can be held either in TALP-Hepes *(36)* with 5% heat-inactivated fetal calf serum (FCS) and heparin (25 IU/mL) pH 7.4 at 37°C or in Tyrode's lactate (TL)-Hepes medium *(37)* at 37°C. Within 10 min of oophorectomy, ovaries are examined under a dissecting microscope for the presence of antral follicles with a size range of ≥300 μm to ≥1 mm *(19,35,38)*. The ovaries are then sectioned in small pieces and the medium and large antral follicles are individually punctured with a 25 gage needle to release oocyte-cumulus complexes (COCs). Follicles showing advanced signs of atresia (dark, dispersed granulosa cells) are discarded. Prior to in vitro maturation, the COCs are collected and pooled at intervals in fresh medium supplemented with 20% FCS before transfer to culture drops. Alternatively, oocytes can be aspirated via laparotomy or laparoscopy following follicular stimulation with gonadotropins (*see* below).

Oocyte Maturation

The maturational status of the oocytes, the expansion of the cumulus and the presence of the first polar body (metaphase II oocyte) are assessed 36-41 h post-culture. The meiotic and developmental capacity of IVM oocytes *(4,11,34,38,39)* is compromised relative to those matured in vivo and obtained from stimulated monkeys *(2,11,36,40)*. While 40%–50% of in vivo matured monkey oocytes develop into blastocysts in vitro *(2,36, 41,42)*, there is only one recent report of IVM/IVF produced embryos developing to the blastocyst stage from nonstimulated rhesus monkeys *(18)*. Schramm and Bavister *(4)* evaluated the role of cumulus cells on meiotic and developmental competence of in vitro matured oocytes from nonstimulated as well as from FSH- primed monkeys. They reported that meiotic and developmental competence was greater for oocytes obtained from ovaries during the luteal versus follicular phase of the macaque menstrual cycle, and that the incidence of nuclear maturation was improved substantially by the presence of granulosa cells and gonadotropins (FSH, LH). Interestingly, granulosa cells or gonadotropins alone did not improve nuclear maturation in oocytes from nonstimulated animals, but had separable effects on cytoplasmic maturation *(38)*. Gonadotropins alone improved oocyte activation and early cleavage events through the 4- to 8-cell stages *(34,38)*. Although granulosa cells increased the proportion of embryos achieving the morula stage, these embryos did not develop further.

Priming of monkeys with FSH for 6-7 d prior to IVM resulted in the production of IVM/IVF blastocysts suggesting that primate oocytes acquire developmental competence relatively late in the follicular growth process; cytoplasmic maturation may begin during folliculogenesis prior to meiotic resumption *(4)*. Nevertheless, the ability to develop into blastocysts remains substantially greater for primate oocytes matured in vivo *(2,18,36,42)* indicating that the follicular environment may be critically important during the last hours of pre-ovulatory development. More recently, Schramm and Bavister *(18)* showed enhancement of IVM of oocytes collected from nonstimulated monkeys when incubated with fresh granulosa cells recovered from FSH-primed monkeys' resulting in the first blastocysts produced in vitro (6.5%) when compared to a control with nonstimulated granulosa cells (0.6%). While it is largely unknown how granulosa cells support cytoplasmic maturation, the simple neutralization or removal of toxic products from the culture medium does not seem responsible as nonstimulated granulosa cells were ineffective in enhancing development beyond the 8- to 16-cell stage. Therefore, it is more likely that the effect is mediated by secretion of granulosa cell-derived products such as steroids *(43–45)*, growth factors, e.g., epidermal growth factor *(46,47)* or insulin like growth factor-I *(48,49)*, or other unidentified components. Recent evidence implicates members of the transforming growth factor-β superfamily of proteins in the regulation of oocyte maturation *(50–54)*. In addition, activin A and inhibin A effectively stimulate human *(54)* and nonhuman primate IVM *(53)*. Early studies have shown that activin and inhibin subunit mRNAs are localized in granulosa cells of murine and primate follicles *(55–57)*. Furthermore, activin A produced by granulosa cells may promote the maturation of enclosed oocytes while supporting their own proliferation and limiting their differentiation *(53)*. In addition, activin A modulates cytoplasmic maturation as suggested by an increase in the proportion of oocytes that reach the blastocyst stage *(58)*. Although the mechanism of action of activin A and inhibin A on oocyte maturation is not known, these two peptides may play an important autocrine-paracrine role. Further studies will be required to improve the culture conditions that support nuclear and cytoplasmic maturation of human and nonhuman primate oocytes and subsequent embryonic development after insemination leading to pregnancy.

IN VITRO FERTILIZATION

Since the report of the first successful pregnancy with IVF-ET by Steptoe and Edwards *(59)*, these techniques, the ARTs, have become an important tool in the treatment of infertility. However, there is a long standing need for animal models, including nonhuman primates, to provide basic information on fertilization and early embryogenesis. This need has become more urgent because of the increasingly invasive clinical applications such as ICSI, nuclear and cytoplasmic transfer and preimplantation genetic diagnosis (PGD). It is important to note, however, that while large numbers of children have been born following application of the ARTs, fewer than twenty nonhuman primates have resulted. Moreover, there are several hundred clinical embryology laboratories and fewer than ten nonhuman primate laboratories. The development of IVF-ET procedures in nonhuman primates could provide a tool to create pools of genetically valuable animals for use in biomedical research and could support efforts to preserve endangered primate species or to propagate primates used as disease models for medical research. Early work on nonhuman primate IVF has been reviewed by Wolf et al. *(9)*. IVF has been reported for oocytes from the squirrel monkey *(60,61)*, marmoset *(62)*, baboon *(63)*, cynomolgus *(12,64)*, rhesus *(1,2,11,36)* and pig-tailed *(7,16)* macaques, chimpanzee *(65)* and the gorilla *(8,13,66)*. The following sections will review the relevant methods associated with the ARTs, including IVF, ICSI and nuclear transfer in nonhuman primates.

Collection of Oocytes Matured In Vivo

Follicular aspiration in anesthetized monkeys can be performed surgically by laparotomy or laparoscopy using equipment similar to that described by Bavister et al. *(40)*. More specifically, a stainless-steel needle attached to a vacuum source is inserted into the base of the follicle (4–7 mm diameter) *(10)* and the follicular contents are aspirated under 80–100mm Hg negative pressure and collected in plastic tubes containing pre-warmed heparinized TALP-Hepes medium. The initial assessment of aspirated eggs is performed with the aid of a stereomicroscope and the quality and density of the surrounding cumulus and corona cell layers are used to grade the oocytes; however, the presence or absence of a polar body cannot be confirmed without first dispersing these layers with brief exposure to hyaluronidase. The appearance of the corona and cumulus cells (number of cell layers, condensed vs loose cells), the zona pellucida, the presence or absence of a perivitelline space, oocyte shape, presence or absence of cytoplasmic vacuoles, as well as the definitive presence of a first polar body are used to classify COCs as containing mature (metaphase-II), maturing (metaphase-I, no GV and no polar body), immature (GV- intact) or atretic oocytes *(36)*. Ovarian stimulation leads to the maturation of multiple follicles and the recovery of approximately 20 oocytes/animal, however, not all of these oocytes are mature and fertilizable.

VandeVoort and Tarantal *(67)* described the first and, to our knowledge, only technique for ultrasound-guided oocyte retrieval via transabdominal follicular aspiration in gonadotropin-stimulated cynomolgus monkeys. A foot-operated vacuum pump was attached to a collection tube fitted with a 22-gage × 3 inch spinal needle with the stylet removed (aspiration needle). The ovaries were imaged with a 7.5 MHz sector scanhead (ATL MK 600, Bothell, Washington), and the aspiration needle positioned 60° to the abdominal wall. With the animals under ketamine immobilization, the needle was introduced into the abdomen with continuous ultrasound guidance using a "free-hand" method for greater flexibility. When the needle tip was imaged near the ovarian wall, it was placed within the ovary and monitored as it entered each follicle during aspiration. The number of times the needle traversed the abdomen/ovary was limited to 3 per side. Ultrasound-guided transabdominal follicle aspiration in macaques is preferred over endovaginal oocyte retrieval, routinely performed in women, because of the thinness of the abdominal wall relative to women, in addition to the lack of endovaginal transducers small enough to accommodate the macaque vagina. This technique resulted in a 77–87% recovery rate of mature oocytes. Although acquisition of the necessary skills for performing this technique may require a considerable investment of time, ultrasound-guided transabdominal follicle aspiration provides an alternative to laparoscopy for nonsurgical recovery of oocytes in macaques *(67)*.

Semen Collection and Sperm Capacitation

Nonhuman primate semen is collected using direct penile or rectal probe stimulation. Penile electroejaculation, with controlled stimulus current optimally requires animal conditioning. While initial data is available from a number of nonhuman primates, extensive studies have been performed only in the rhesus monkey *(68,69)*. Semen in most nonhuman primates is characterized by the presence of a large coagulum, therefore, the sample should liquefy at $37^{\circ}C$ for approximately 30 min before the liquid portion is removed by aspiration. The resultant sperm population in macaques is remarkably uniform in structure and morphology *(68)*. The conventional semen parameters used to assess the fertility potential of a semen sample include semen volume, sperm concentration, motility and morphology. For the rhesus macaque at the Oregon Regional Primate Research Center, semen volumes range from 0.2–0.6 mL with sperm concentrations of 100–500 million sperm/mL and motile sperm percentages of 75–95% *(70)*.

For IVF and ICSI, sperm processing involves semen dilution with 3 or more volumes of TALP-Hepes, followed by centrifugation ($360 \times g$ for 7 min) and supernatant removal. This process may be repeated before the final sperm pellet is resuspended in TALP medium containing 0.3% BSA at 20 million sperm/mL and held at $37^{\circ}C$ in 5% CO_2 in humidified air. High quality, washed sperm preparations free of seminal plasma are a prerequisite for IVF/ICSI since the latter contains putative decapacitating factors *(71)*. Furthermore, head-to-head sperm agglutination is a significant problem in some males, especially after exposure to capacitation/activation agents such as dibutyryl cyclic AMP and caffeine at 1m*M (40,72)*. Our current experience indicates that male-dependent agglutination is significantly alleviated with proper dilution of semen. Capacitation/activation treatment of rhesus monkey sperm can be carried out from 30 min up to 3–4 h prior to insemination, and is not necessary for ICSI.

Sperm Cryopreservation

Semen cryopreservation in nonhuman primates remains problematic, despite attempts in several Old and New World monkeys, and great apes *(9)*. Nonetheless, the first live births following insemination with frozen-thawed sperm have been reported in the gorilla *(73)*, chimpanzee *(74)*, and cynomolgus monkey *(3)*. Studies on nonhuman primate semen cryopreservation including comparisons of cryoprotectants, buffers and extenders, freezing methods, and evaluation of post-thaw fertilizing ability have been reviewed (71; *see* Chapter 10). The percent motility (56–67%), viability (72%), and acrosome-intactness (31–38%) of frozen-thawed cynomolgus monkey semen was highest in TES-Tris or TES-Tris-20% skim milk buffer when the glycerol concentration was 2–3%; in contrast, egg yolk extender reduced these parameters (12%, 57%, and 16%, respectively; *3*). Post-thaw motility and survival of rhesus monkey sperm decreased dramatically relative to unfrozen sperm despite the use of a controlled-rate freezer and varying concentrations of glycerol as the cryoprotectant in either TES-Tris or egg yolk buffer *(71)*. Macaque sperm are generally more susceptible to acrosomal damage than are human sperm treated in a similar manner. Despite the advances made, a clearer understanding of how and when sperm cryodamage occurs is necessary for this procedure to become routinely used in nonhuman primate species. Optimization of this technique has important implications for breeding management of captive primates as well as for the propagation of endangered species.

Insemination and Evaluation of Fertilization

Metaphase-II oocytes that are matured at the time of follicular aspiration or have matured in vitro are usually incubated with relatively high sperm concentrations (1 to 2 $\times 10^6$ motile sperm/mL) in TALP medium supplemented with 0.3% BSA *(75)*. In vitro fertilization is evaluated 12 to 16 h after insemination when the presence of two well developed pronuclei and two polar bodies is taken as evidence of sperm penetration and egg activation. If polyspermy occurs this should result in the formation of more than two pronuclei, while spontaneous activation should be associated with the presence of a single pronucleus. In the rhesus monkey, pronuclei are less distinct when compared to the human. Removal of any residual cumulus or corona cells is often critical when visualizing pronucleus formation, even with an inverted microscope equipped with the highest quality optical system. The fertilization rate for rhesus monkey oocytes is typically in the 50-75% range *(2,12)* depending on the state of maturity and quality of the inseminated oocytes; values as high as 93% *(11)* have been reported. Eighteen hours or more after insemination, pronuclei may no longer be visible and by 24 h, most embryos have cleaved and, at this point, polyploidy based on pronuclear number can no longer be detected. Lower fertilization rates have been associated with in vitro matured oocytes where zona hardening during maturation may be a problem *(76)*. Moreover, it is not possible to predict in advance which oocytes will fertilize. Johnson and co-workers *(76)* noted that serum estradiol response, follicle size and cumulus morphology, which are commonly used to determine in vivo oocyte maturation, were inadequate predictors of oocyte quality.

EMBRYO TRANSFER AND CRYOPRESERVATION

The success of IVF ultimately depends on evidence of live births following the transfer of IVF-derived embryos. Approximately a decade has passed since the first reports of transfer of nonfrozen or frozen-thawed IVF-derived embryos in various nonhuman primate species *(1,9,36,71)*. Embryo transfers have been conducted using surgical (oviductal) and nonsurgical (transcervical, intrauterine) methods. In macaques, the surgical method is most commonly reported since the tortuous anatomy of the cervix makes the nonsurgical approach quite challenging. The embryo transfer technique evolved from initial attempts at transferring nonfrozen embryos to those involving cryopreserved, thawed embryos *(9,36,71)*, and has recently been extended to the transfer of ICSI-derived embryos *(5)*. Despite the limited experience in macaques up until 1990, an overall implantation rate of 14% and pregnancy rate of 20% were comparable to human IVF outcomes *(71)*. This section will describe the procedures currently used for oviductal and transcervical embryo transfers in rhesus monkeys, and will summarize the most recent embryo transfer reports in nonhuman primates (since 1990).

The focus of more recent studies on embryo transfer has not been on propagating large numbers of nonhuman primates, but to demonstrate live births in validation of the nonhuman primate as a model for IVF-ET following recombinant gonadotropin stimulation, ICSI, or nuclear transfer as well as in the development of techniques for conserving endangered species. Table 2 summarizes the implantation and pregnancy rates following oviductal and intrauterine embryo transfers which will be discussed in more detail in the

Table 2

Implantation and Pregnancy Rates in Nonhuman Primates Following Oviductal and Intrauterine Embryo Transfer to Recipients During the Early Luteal Phase of Spontaneous Menstrual Cycles

Species	Oocyte Donor stimulation	Embryo source	Nonfrozen (NF) Frozen/Thawed (F/T)	Stage frozen	Post-thaw viability (%)	Type transfer	Stage at transfer	Implantation rate (%)[a]	Pregnancy rate (%)[b]	Ref.
Rhesus	r-hFSH	IVF	F/T	2-7 cell	56	Oviductal	2-7 cell	2/16 (12)	1/8 (12)	23
	r-hFSH/LH	IVF	F/T	2-7 cell	78	Oviductal	2-7 cell	2/6 (33)	2/3 (66)	
Rhesus	r-hFSH/LH	ICSI	NF	—	—	Oviductal	2-8 cell	6/14 (66)	5/9 (55)	5
Rhesus	r-hFSH/LH	Nuclear Transfer	F/T	2-16 cell	nr[c]	Oviductal	2-16 cell	4/53 (7)	2/17 (12)	6
Rhesus	Natural cycle	In vivo Blastocyst	NF	—	—	Intrauterine	Hatched	2/14 (14)	1/14 (7)	84
Rhesus	u-hFSH/LH	IVF	F/T	pronuclear	nr	Intrauterine	2-6 cell	1/7 (14)	1/7 (14)	Unpub.
Gorilla	u-hFSH	IVF	NF	—	—	Intrauterine	6-8 cell	1/3 (33)	1/1 (100)	8
Marmoset	Natural cycle	In vivo	NF	—	—	Intrauterine	Asynch.	6/17 (35)	6/9 (44)	86
							Synch.	1/22 (5)	1/11 (9)	

[a] Number of fetuses/number of embryos transferred
[b] Number of infants born/number of recipients
[c] nr = not reported

263

appropriate sections below. Although direct comparisons cannot be made between these data sets, the results are promising and prove that current transfer techniques will, for the most part, be adequate for advancing the ARTs in nonhuman primates.

Oviductal Embryo Transfer

Rhesus monkey recipients are chosen for surgical embryo transfer based on the following criteria: health and physical condition, a record of previous pregnancy and live births, demonstration of normal ovarian cycles indicated by the typical patterns of estradiol in the follicular phase and progesterone in the luteal phase as measured by radioimmunoassay (RIA) and menstrual cyclicity based on a regular pattern of menses every 28–30 d. Beginning 8 d after menses during a spontaneous menstrual cycle, blood samples are collected daily from the saphenous vein for determination of estradiol by RIA. The LH surge is estimated to occur one day prior to the precipitous decline in serum estradiol, typically to levels <100 pg/mL. If progesterone levels are measured simultaneously, a transient increase in progesterone from baseline levels during the late follicular phase (<0.5 ng/mL) to 1.0–1.5 ng/mL will be observed in some animals; the day of this increase in progesterone can be estimated as the LH surge. The actual LH surge can be measured retrospectively using an in vitro mouse Leydig cell bioassay validated for macaque serum. Two to four days after the estimated LH surge, fresh or frozen-thawed embryos, typically 2/recipient, are surgically transferred to the oviduct ipsilateral to the ovary bearing the ovulatory stigma in anesthetized recipients (2). The embryos are loaded into a syringe driven catheter of flexible silicon tubing (Dow-Corning, Midland, MI; 0.5 mm ID × 1.0 mm OD or 0.6 mm ID × 1.2 mm OD, the largest size possible dictated by oviduct size), the tip of the catheter placed in the fimbrial os, and the embryos expelled. The catheter is checked for retained embryos after transfer. No hormonal supplementation is used before or after embryo transfer. To confirm implantation following embryo transfer, daily blood samples are collected to monitor serum estradiol and progesterone levels and bioactive LH/chorionic gonadotropin through d 28–32 post-LH surge (23). At this time, clinical pregnancies are confirmed by fetal cardiac activity as determined by ultrasonography. Embryonic gestational age is estimated using values for gestational sac and embryo length as described for rhesus monkeys by Tarantal and Hendrickx (77). Ultrasonography at later times can be used to monitor fetal viability and gestational age by measuring femur length and biparietal diameter (77). If characterization of hormone levels throughout gestation is desired, blood samples can be obtained three times a week without adverse effects on fetal outcome and birth (11).

Transcervical Intrauterine Embryo Transfer

The first IVF-derived rhesus monkey, Petri, resulted from the nonsurgical technique of transcervical embryo transfer (1). Since that time, progress in the development of nonsurgical embryo transfer for obtaining successful pregnancies has been limited; the tortuous cervical canal of the rhesus monkey provides a difficult barrier for routine transcervical cannulation. Nonetheless, the surgical technique used for flushing embryos from the macaque uterus (78,79) was modified to a nonsurgical procedure by Goodeaux (80,81) and Seshagiri (82), and has been adapted for transcervical intrauterine embryo transfer in rhesus monkeys. Females are anesthetized with ketamine and positioned in sternal recumbency. A stainless steel stylet (0.0655 inches o.d., 6 inches long) is inserted into the vagina and, using rectal palpation, guided through the cervix and into the uterus.

A stainless steel cannula (0.1048 inches o.d., 4 inches long) is placed directly over the stylet until positioned in the uterus. Embryos are loaded into a polyvinyl catheter (PV-4, 0.30 inches i.d., 0.48 inches o.d., 12 inches long; Bolab Inc. Lake Havasu City, AZ) connected to a 20 gage blunt-tipped needle on a 1 cc syringe, in the order of medium, air, embryos/medium, air, and medium, not to exceed 20 µL of medium. The catheter containing the embryos is threaded through the cannula via the external cervical os with subsequent passage into the uterus. Prior to expelling the embryos, the cannula is pulled back approximately 0.5 inch so that the tip of the catheter is exposed in the uterus, making sure that the catheter is kept stationary during cannula movement. The embryos are slowly expelled, and the catheter is removed, and rinsed with media that is subsequently examined for retained embryos. Once embryo transfer is assured, the cannula is removed. Pregnancy is monitored by ultrasound and serum steroids as described above for oviductal embryo transfers.

To enhance selection of female macaques for successful transcervical cannulation, Iliff-Sizemore and associates (83) investigated the effects of parity, stage of the menstrual cycle and season of the year in 76 adult rhesus monkeys and 4 Celebes macaques (*Macaca nigra*). Overall, a 51% cannulation success rate, based on a single attempt per animal, was observed. The reproductive tract of multiparous females is more conducive to successful cannulation, while menstrual cycle stage and season did not affect success rate. Currently at ORPRC, rhesus females are screened for successful cannulation prior to assignment as recipients for transcervical, intrauterine embryo transfers.

Only a few successful pregnancies following transcervical intrauterine embryo transfer in macaques have been reported in the past decade (Table 2). Fourteen embryos recovered nonsurgically from rhesus females by Goodeaux and colleagues (84) were transferred into recipients that had undergone uterine flushing during the transfer cycle (n = 12) or into recipients that had not been previously flushed (n = 2). Eleven of the 14 embryos were co-cultured to blastocysts on rhesus uterine epithelial cells in CMRL or Menezo's B2 media; 2 pregnancies resulted after transfer to flushed recipients. One pregnancy following transfer of an embryo co-cultured in Menezo's B2 was lost between 40–50 d of gestation. The other pregnancy established from an embryo co-cultured in CMRL yielded a normal, healthy infant. No pregnancies resulted from 3 embryos not cultured prior to transfer.

In a small unpublished trial at ORPRC (Table 2), 7 rhesus female recipients underwent transcervical transfer on d 4 of the luteal phase and received 2- to 6-cell embryos previously frozen at the pronuclear stage. One singleton biochemical pregnancy occurred; bioactive mCG in serum began to rise on d 19 of gestation, but the pregnancy was lost by d 38. Current efforts are directed at optimizing embryo quality, synchrony between embryo and endometrium and the transfer technique with the goal of using nonsurgical embryo transfers routinely in rhesus monkeys.

Transcervical embryo transfer appears to be less problematic in the gorilla relative to macaques. The linear orientation between the uterus, cervix and vagina of the gorilla reproductive tract (85) allows for easier access to the uterus. Pope and associates (8) reported the first birth of a Western lowland gorilla, Timu, following transcervical transfer 47 h postinsemination of three IVF-derived embryos cultured in vitro to the 6- to 8 cell stage. This landmark achievement provides encouraging evidence that the ARTs can be used in the development of captive breeding programs to enhance propagation of endangered great apes.

Nonsurgical, intrauterine embryo transfer in common marmosets was reported for the first time by Marshall and colleagues (*86*; Table 2). Synchronous transfers, wherein the oocyte donor and recipient ovulated on the same day, performed on d 5–8 postovulation resulted in one pregnancy from 11 transfers (9%); the pregnancy was lost by d 40 of gestation. Asynchronous transfers, between oocyte donors that ovulated 2 d before the recipient, performed when the recipient was 2–4 d post-ovulation yielded four pregnancies from nine transfers (44%), with three carried to term (6 infants from 17 embryos). Although somewhat lower than transfer of morulae or blastocysts using a surgical technique (66%), the high pregnancy rate after nonsurgical transfer most likely reflects the fecundity of the marmoset species, the ability to synchronize ovarian cycles with prostaglandins and the high quality of the in vivo-produced embryos used for transfer *(86)*. The greater success rate following asynchronous transfer may be due to transfer of embryos 4–6 d before implantation in the marmoset. At this uterine stage, damage of the potential implantation site due to cannulation is less likely, and the endometrium has time to recover prior to implantation. Conversely, manipulation of a cannula in the uterine lumen during synchronous transfers which were carried out closer to the time of implantation may have disrupted the peri-implantation endometrial milieu *(86)*. The proven success of this technique will aid the conservation of endangered Callithrichid species as well as advance knowledge of postimplantation embryonic development in nonhuman primates.

Improved pregnancy outcome in nonhuman primates may be obtained following intrauterine transfer of advanced preimplantation-stage embryos (i.e., morula and blastocyst) exhibiting developmental synchrony with the endometrium of the recipient. In rhesus monkeys, nonsurgical collection via transcervical cannulation and uterine flushing on d 4, 5, and 6 postovulation of embryos derived from natural matings yielded morula, early blastocysts and expanded blastocysts, respectively *(81)*. Likewise, the majority of embryos recovered surgically from rhesus monkey uteri on d 4–5 of the luteal phase were 8- to 16-cell and morula *(87)*, while zona-encased and zona-free blastocysts were more frequently recovered during the midluteal phase (d 6–7) of the spontaneous menstrual cycle *(82,88)*. Determination of the optimal embryo stage for transfer following in vitro culture (*see* below) and the interval of uterine receptivity at transfer is a priority before consistent success can be realized from transcervical embryo transfers in macaques.

Synchronization of Ovarian Cycles in Recipients

Ovarian cycles are routinely synchronized in marmosets with exogenous administration of a prostaglandin $F_{2\alpha}$ analog between d 17-21 of the luteal phase which causes premature luteolysis and initiation of the follicular phase *(89)*. Unlike the marmoset, prostaglandin $F_{2\alpha}$ is ineffective when given systemically to rhesus monkeys, but will cause luteal regression in some cases when delivered directly into the corpus luteum *(90)*. This latter method requires surgical intervention and is therefore inappropriate for routine use during embryo transfer protocols in macaque recipients. Thus, current methods for determining the time of embryo transfer in macaques (*see* above), while time-consuming, and requiring large numbers of animals to increase the probability of having a recipient available at the appropriate time, rely on determination of the midcycle estradiol surge in serum or urine collected daily during spontaneous menstrual cycles.

Oocyte and embryo donation in women has been used in the treatment of a variety of disorders, e.g. premature ovarian failure, poor oocyte quality, and age-related infertility. Pregnancies are achieved when suppression of ovarian function with a GnRH agonist is followed by sequential administration of estradiol and progesterone for synchronization of the recipient endometrium with the time required for donor oocyte collection, fertilization and embryonic development prior to embryo transfer (*see* Chapter 9). Pioneering studies by Hodgen *(91)* were the first to show that a sequential estradiol-progesterone regimen of silastic implants in ovariectomized rhesus monkeys, designed to mimic the levels and patterns of these steroids during the natural cycle, could support implantation and pregnancy of donor embryos removed from naturally mated animals. However, this model has received little attention for the synchronization of ovarian-intact recipients prior to transfer of either nonfrozen or frozen-thawed embryos in nonhuman primates, particularly macaques. Cranfield *(7)* reported two pregnancies in steroid-treated, synchronized pig-tail macaque recipients following four oviductal transfers of nonfrozen 2-cell embryos derived from IVF; one resulted in the live birth of a singleton and the other carried twins that were lost on d 93 of gestation. Synchronization of endometrial receptivity in recipients undergoing embryo transfer is an area clearly in need of further development for increasing the propagation of nonhuman primates for basic research or in preserving biodiversity.

Embryo Cryopreservation

At the Oregon Regional Research Primate Center's (ORPRC) ART program, IVF freezing, thawing and surgical embryo transfer have been successfully achieved with the delivery of the world first rhesus monkey twins *(11)*. The ability to reliably freeze-thaw nonhuman primate embryos should benefit research in genetic manipulation of these embryos, since the supply of embryos and synchronized recipients could be dissociated in time (*see* Chapter 10).

Cryopreservation of IVF-derived embryos at the pronuclear to 8-cell stages is performed at the ORPRC using protocol II of Kuzan and Quinn *(92)* in phosphate-buffered saline containing 20% heat-inactivated fetal bovine serum (FBS) and 1,2-propanediol (1.5 M) as the cryoprotectant, as described by Lanzendorf and colleagues *(11)*. After the stepwise introduction of cryoprotectant, embryos are transported on wet ice in 2.0 mL cryo-vials for freezing in a controlled-rate freezer (BioCool; FTS Systems, Stoneridge, NY). Samples are seeded at $-7°C$, held for 5 min before cooling at $0.3°C$/min to $-30°C$, then plunged into and stored in liquid nitrogen. Embryos are thawed in a $37°C$ water bath followed by stepwise dilution of the cryoprotectant at room temperature in the presence of 0.2 M sucrose. Thawed embryos are cultured in TALP medium containing 20% heat-inactivated fetal bovine serum for approximately 2 h prior to the surgical transfer procedure. Embryos frozen at the pronuclear stage are cultured in TALP containing 20% FBS without bovine serum albumin or in CRML with co-culture for an additional 24 h prior to transfer.

EMBRYO CULTURE AND DEVELOPMENT IN VITRO

The developmental potential of IVF-produced embryos from rhesus monkeys is relatively poor and inconsistent, and remains a major limitation for advancement of the ARTs in macaques. Suboptimal culture conditions contribute greatly to the impaired development of nonhuman primate embryos. The benefits of serum relative to BSA as a protein source during culture of IVF-derived embryos from cynomolgus monkeys was noted by Fujisaki *(93)*. Embryonic development was blocked at the 4-cell stage in BSA-supplemented

Whitten's medium without serum, however, development continued to the morula stage in Ham's F12 with serum *(93)*. In contrast, blastulation was achieved during culture with modified CMRL-1066 medium containing serum from IVF-derived zygotes obtained after in vivo *(2,36,41,72,94)* and in vitro *(4)* oocyte maturation in the rhesus monkey, as well as in the baboon *(95)*. Boatman *(36)* also noted that rhesus monkey embryos developed better in CMRL than in TALP medium. Thus, modified CMRL plus serum has been employed by the majority of investigators attempting nonhuman primate embryo culture (*see* Table 3). Successful development to blastocysts in this medium occurred in 22% of nonfrozen *(36)* and only 8% of frozen-thawed *(41)* rhesus macaque embryos, whereas 90% of morulae obtained via uterine lavage of pregnant rhesus macaques became blastocysts in vitro *(87)*. Weston and Wolf *(96)* compared developmental efficiencies of IVF-produced rhesus monkey embryos cultured in KSOM plus amino acids (KSOM/AA; *97,98*) or CMRL, both supplemented with serum, and found no significant differences between the two media (Table 3). Low blastulation rates in vitro may be related to inadequate development of the inner cell mass at the hatched blastocyst stage as noted by Enders and colleagues *(99)* in IVF-derived rhesus embryos relative to those produced in vivo.

Developmental efficiencies of IVF-produced embryos of nonprimate species as well as humans can be improved with co-culture on somatic cells (reviewed in ref. *41*). Goodeaux and associates *(84)* were the first to observe in rhesus macaques that transient exposure of uterine-stage embryos, collected by lavage, to uterine epithelial cells in vitro improved developmental efficiencies to hatching from 17% to 63% (CMRL alone, CMRL with co-culture, respectively). Co-culture was associated with embryos containing higher inner cell mass cell numbers and resulted in successful pregnancy following intrauterine embryo transfer (*see* Table 2). Subsequently, Zhang et al *(41)* examined the developmental potential of frozen-thawed, IVF-derived rhesus monkey embryos cultured in CMRL plus serum alone, or co-cultured with primary cultures, (bovine oviductal epithelial and bovine cumulus cells), or established cell lines, (Vero and buffalo rat liver (BRL) cells) (Table 3). Co-culture with BRL cells resulted in the greatest development to hatched blastocyst (Table 3). However, co-culture did not improve embryo quality since well-developed ICMs were noted in the majority of hatched blastocysts derived from all treatment groups *(41)*. The BRL cell co-culture system was subsequently used to investigate whether LH was required during the preovulatory interval for normal embryonic development *(23)*. A similar proportion of frozen-thawed, IVF-derived embryos, from gonadotropin releasing hormone antagonist-treated rhesus macaques that received r-hFSH alone for follicular stimulation, developed to the hatched blastocyst stage with a definitive ICM during co-culture, relative to animals that received r-hFSH + r-hLH *(23*; Table 3). The developmental efficiency to hatched blastocyst ranged from 28-31% which was somewhat lower than the 45% observed following culture of embryos derived after urinary gonadotropin treatment during the preovulatory interval *(41)*.

Bavister *(100)* has speculated that co-culture systems compensate for deficiencies in currently used culture media, e.g. somatic cells benefit embryonic development by providing nutrients or stabilizing the pH that might change as a consequence of the metabolic activity of both the embryo and cells. While co-culture technology can produce more viable embryos under certain conditions relative to medium alone, it precludes studies on the specific components that regulate embryonic development in primates. Schramm and Bavister *(101)* developed a chemically-defined, protein-free culture medium, hamster embryo culture medium-6 (HECM-6), that was able to support rhesus monkey embryonic development to

Table 3
Developmental Efficiency of Rhesus Monkey Embryos Under Various In Vitro Culture Conditions

Medium	Embryo source	Nonfrozen (NF) Frozen/thawed (FT)	Stage frozen or at culture initiation	Viable embryos achieving indicated stage (%)[e]					
				8c-EM	M	B	XB	HB	Ref.
CMRL[a]	Spont. cycle d 5 post-ov.	NF	M					90	87
	d 6 post-ov.	NF	B					90	
	IVF	FT	1-4 cell	77	23		8	8	41
	IVF	NF	1 cell			55	53	49	96
	IVF	NF	1 cell			75	64	55	96
KSOM/AA[a]	IVF	NF	1 cell	93	73		40	33	41
CMRL[a] + Bovine Oviduct	IVF	NF	1 cell	85	65		15	15	
CMRL[a] + Bovine Cumulus	IVF	NF	1 cell	73	73		36	9	
CMRL[a] + Vero	IVF	NF	1 cell	100	73		55	45	
CMRL[a] + BRL	IVF r-hFSH	FT	1-4 cell		64	36	36	28	23
CMRL[a] + BRL	IVF r-hFSH + r-hLH	FT	1-4 cell		62	41	31	31	
HECM-6	IVF	NF	1 cell	85	72	22	7	2	101
CMRL[a]	IVF	NF	1 cell	95	80	48	45	31	
HECM-6/CMRL[b]	IVF	NF	1 cell	78	69	61	54	44	
HCEM-6/CMRL 8c[c,d]	IVF	NF	1 cell			60	55	55	
HCEM-6/HCEM-6 8c	IVF	NF	1 cell			50	50	40	
HCEM-6/CMRL M[b,d]	IVF	NF	1 cell			20	20	18	
HCEM-6/HCEM-6 M	IVF	NF	1 cell			35	35	30	

[a] Medium contains serum.
[b] Embryos were cultured in 2-step sequential media; step 1 = no serum; step 2 = contains serum; media changed at the morula stage.
[c] Embryos were cultured in 2-step sequential media; step 1 = no serum; step 2 = contains serum; media changed at the 8-cell stage.
[d] Percentages estimated from the reported means in reference 101.
[e] M = Morula; B = Blastocyst; XB = Expanded blastocyst; HB = Hatched blastocyst.

the morula stage in a proportion similar to CMRL plus serum, however, they discovered that a 2-component culture system, i.e., culture in HECM-6 through the 8-cell stage followed by CMRL plus serum, was required for blastulation and hatching (*see* Table 3). To ascertain stage-specific requirements for serum-containing media, IVF-derived zygotes were incubated through the 8-cell stage with HECM-6 alone, followed by either CMRL plus serum or HECM-6 plus serum. The same combinations were tested with the second medium introduced at the morula stage. Embryos cultured initially in HECM-6 to the 8-cell stage, developed into blastocysts and hatched in similar proportions to those exposed to either serum-supplemented CMRL or HECM-6. In contrast, embryos transferred at the morula stage to serum-containing medium were severely compromised in their capacity to develop into blastocysts (Table 3). These results suggest that neither protein nor serum are required for macaque embryo development through the early cleavage stages in vitro, but that culture through the morula stage in protein-free media is detrimental to further development *(101)*. Furthermore, the developmental requirements for blastulation and hatching of macaque embryos appear to be acquired between the 8-cell and early morula stages. In contrast to humans, macaque embryos may not require glucose or pyruvate for progression to morula (absent in HECM-6), but these energy sources may be essential for blastulation. In addition, this study suggests that macaque embryos require some unknown components present in serum for blastulation *(101)*.

Developmental rates of morula and blastocyst stages in vitro are generally slower than those seen in vivo, based on comparisons with embryos recovered from oviductal or uterine lavages (*see* Table 4). However, rhesus macaque embryos cultured in KSOM/AA developed significantly faster, reaching the expanded and hatched blastocyst stages a day earlier than those in CMRL.

Further refinements in media used for culturing nonhuman primate embryos will hopefully allow the elimination of protein or serum sources and the use of co-culture on somatic cells. Based on the robust success rates following blastocyst transfers in women, sequential media exposure should be evaluated further. If development to the blastocyst stage becomes routine and can be combined with nonsurgical, intrauterine embryo transfers, a significant improvement in the production of nonhuman primates could be realized.

INTRACYTOPLASMIC SPERM INJECTION

In mammals, successful fertilization has been reported in rabbit *(102)*, cattle *(103)*, mice *(104)* and more recently in nonhuman primates using partial zona drilling *(13)* or ICSI *(5,105–107)*. During the conventional process of fertilization only the capacitated sperm progress through the cumulus oophorus, bind to the zona pellucida and penetrate into the cytoplasm of mature oocytes *(108)*. The fusion of the male and female gametes initiates a cascade of events resulting in oocyte activation which includes the cortical reaction, the triggering of the polyspermy preventing mechanisms *(109)*, resumption of meiosis, increased metabolic activity and cytoskeletal remodeling *(110–112)*. The process of ICSI obviously bypasses the sperm-oocyte membrane fusion process along with an undefined number of the other events listed here that are associated with fertilization.

The ICSI Procedure

ICSI is performed with the aid of an inverted microscope equipped with Hoffman modulation contrast Nomarski or DIC optics, hydraulic manipulators (X-, Y-, and Z

Table 4
Developmental Rates of Rhesus Monkey Embryos In Vivo and In Vitro

Source or medium	Nonfrozen (NF) Frozen/thawed (FT)	Stage at initiation in culture	Days to reach indicated stage post-ovulation or in culture[d]				Ref.
			M	B	XB	HB	
Oviductal lavage	NF	—	4	5			35
Uterine lavage	NF	—	4	5	6		81
Uterine lavage	NF	—	4-5	4-5	5-6		87
Uterine lavage/CMRL[a]	NF	M[b]				7.8	82
	NF	B[b]				7.5	
	FT	1-4 cell	5.6	8.9	9.5	10.8	41
	NF	1 cell	5.8	7.4	9.0	9.9	96
KSOM/AA[a]	NF	1 cell	5.4	6.7	7.9	8.8	96
CMRL[a] + BRL[b]	FT r-hFSH	1-7 cell	5.9	8.5	10.0	12.0	23
	FT r-hFSH + r-hLH	1-7 cell	5.6	7.8	8.5	10.0	
HCEM-6/CMRL[a] or HCEM-6/HCEM-6[a]	NF	1 cell	6 (5-8)[c]		8 (7-10)[c]		101

[a] Medium contains serum.
[b] Embryos co-cultured on BRL cells.
[c] Range of developmental rates observed in reference 101.
[d] M = Morula; B = Blastocyst; XB = Expanded blastocyst; HB = Hatched blastocyst.

271

axis), and joysticks for both the injection and holding pipettes. In our system, each manipulator set is coupled with a microinjector, used either to hold and release the oocyte or to aspirate and inject a sperm. The injector consists of a 800 μL syringe and Teflon tubing with a micrometer driven plunger. The syringe and tubing lines are filled with sterile Milli-Q water with care taken to avoid the presence of air bubbles in the system. The microscope is equipped with a video camera, and all manipulations can be followed on a monitor. The holding and microinjector pipettes are prepared from borosilicate glass capillaries. The holding pipet has an external diameter of 150 μm and an internal diameter of 40 μm. The injection pipette is bevelled to an angle of 45° using a micro grinder and has external and internal diameters of 7 μm and 5 μm, respectively. A spike (~3 μm) is pulled using a microforge. The micropipettes are filled with mineral oil and connected to the tubing of each microinjector. Typically, this working station is set up prior to oocyte manipulation. All oocytes are then treated with 0.1% hyaluronidase in TALP-Hepes medium for approx 2–3 min to remove cumulus and corona cells and allow visualization of the polar body. ICSI is performed 2–6 h after the presence of the polar body is confirmed, and is in a 32–33°C prewarmed room. A plastic petri dish containing 50 μL microdrops of TALP-Hepes supplemented with 0.3% BSA is used. A drop of sperm in TALP-Hepes-0.3% BSA supplemented with 10% polyvinyl pyrrolidone (PVP: MW 360,000) is also added and all drops are covered with mineral oil. The sperm suspension is typically diluted 1:4 in 10% PVP which facilitates sperm manipulation and allows good control of the fluid in the injection pipette. Sperm immobilization involves aspiration of a single motile sperm into the injection pipette and gently expelling it from the pipette near the medium-oil interface; the sperm is then placed perpendicular to the injection pipette, which is moved over the tail, lowered, and the tail is crushed or compressed between the pipette and the bottom of the dish. After immobilization, the sperm is again aspirated tail first into the injection pipette. The injection pipette with the sperm is then moved to the oocyte drop. The holding pipette is lowered, an oocyte is rotated slowly to locate the polar body and the oocyte is grasped and held in place by gentle suction from the holding pipette with the polar body at the 12 or 6 o'clock position. To avoid damage to the meiotic spindle during ICSI, oocytes are always injected with the polar body as far away from the injection site as possible, however it has been noted that the position of the polar body is not always a reliable guide to locate the metaphase plate *(113)*. The injection pipette is brought into the same focal plane as the outer border of the oolemma on an equatorial plane at 3 o'clock. The immobilized sperm is carefully positioned in the tip of the pipette, and the pipette is pushed through the zona almost to the opposite side of the oocyte. At this point, a break in the membrane should occur, visualized by disruption of the funnel shaped oolemma around the injection pipette above and below the penetration point, as well as by flow of cytoplasm and sperm inside the injection pipette. Additional aspiration of the cytoplasm into the pipette confirms oolemma rupture. The cytoplasm and the sperm are then injected into the egg. Following ICSI, injected oocytes are placed in culture in TALP medium supplemented with 10% FCS or in CMRL on BRL co-culture at 37°C in 5% CO_2 in humidified air.

Evaluation of Fertilization and Embryonic Development

Similar to conventional insemination, assessment of fertilization following ICSI is carried out 12–16 h postsperm exposure. Pronuclear formation and extrusion of the second polar body are recorded as evidence of fertilization. Using these criteria, Lanzendorf and Wolf *(105)* first reported successful fertilization of rhesus monkey oocytes following ICSI . Oocyte activation was improved upon exposure of macaque oocytes to calcium ionophore post-microinjection *(105)*, a finding that was later corroborated by Hewitson and colleagues using IVM oocytes retrieved from unstimulated females *(107)*. Microinjection of a rhesus monkey sperm extract into mature oocytes induced oocyte activation, suggesting that sperm contain an oocyte-activating factor, perhaps localized in the sperm head that could be used instead of ionophores *(114)*. However, activation of higher quality oocytes obtained via laparoscopy from gonadotropin-stimulated rhesus monkeys does not require a chemical stimulus *(106,114)*. Initial fertilization rates following ICSI of oocytes matured in vitro were relatively low *(107)*, while those for in vivo matured oocytes were comparable *(106)* to conventional in vitro insemination under similar conditions *(9)*. ICSI-produced rhesus monkey embryos co-cultured on BRL cells in CMRL medium containing 10% FCS undergo successive cleavage divisions culminating in hatched blastocysts within 10 d *(106)*, a developmental rate similar to embryos derived from IVF oocytes *(36)*. We are currently using ICSI and in vitro embryonic development to the blastocyst stage as a means of assessing oocyte quality.

Oviductal transfer of nonfrozen 3- to 8-cell stage rhesus monkey embryos produced by ICSI to recipients during the early luteal phase of spontaneous menstrual cycles resulted in 6 pregnancies; one biochemical, one stillborn and 4 live births, the first reported in this species *(5)*. Despite these successes, numerous abnormalities in the fertilization by ICSI process were observed when compared to fertilization following conventional insemination. Although hundreds of human infants have been born following ICSI, serious concerns regarding the possibility of increased chromosomal and physical abnormalities in these children have been raised (*see* Chapters 7 and 17). The rhesus monkey may provide a suitable model for further evaluation of the safety and effectiveness of ICSI.

NUCLEAR TRANSFER

Nuclear transfer was proposed as early as 1938 by Spemann *(115)* as a method of studying cellular differentiation. Basically the procedure of nuclear transfer involves the transfer of a donor nucleus into an enucleated, mature, metaphase-II oocyte called a cytoplast. Nuclear transfer in other species is described in detail in Chapters 13, 14 and 15. A description of primate embryonic stem cells and their potential precedes a detailed discussion of nuclear transfer as practiced in the monkey.

Primate Embryonic Stem Cells as Nuclear Donors

Primate embryonic stem (ES) cells, derived from preimplantation embryos, are capable of prolonged undifferentiated proliferation, and yet even after prolonged culture, are capable of forming advanced derivatives of all three embryonic germ layers. Primate ES cells have been derived from rhesus monkeys, common marmosets, and humans *(116–119)*. The procedures for isolating primate and mouse cells are similar, but the properties of the resulting primate and mouse ES cells differ significantly. The inner cell mass (ICM) of the blastocyst is isolated by immunosurgery and plated on mouse embryonic fibroblasts. After approximately one week of culture, the ICM is split and replated. With careful attention to water and serum quality, undifferentiated colonies with a distinct morphology appear, which are individually selected and expanded. The morphology of rhesus ES and human ES cell colonies are quite similar, but marmoset ES cell colonies are somewhat distinct (Fig. 1). Marmoset ES cells have a morphology more intermediate

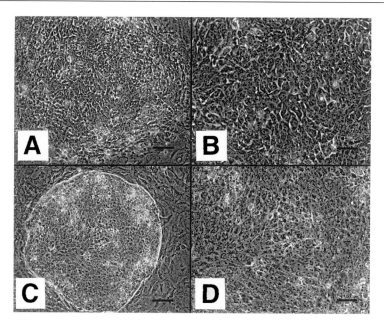

Fig. 1. Undifferentiated colony morphology of primate ES cells. (**A**) Rhesus monkey ES cell colony, phase contrast. Bar = 200 μ. (**B**) Rhesus monkey ES cell colony, phase contrast. Bar = 100 μ. (**C**) Common marmoset ES cell colony, phase contrast. Bar = 200 μ. (**D**) Common marmoset ES cell colony, phase contrast. Bar = 100 μ.

between human ES cells and mouse ES cells, probably reflecting the greater evolutionary distance of marmosets from humans. Primate ES cells all have a high nuclear-cytoplasmic ratio and contain multiple prominent nucleoli. Electron microscopy of rhesus ES cells reveals a highly convoluted nucleus, prominent nucleoli and sparse microvilli at the surface—an ultrastructure very similar to human EC cells *(117)*. Rhesus ES, marmoset ES, human ES, and human EC cells all share characteristic cell surface markers, including stage specific embryonic antigen (SSEA)-3, SSEA-4, TRA-1-60, and TRA-1-81, but not SSEA-1. This contrasts with the pattern of expression of mouse ES cells, which express SSEA-1, but don't express SSEA-3, SSEA-4, TRA-1-60, or TRA-1-81 *(120–125)*. The shared pattern of expression of cell surface markers by all described primate ES cells, and differing pattern of expression by mouse ES cells, likely reflects fundamental embryological differences between primates and mice.

When removed from fibroblast feeder layers, primate ES cells differentiate into a variety of cell types. Leukemia inhibitory factor (LIF), which prevents the differentiation of mouse ES cells, fails to prevent the differentiation of primate ES cells in the absence of fibroblasts *(116,118,119)*. When primate ES cells are allowed to differentiate in the absence of fibroblasts, endoderm differentiation is indicated by the expression of α-fetoprotein m-RNA and by the secretion of α-fetoprotein into the medium *(116,118,119)*. Trophoblast differentiation is indicated by the expression of chorionic gonadotropin (CG) -α and -β subunit m-RNA, and by the secretion of CG into the culture medium. When rhesus ES and human ES cells are injected into SCID mice, they form teratomas with advanced differentiation of all three embryonic germ layers *(116,118,119)*. Differentiation of rhesus ES cells includes ciliated respiratory epithelium, gut epithelium, and hepatocytes (endoderm); striated muscle, smooth muscle, cartilage, bone, and connective

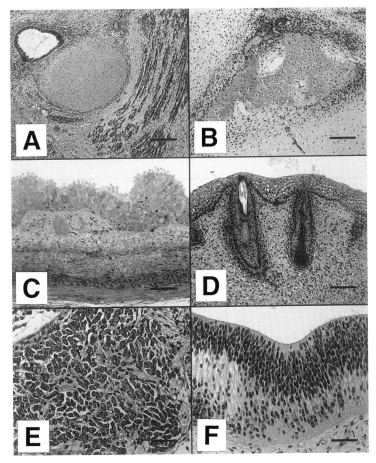

Fig. 2. Rhesus ES cell teratomas formed in SCID mice. (**A**) Cartilage (center) and striated muscle (lower right). Bar = 250 μ. (**B**) Bone. Bar = 100 μ. (**C**) Gut epithelium (top) and smooth muscle wall formation (bottom). Bar = 66 μ. (**D**) Hair follicles. Bar = 100 μ. (**E**) Embryonic ganglion. Bar = 50 μ. (**F**) Neural tube. Bar = 50 μ.

tissue (mesoderm); neural tissue, skin, hair, and teeth (ectoderm); and numerous uniden-tified cell types (Fig. 2). Within rhesus ES cell teratomas, there is abundant evidence of coordinated interactions between cells, and even between cells originating from different embryonic germ layers. For example, in some gut-like structures there is regional differ-entiation of small intestine, complete with villi lined by goblet cells and absorptive enter-ocytes (endoderm). Encircling these gut like structures there is often developing smooth muscle layers (mesoderm) which are found in the appropriate location and orientation for muscularis externa and interna. Similarly, the development of hair and teeth require coordinated interactions between the overlying ectoderm and underlying mesenchyme. In neural differentiation, there are organized neural tubes, with stratification of layers. A ventricular layer with mitotic figures over-lies a mantle layer with maturing neurons and glial cells. The expression of a series of neural markers in rhesus ES cell teratomas recapitulates normal neural development in many respects *(117)*. Human ES cells in tera-tomas exhibit a similar range of differentiation as rhesus ES cells, but have not yet been as extensively studied *(116)*.

Significance of Nonhuman Primate ES Cells

Primate ES cells, including human ES cells, offer a powerful new model for studying primate development. Most of what is known about human development, especially in the early postimplantation period, is based on histological sections of a limited number of human embryos and on analogy to the experimental embryology of the mouse. However, human and mouse embryos differ significantly, for example in the formation, structure, and function of the fetal membranes and placenta *(126–128)*. In the mouse, the yolk sac is a well-vascularized robust extraembryonic organ throughout gestation and has important nutrient exchange functions. In humans, the yolk sac has important early functions, including the initiation of hematopoiesis and germ cell migration, but later in gestation it is essentially a vestigial structure. Similarly, there are dramatic differences between the mouse and the human placenta, both in structure and function. Even the basic embryonic molecules that signal to the mother that she is pregnant differ between the mouse and the human. In the human, the outer trophoblast layer of the placenta human hCG, which causes the corpus luteum of pregnancy to be maintained. Without hCG, the corpus luteum regresses, and another ovarian cycle is initiated. In the mouse there is no homologous placental molecule to hCG. Thus, for understanding the developmental events that support the initiation and maintenance of human pregnancy, mice can provide only a limited understanding. Primate ES cells provide an in vitro developmental model that complements our limited access to intact primate embryos. Nonhuman primate ES cell lines will improve our understanding of the differentiation of human tissues, and thus provide important insights into such processes as infertility, pregnancy loss, and birth defects.

Nonhuman primate ES cells have a potential application in the development of transgenic primates. The major current use of mouse ES cells is to generate mice that carry specific genetic changes generated by homologous recombination. This is accomplished by introducing genetic changes into ES cells in culture, injecting these genetically modified ES cells into blastocysts, and allowing the resulting chimera to develop to term in a foster mother *(129)*. If the resulting chimeric progeny has a contribution to the germ line by the ES cells, then in the next generation, a non-chimeric mouse can be generated with the genetic change of interest. It would be unrealistic to propose using rhesus cells to modify the rhesus monkey genetically by the same ES cell strategy used for mice; the reproductive biology of the species simply makes it impractical. Because rhesus monkeys generally only give birth to single young, and because the age at sexual maturity in male rhesus monkeys is 4–5 years, if the mouse chimera strategy were employed, it could take most of a decade to generate a useful animal. The reproductive biology of the common marmoset, on the other hand, may allow the use of marmoset ES cells for the generation of transgenic marmosets. Common marmosets are small, reach sexual maturity at an early age (about 18 months), and have naturally occurring twins, triplets, and even occasionally quadruplets. Importantly, marmoset ovarian cycles can be synchronized by the administration of prostaglandins which means that embryo transfers can be performed extremely efficiently, with up to 80% of embryos transferred surgically surviving to term *(62,89,97)*. However, even generating transgenic common marmosets using ES cells in chimeras will be extremely difficult and expensive due to the need to wait to breed the resulting chimera to obtain a useful animal. The nuclear transfer strategies discussed elsewhere in this chapter would allow the direct generation of a transgenic primate, without the need to wait for a second generation. Genetically modified ES cells might be used as nuclear donors for this purpose, but it is presently unknown whether their use would offer any advantage over the use of nuclei from differentiated cells.

In addition to providing important insights into human development, human ES cells could have a more direct role in the treatment of human disease. Disease ultimately involves the death or dysfunction of cells. Because certain diseases result from the death or dysfunction of just one or a few cell types, the replacement of those cells by transplantation can be envisioned as a potentially life-long treatment. Human ES cells have the ability to proliferate indefinitely and the ability to differentiate to many, if not all, cells of the body. Human ES cells therefore have the potential to provide a limitless source of specific cell types for transplantation. Diseases that might be treated by this approach include heart disease, juvenile onset diabetes, Parkinson's disease, and leukemia. Large banks of human ES cell lines could be MHC-typed so that close matching between patient and donor cells could be obtained, and because ES cells can proliferate indefinitely, they could also be genetically altered to reduce immunogenicity. However, malignant transformation of transplanted cells could be a concern because of the necessary extended culture of ES cells prior to differentiation and transplantation. Strategies will be needed to kill transplanted cells that do become malignantly transformed. Because of these concerns, the long-term clinical importance of rhesus ES cells will be for developing safe and effective transplantation strategies in the rhesus monkey prior to the clinical use of human ES cells. Indeed, many important diseases that might be treated by this approach, including Parkinson's disease and diabetes mellitus, have extremely accurate rhesus monkey models *(130,131)*. For many diseases, more sophisticated methods of modulating either the host's immune system or the immunogenicity of the ES cell derivatives will have to be developed, as the consequences of immunosuppressive therapies could actually be worse then the disease being treated.

The Nuclear Transfer Procedure

Nuclear transfer is performed with the aid of an inverted microscope in much the same manner as previously described for intracytoplasmic sperm injection *(6)*. The injection pipette can be either straight or bent, and sharply beveled at the tip with dimensions tailored to the size of the donor cell. For instance, if the donor cell is a blastomere, an inner cell mass or a granulosa cell, the inner diameters of the injection pipettes are 25 μm *(64)*, 8 μm and 4 μm, respectively *(132)*. Briefly, the nuclear transfer procedure includes the recovery of matured metaphase-II oocytes, enucleation and the preparation of cytoplasts, and the preparation and isolation of donor nuclei. Donor cell injection into the perivitelline space is the next step, followed by chemical activation of the cytoplasts. Unfused pairs are fused and nuclear transfer embryos are placed in culture. Finally, embryo transfers can be conducted to the oviduct or uterus of a synchronized recipient either with or without prior embryo cryopreservation and low temperature storage.

Nuclear Transfer Experimentation

In first approaching the possibility of conducting nuclear transfer in rhesus monkey, isolated blastomeres from IVF-produced embryos were used as the source of donor nuclei *(6)*. Enucleation procedures were established and chemical activation of the cytoplast was first assessed in parthenote experiments. Activation of intact oocytes by a combination of electropulse, cycloheximide and cytochalasin B resulted in parthenote development to expanded blastocyst and hatching stages (75%) at a rate similar to that observed for normal IVF-produced embryos *(133)*. This validated the cytoplast activation and cell fusion steps in the nuclear transfer process. The developmental viability of cloned, nuclear transfer (NT) embryos was successfully proven with four pregnancies initiated and two live births following the transfers of 53 frozen thawed, embryos into 17 recipients *(6)*. In the rhesus monkey, synchronization between donor nuclei and recipient cytoplast or between reconstituted embryos and surrogate mothers for embryo transfer is a significant challenge, since the number of available animals is limiting. Embryo cryopreservation alleviates this problem but not without a downside.

With the advent of the first clonally derived sheep *(134)* and the realization that fetal as well as adult cells could be used for nuclear transfer, somatic cell cloning became an objective of our research efforts. Initially, embryonic stem cells (discussed above) and fetal fibroblasts were used as the source of donor nuclei, with or without the imposition of a serum starvation step to synchronize donor cells in G_0. G_0 cells, arrested in a post-M or pre-S-state with a diploid DNA content, may be more appropriate for transfer into metaphase-II enucleated oocytes with high MPF activity *(134,135)*. We have produced 166 reconstructed embryos with no evidence that the source or cell cycle stage of donor cells is critical to early development of NT embryos. However, we have not yet succeeded in establishing a pregnancy following the transfer of NT embryos into synchronized recipients *(32)*. In 1998/1999, over 100 NT embryos, without prior cryopreservation, from the 4-16-cell stage of development, containing donor nuclei from either ES cells or fibroblasts, were surgically transferred into the oviducts of 23 females during spontaneous menstrual cycles without a pregnancy.

CONCLUSIONS

While the protocols are now available for IVF, ICSI, sperm processing and capacitation, embryo culture and embryo cryopreservation in nonhuman primates, they are far from optimized and in many cases are based on experience with human oocytes and embryos. This point becomes especially critical in the definition of culture systems for preimplantation development and in the optimization of protocols for non-surgical embryo transfer. Despite these caveats, significant progress has been made as described herein. In fact, we would like to believe that the production of clonally-derived rhesus monkey is a realistic expectation where success will be largely dependent upon the strength of the available protocols. Cloning from cell lines or ES cells offers the possibility in conjunction with gene targeting technology, of creating disease models for biomedical research. The production of genetically identical rhesus monkeys by nuclear transfer would also provide valuable animal models for use in vaccine development as well as for propagating endangered species.

ACKNOWLEDGMENTS

The numerous contributions made by the talented post-doctoral fellows, research assistants and animal technicians at ORPRC and WRPRC to studies from the authors' laboratories are acknowledged. We also thank Ares Advanced Technology, Inc. (Ares Serono) for their donation of Antide and human gonadotropins. Studies conducted at ORPRC were supported by the National Cooperative Program on Nonhuman In vitro Fertilization and Preimplantation Development (HD28484), RR12804, A142709, HD18185 and RR00163. Research at WRPRC was supported by NIH grants RR00167 and RR11571.

REFERENCES

1. Bavister BD, Boatman DE, Collins K, Dierschke DJ, Eisele SG. Birth of rhesus monkey infant after *in vitro* fertilization and non surgical embryo transfer. PNAS 1984;81:2218–2222.
2. Wolf DP, VandeVoort CA, Meyer-Haas GR, Zelinski-Wooten MB, Hess DL, Baughman WL, Stouffer RL. *In vitro* fertilization and embryo transfer in the rhesus monkey. Biol Reprod 1989;41:335–346.
3. Tollner TL, VandeVoort CA, Overstreet JW, Drobniz EZ. Cryopreservation of spermatozoa from cynomolgus monkeys (*Macaca fascicularis*). J Reprod Fert 1990;90:347–352.
4. Schramm RD, Bavister BD. FSH-priming of rhesus monkeys enhances meiotic and developmental competence of oocytes *in vitro*. Biol Reprod 1994;51:904–912.
5. Hewitson L, Dominko T, Takahashi D, Martinovich C, Ramalho-Santos J, Sutovsky P, et al. Unique checkpoints during the first cell cycle of fertilization after intracytoplasmic sperm injection in rhesus monkeys. Nature Med 1999;5:431–433.
6. Meng L, Ely JJ, Stouffer RL, Wolf DP. Rhesus monkeys produced by nuclear transfer. Biol Reprod 1997;57:454–459.
7. Cranfield MR, Bavister BD, Boatman DE, Berger NG, Schaffer N, Kempske SE, et al. Assisted reproduction in the propagation management of the endangered lion-tailed macaque (*Macaca silenus*). In: Wolf DP, Stouffer RL, Brenner RM, eds. *In vitro* Fertilization and Embryo Transfer in Primates. Springer-Verlag, New York, NY, 1993, pp. 331–348.
8. Pope CE, Dresser BL, Chin NW, Liu JH, Loskutoff NM, Behnke EJ, et al. Birth of a Western lowland gorilla (*Gorilla gorilla gorilla*) following *in vitro* fertilization and embryo transfer. Am J Primatol 1997;41:247–260.
9. Wolf DP, Thomson JA, Zelinski-Wooten MB, Stouffer RL. *In vitro* fertilization-embryo transfer in nonhuman primates: The technique and its application. Mol Reprod Dev 1990;27:261–280.
10. Stouffer RL, Zelinski-Wooten MB, Aladin Chandrasekher Y, Wolf DP. Stimulation of follicle and oocyte development in macaques for IVF procedures. In: Wolf DP, Stouffer RL, Brenner RM, eds. *In vitro* Fertilization and Embryo Transfer in Primates. Springer-Verlag, New York, NY, 1993, pp. 124–141.
11. Lanzendorf SE, Zelinski-Wooten MB, Stouffer RL, Wolf DP. Maturity at collection and developmental potential of rhesus monkey oocytes. Biol Reprod 1990;42:703–711.
12. Balmaceda JP, Pool TB, Arana JB, Heitman TS, Asch RH. Successful *in vitro* fertilization and embryo transfer in cynomolgus monkeys. Fertil Steril 1984;42:791–795.
13. Lanzendorf SE, Holmgren WJ, Schaffer N, Hatasaka H, Wentz AC, Jeyendran RS. *In vitro* fertilization and gamete micromanipulation in lowland gorilla. J Assist Reprod Gen 1992;9:358–364.
14. Zelinski-Wooten MB, Alexander M, Christensen CL, Wolf DP, Hess DL, Stouffer RL. Individualized gonadotropin regimens for follicular stimulation in macaques during *in vitro* fertilization cycles. J Med Primatol 1994;23:367–374.
15. Lopata A, Summers PM, Hearn JP. Births following the transfer of cultured embryos obtained by *in vitro* and *in vivo* fertilization in the marmoset monkey (Callithrix jacchus). Fertil Steril 1988;50:503–509.
16. Cranfield MR, Schaffer N, Bavister BD, Berger N, Boatman DE, Kempske S, et al. Assessment of oocytes retrieved from stimulated and unstimulated ovaries of pig-tailed macaques (Macaca nemestrina) as a model to enhance the genetic diversity of captive lion-tailed macaques (Macaca silenus). Zool Biol 1989;(Suppl 1):33–46.
17. McCarthy TJ, Fortman JD, Boice ML, Fazleabas AT, Verhage HG. Induction of multiple follicular development and superovulation in the olive baboon, *Papio anubis*. J Med Primatol 1991;20:308–314.
18. Schramm RD, Bavister BD. Granulosa cells from follicle stimulating hormone-primed monkeys enhance the developmental competence of *in vitro* matured oocytes from non-stimulated rhesus monkeys. Hum Reprod 1996;11:1698–1702.
19. Younis AI, Sehgal PK, Biggers JD. Antral follicle development and in-vitro maturation of oocytes from macaques stimulated with a single subcutaneous injection of pregnant mare's serum gonadotrophin. Hum Reprod 1994;9:2130–2134.
20. VandeVoort CA, Baughman WL, Stouffer RL. Comparison of different regimens of human gonadotropins for superovulation of rhesus monkeys: Ovulatory response and subsequent luteal function. *In vitro* Fert Embryo Transfer 1989;6:85–91.
21. Stouffer RL, Aladin Chandrasekher Y, Zelinski-Wooten MB. Recombinant gonadotropins: induction of the mid-cycle surge in IVF-related cycles. In: Filicori M, Flamigni C, eds. Ovulation Induction Update '98. Elsevier Science BV, New York, NY, 1988, pp. 147–157.
22. Zelinski-Wooten MB, Weston AM, Wolf DP, Stouffer RL. Specific roles of luteinizing hormone (LH) and follicle stimulating hormone (FSH) in folliculogenesis and ovulation. In: Filicori M, ed. The Role

of Luteinizing Hormone in Folliculogenesis and Ovulation Induction. Monduzzi Editore, Bologna, Italy, 1999, pp. 21–36.

23. Weston AM, Zelinski-Wooten MB, Hutchison JS, Stouffer RL, Wolf DP. Developmental potential of embryos produced by *in vitro* fertilization from gonadotrophin-releasing hormone antagonist-treated macaques stimulated with recombinant human follicle stimulating hormone alone or in combination with luteinizing hormone. Hum Reprod 1996;11:608–613.

24. Bavister BD, Dees C, Schultz RD. Refractoriness of rhesus monkeys to repeated ovarian stimulation by exogenous gonadotropins is caused by nonprecipitating antibodies. Am J Reprod Immunol Microbiol 1986;11:11–16.

25. Iliff SA, Molskness TA, Stouffer RL. Anti-human gonadotropin antibodies generated during *in vitro* fertilization (IVF)-related cycles: Effect on fertility of rhesus monkeys. J Med Primatol 1995;24:7–11.

26. Zelinski-Wooten MB, Hutchison JS, Hess DL, Wolf DP, Stouffer RL. Follicle-stimulating hormone alone supports follicle growth and oocyte development in gonadotrophin-releasing hormone antagonist-treated monkeys. Hum Reprod 1995;10:1658–1666.

27. Zelinski-Wooten MB, Alexander MA, Hess DL, Wolf DP, Stouffer RL. Combined regimen of GnRH antagonist and sequential human gonadotropins for follicular stimulation in macaque *in vitro* fertilization (IVF) cycles. Am J Primatol 1994;33(3):254.

28. Byrd S, Iskovitz J, Chillik C, Hodgen GD. Flexible protocol for administration of human follicle-stimulating hormone with gonadotropin-releasing hormone antagonist. Fertil Steril 1992;57:209–214.

29. Zelinski-Wooten MB, Hutchison JS, Trinchard-Lugan I, Hess DL, Wolf DP, Stouffer RL. Initiation of periovulatory events in gonadotrophin-stimulated macaques with varying doses of recombinant human chorionic gonadotrophin. Hum Reprod 1997;12:1877–1885.

30. Zelinski-Wooten MB, Hutchison JS, Hess DL, Wolf DP, Stouffer RL. A bolus of recombinant human follicle stimulating hormone at mid-cycle induces periovulatory events following multiple follicular development in macaques. Hum Reprod 1998;13:554–560.

31. Zelinski-Wooten MB, Alexander M, Molskness TA, Stouffer RL, Wolf DP. Use of recombinant human gonadotropins for repeated follicular stimulation in rhesus monkeys. XVth Congress of the International Primatology Society/XIXth Conference of the American Society of Primatologists, 1996, Abstract Book, #133.

32. Wolf DP, Meng L, Ouhibi N, Zelinski-Wooten M. Nuclear transfer in rhesus monkey: practical and basic implications. Biol Reprod 1999;60:199–204.

33. Wolf PD, Alexander M, Zelinski-Wooten MB, Stouffer RL. Maturity and fertility of rhesus monkey oocytes collected at different intervals after an ovulatory stimulus (human chorionic gonadotropin) in *in vitro* fertilization cycles. Mol Reprod Dev 1996;43:76–81.

34. Morgan PM, Warikoo PK, Bavister BD. *In vitro* maturation of ovarian oocytes from unstimulated rhesus monkeys: assessment of cytoplasmic maturity by embryonic development after *in vitro* fertilization. Biol Reprod 1991;45:89–93.

35. Alak BM, Wolf DP. Rhesus monkey oocyte maturation and fertilization *in vitro*: roles of the menstrual cycle phase and exogenous gonadotropins. Biol Reprod 1994;51:879–887.

36. Boatman DE. *In vitro* growth of nonhuman primate pre- and peri-implantation embryos. In: Bavister BD, ed. The Mammalian Preimplantation Embryo: Regulation of Growth and Differentiation *In Vitro*. Plenum, New York, NY, 1987, pp. 273–308.

37. Bavister BD. A consistently successful procedure for *in vitro* fertilization of golden hamster eggs. Gamete Res 1989;23:139–158.

38. Schramm RD, Bavister BD. Effects of granulosa cells and gonadotrophins on meiotic and developmental competence of oocytes *in vitro* in non-stimulated rhesus monkeys. Hum Reprod 1995;10:887–895.

39. Schramm RD, Tennier MT, Boatman DE, Bavister BD. Effects of gonadotropins upon the incidence and kinetics of meiotic maturation of macaque oocytes *in vitro*. Mol Reprod Dev 1994;37:467–472.

40. Bavister BD, Boatman DE, Leibfried ML, Loose M, Vernon MW. Fertilization and cleavage of rhesus monkey oocytes *in vitro*. Biol Reprod 1983;28:983–999.

41. Zhang L, Weston AM, Denniston RS, Goodeaux LL, Godke RA, Wolf DP. Developmental potential of rhesus monkey embryos produced by *in vitro* fertilization. Biol Reprod 1994;51:433–440.

42. Boatman DE, Morgan PM, Bavister BD. Variables affecting the yield and developmental potential of embryos following superstimulation and *in vitro* fertilization in rhesus monkeys. Gamete Res 1986:13:327–338.

43. Moor RM, Trounson AO. Hormonal and follicular factors affecting maturation of sheep oocytes *in vitro* and their subsequent developmental capacity. J Reprod Fertil 1977;49:101–109.

44. Osborn JC, Moor RM. The role of steroid signals in the maturation of mammalian oocytes. J Steroid Biochem 1983;19:133–137.

45. Tornell J, Bergh C, Selleskog U, Hillensjo T. Effect of recombinant human gonadotrophins on oocyte meiosis and steroidogenesis in isolated pre-ovulatory rat follicles. Hum Reprod 1995;10:1619–1622.

46. Maruo T, Ladines-Llave CA, Samoto T, Matsuo H, Manolo AS, Itoh H, Mochizuki M. Expression of epidermal growth factor and its receptor in the human ovary during follicular growth and regression. Endocrinol 1993;132:924–931.

47. Harper KM, Brackett BG. Bovine blastocyst development after *in vitro* maturation in a defined medium with epidermal growth factor and low concentrations of gonadotropins. Biol Reprod 1993;48:409–416.

48. Hammond JM, Baraneo JL, Skaleris D, Knight AB, Romanus JA, Rechler MM. Production of insulin-like growth factors by ovarian granulosa cells. Endocrinology 1985;117:2553–2555.

49. Xia P, Tekpetey FR, Armstrong DT. Effect of IGF-I on pig oocyte maturation, fertilization and early embryonic development *in vitro* and on granulosa and cumulus cell biosynthetic activity. Mol Reprod Dev 1994;38:373–379.

50. O WS, Robertson DM, deKrester DM. Inhibin as an oocyte meiotic inhibitor. Mol Cell Endocrinol 1989;62:307–311.

51. Sadatsuki M, Tsutsumui O, Yamada R, Muramatsu M, Taketani Y. Local regulatory effects of activin A and follistatin on meiotic maturation of rat oocytes. Biochem Biophys Res Commun 1993;196:388–395.

52. Feng P, Catt KJ, Knecht M. Transforming growth factor-β stimulates meiotic maturation of the rat oocyte. Endocrinol 1998;122:181–186.

53. Alak BM, Smith GD, Woodruff TK, Stouffer RL, Wolf DP. Enhancement of primate oocyte maturation and fertilization *in vitro* by inhibin A and activin A. Fertil Steril 1996;66:646–653.

54. Alak BM, Coskun S, Friedman CI, Kennard EA, Kim MH, Seifer DB. Activin A stimulates meiotic maturation of human oocytes and modulates granulosa cell steroidogenesis *in vitro*. Fertil Steril 1998; 70:1126–1130.

55. Woodruff TK, D'Asgotino JB, Schwartz NB, Mayo KE. Dynamic changes in inhibin messenger RNAs in rat ovarian follicles during the reproductive cycle. Science 1988;239:1269–1299.

56. Schwall RH, Mason AJ, Wilcox JN, Bassett SG, Zeleznik AJ. Localization of inhibin activin subunit mRNAs within the primate ovary. Mol Endocrinol 1990;4:75–79.

57. Yamoto M, Minami S, Nakano R, Kobayashi M. Immunohistochemical localization of inhibin/activin subunits in human ovarian follicles during the menstrual cycle. J Clin Endocrinol Metab 1992;74:989–993.

58. Silva CC, Knight PG. Modulatory action of activin-A and follistatin on the developmental competence of *in vitro* matured bovine oocyte. Biol Reprod 1998;58:558–565.

59. Steptoe PC, Edwards RG. Birth after reimplantation of a human embryo. Lancet 1978;2:366–369.

60. Gould KG, Cline EM, Williams WL. Observations on the induction of ovulation and fertilization *in vitro* in the squirrel monkey (Saimiri sciureus). Fertil Steril 1973;24:260–268.

61. Kuehl TJ, Dukelow WR. Time relations of squirrel monkey (Saimiri sciureus) sperm capacitation and ovum maturation in an *in vitro* fertilization system. J Reprod Fertil 1982;64:135–137.

62. Lopata A, Summers PM, Hearn JP. Births following the transfer of cultured embryos obtained by *in vitro* and *in vivo* fertilization in the marmoset monkey (*Callithrix jacchus*). Fertil Steril 1988;50:503–509.

63. Clayton O, Kuehl TJ. The first successful *in vitro* fertilization and embryo transfer in a nonhuman primate. Theriogenology 1984;21:228.

64. Kreitman O, Lynch A, Nixon WE, Hodgen GD. Ovum collection, induced luteal dysfunction, *in vitro* fertilization, embryo development and low tubal ovum transfer in primates. In: Hafez ESE, Semm K, eds. In Vitro Fertilization and Embryo Transfer. Lancaster, UK, MTP Press Ltd, 1982, pp. 303–324.

65. Gould KG. Ovum recovery and *in vitro* fertilization in the chimpanzee. Fertil Steril 1983;40:378–383.

66. Huntress SL, Loskutoff NM, Raphael BL, Yee B, Bowsher TR, Putman JM, Kraemer DC. Pronucleus formation following *in vitro* fertilization of oocytes recovered from a gorilla (*Gorilla gorilla gorilla*) with unilateral endometrioid adenocarcinoma of the ovary. Am J Primatol 1989;18:259–266.

67. VandeVoort CA, Tarantal AF. The macaque model for *in vitro* fertilization: superovulation techniques and ultrasound-guided follicular aspiration. J Med Primatol 1991;20:110–116.

68. Harrisson RM. Semen parameters in *Macaca mulatta*: ejaculates from random and selected monkeys. J Med Primatol 1980;9:265–273.

69. Gould KG, Martin DE. Artificial insemination of nonhuman primates. In: Bernirschke K, ed. Primates: The Road to Self-Sustaining Populations. Springer-Verlag, New York, NY, 1986, pp. 425–443.

70. Lanzendorf SE, Gliessman PM, Archibong AE, Alexander M, Wolf DP. Collection and quality of rhesus monkey semen. Mol Reprod Dev 1990;25:61–66.

71. Wolf DP, Stouffer RL. IVF-ET in Old World monkeys. In: Wolf DP, Stouffer RL, Brenner RM, eds. *In vitro* Fertlization and Embryo Transfer in Primates. Serono Symposia, Springer-Verlag, New York, NY, 1993, pp. 85–99.

72. Boatman DE, Bavister BD. Stimulation of rhesus monkey sperm capacitation by cyclic nucleotide mediators. J Reprod Fertil 1984;71:357–366.

73. Douglass EM. First gorilla born using artificial insemination. Int Zoo News 1981;28:9–15.

74. Gould KG, Styperek RP. Improved methods for freeze preservation of chimpanzee sperm. Am J Primatol 1989;18:275–284.

75. Bavister BD, Yanagimachi R. The effects of sperm extracts and energy sources on the motility and acrosome reaction of hamster spermatozoa *in vitro*. Biol Reprod 1977;18:228–237.

76. Johnson LD, Mattson BA, Albertini DF, Sehgal PK, Becker RA, Avis J, Biggers JD. Quality of oocytes from superovulated rhesus monkeys. Hum Reprod 1991;6:623–631.

77. Tarantal AF, Hendrickx AG. Prenatal growth in the cynomolgus and rhesus macaque (*Macaca fascicularis* and *Macaca mulatta*): A comparison by ultrasonography. Am J Primatol 1988;15:309–323.

78. Eddy CA, Garcia RG, Kraemer DC, Pauerstein CJ. Detailed time course of ovum transport in the rhesus monkey (*Macaca mulatta*). Biol Reprod 1975;13:363–369.

79. Hurst PR, Jefferies K, Eckstein P, Wheeler AG. Recovery of uterine embryos in rhesus monkeys. Biol Reprod 1976;15:429–434.

80. Goodeaux LL, Anzalone CA, Webre MK, Graves KH, Voelkel SA. Nonsurgical technique for flushing the *Macaca mulatta* uterus. J Med Primatol 1990;19:59–67.

81. Goodeaux LL, Anzalone CA, Thibodeaux JK, Menezo Y, Roussel JD, Voelkel SA. Successful non-surgical collection of *Macaca mulatta* embryos. Theriogenology 1990;34:1159–1167.

82. Seshagiri PB, Dierschke DJ, Eisele SG, Scheffler J, Hearn JP. Recovery of rhesus monkey preimplantation embryos by non-surgical uterine flushing. Biol Reprod 1991;44(Suppl 1):157.

83. Iliff-Sizemore SA, Thomson JA, Wolf DP. Effect of parity and menstrual cycle stage on transcervical uterine cannulation of macaques. Cont Topics Lab Anim Sci 1993;32:12–13.

84. Goodeaux LL, Thibodeaux JK, Voelkel SA, Anzalone CA, Roussel JD, Cohen JC, Menezo Y. Collection, co-culture and transfer of rhesus preimplantation embryos. ARTA 1990;1:370–379.

85. Gould KG, Martin DE. The female ape genital tract and its secretions. In: Graham CE, ed. Reproductive Biology of the Great Apes: Comparative and Biomedical Perspectives. Academic Press, New York, NY, 1981, pp. 105–125.

86. Marshall VS, Kalishman J, Thomson JA. Nonsurgical embryo transfer in the common marmoset monkey. J Med Primatol 1997;26:241–247.

87. Seshagiri PB, Hearn JP. In-vitro development of in-vivo produced rhesus monkey morulae and blastocysts to hatched, attached and post-attached blastocyst stages: morphology and early secretion of chorionic gonadotropin. Hum Reprod 1993;8:279–287.

88. Ghosh D, Kumar PG, Sengupta J. Early luteal phase administration of mifepristone inhibits preimplantation embryo development and viability in the rhesus monkey. Hum Reprod 1997;12:575–582.

89. Summers PM, Wennink CJ, Hodges JK. Cloprostenol-induced luteolysis in the marmoset monkey (*Callithrix jacchus*). J Reprod Fertil 1985;73:133–138.

90. Zelinski-Wooten MB, Stouffer RL. Intraluteal infusion of prostaglandins of the E, D, I and A series prevent $PGF_{2\alpha}$-induced, but not spontaneous luteal regression in rhesus monkeys. Biol Reprod 1990; 43:507–516.

91. Hodgen GD. Surrogate embryo transfer combined with estrogen-progesterone therapy in monkeys. Implantation, gestation, and delivery without ovaries. JAMA 1983;250:2167–2171.

92. Kuzan FB, Quinn P. Cryopreservation of mammalian embryos. In: Wolf DP, ed. *In vitro* Fertilization and Embryo Transfer: A Manual of Basic Techniques. Plenum, New York, NY, 1988, pp. 301–347.

93. Fujisaki M, Suzuki M, Kohno M, Cho F, Honjo S. Early embryonal culture of the cynomolgus monkey (*Macaca fascicularis*). Am J Primatol 1989;18:303–313.

94. Morgan PM, Boatman DE, Bavister BD. Relationships between follicular fluid steroid hormone concentrations, oocyte maturity, *in vitro* fertilization and embryonic development in the rhesus monkey. Mol Reprod Dev 1990;27:145–151.

95. Pope V, Pope E, Beck L. *In vitro* development of the primate embryo. In: Brans YW, Kuehl TJ, eds. Nonhuman Primates in Perinatal Research. John Wiley and Sons, New York, NY, 1988, pp. 161–174.

96. Weston AM, Wolf DP. Differential preimplantation development of rhesus monkey embryos in serum-supplemented media. Mol Reprod Dev 1996;44:88–92.

97. Lawitts JA, Biggers JD. Joint effects of sodium chloride, glutamine, and glucose in mouse preimplantation embryo culture media. Mol Reprod Dev 1992;31:189–194.

98. Ho Y, Wigglesworth K, Eppig JJ, Schultz RM. Preimplantation development of mouse embryos in KSOM: augmentation by amino acids and analysis of gene expression. Mol Reprod Dev 1995;41:232–238.

99. Enders AC, Boatman D, Morgan P, Bavister BD. Differentiation of blastocysts derived from *in vitro*-fertilized rhesus monkey ova. Biol Reprod 1989;41:715–727.

100. Bavister BD. Co-culture for embryo development: is it really necessary? Hum Reprod 1992;7:1339–1341.

101. Schramm RD, Bavister BD. Development of in-vitro-fertilized primate embryos into blastocysts in a chemically defined, protein-free culture medium. Hum Reprod 1996;11:1690–1697.

102. Hosoi Y, Miyake M, Utsumi K, Iritani A. Development of rabbit oocytes after microinjection of spermatozoon. 11th Int Congr Anim Reprod Artif Insem 1988;3:331–333.

103. Goto K, Kinoshita A, Takuma Y, Ogawa K. Fertilization of bovine oocytes by injection of immobilized, killed spermatozoa. Vet Rec 1990;127:517–520.

104. Kimura T, Yanagimachi R. Intracytoplasmic sperm injection in the mouse. Biol Reprod 1995;52:709–720.

105. Lanzendorf S, Wolf DP. Microinjection of rhesus monkey eggs. 45th Ann Mtg Amer Fertil Soc 1989; Program Suppl:S14, Abstract O–032.

106. Hewitson L, Takahashi D, Dominko T, Simerly C, Schatten G. Fertilization and embryo development to blastocysts after intracytoplasmic sperm injection in the rhesus monkey. Hum Reprod 1998;13:3449–3455.

107. Hewitson LC, Simerly CR, Tengowski MW, Sutovsky P, Navara CS, Haavisto AJ, Schatten G. Microtubule and chromatin configurations during rhesus monkey intracytoplasmic spern injection: successes and failures. Biol Reprod 1996;55:271–280.

108. Yanagimachi R. Mammalian fertilization. In: Knobil E, Neill JD, eds. The Physiology of Reproduction, 2nd edition. Raven, New York, NY, 1994, pp. 189–317.

109. Soupart P, Strong PA. Ultrastructural observations on polyspermic penetration of zona pellucida-free human oocytes inseminated *in vitro*. Fertil Steril 1975;26:523–527.

110. Albertini DF. Cytoplasmic reorganization during the resumption of meiosis in cultured preovulatory rat oocytes. Dev Biol 1987;120:121–131.

111. Albertini DF. Regulation of meiotic maturation in the mammalian oocyte: interplay between exogenous cues and the microtubule cytoskeleton. Bioessays 1992;12:97–103.

112. Van Blerkom J, Davis P, Merriam J, Sinclair J. Nuclear and cytoplasmic dynamics of sperm penetration, pronuclear formation and microtubule organization during fertilization and early preimplantation development in the human. Hum Reprod Update 1995;1:429–461.

113. Palermo GD, Cohen J, Alikani M, Adler A, Rosenwaks Z. Intracytoplasmic sperm injection: a novel treatment for all forms of male factor infertility. Fertil Steril 1995;63:1231–1240.

114. Meng L, Wolf DP. Sperm-induced oocyte activation in the rhesus monkey: nuclear and cytoplasmic changes following intracytoplasmic sperm injection. Hum Reprod 1997;12:1062–1068

115. Spemann H. Embryonic development and induction. Hafner Publishing Company, New York, NY, 1938, pp. 210–211.

116. Thomson JA, Iskovitz-Eldor J, Shapiro SS, Waknitz MA, Swiergel JJ, Marshall VS, Jones JM. Embryonic stem cell lines derived from human blastocysts. Science 1998;282:1145–1147.

117. Thomson JA, Marshall VS. Primate embryonic stem cells. Curr Top Dev Biol 1998;38:133–165.

118. Thomson JA, Kalishman J, Golos TG, Durning M, Harris CP, Becker RA, Hearn JP. Isolation of a primate embryonic stem cell line. Proc Natl Acad Sci USA 1995;92:7844–7848.

119. Thomson JA, Kalishman J, Golos TG, Durning M, Harris CP, Hearn JP. Pluripotent cell lines derived from common marmoset (*Callithrix jacchus*) blastocysts. Biol Reprod 1996;55:254–259.

120. Andrews PW, Damjanov I, Simon D, Banting G, Carlin C, Dracopoli N, Fogh J. Pluripotent embryonal carcinoma clones derived from the human teratocarcinoma cell line Tera-2. Lab Invest 1984;50:147–162.

121. Andrews PW, Banting G, Damjanov I, Arnaud D, Avner P. Three monoclonal antibodies defining distinct differentiation antigens associated with different high molecular weight polypeptides on the surface of human embryonal carcinoma cells. Hybridoma 1984;3:347–361.

122. Andrews PW, Oosterhuis J, Damjanov I. In: Robertson E, ed. Teratocarcinomas and Embryonic Stem Cells: A Practical Approach. IRL Press, Oxford, 1987, pp. 207–246.

123. Wenk J, Andrews PW, Casper J, Hata J, Pera MF, von Keitz A, et al. Glycolipids of germ cell tumors: extended globo-series glycolipids are a hallmark of human embryonal carcinoma cells. Int J Cancer 1994;58:108–115.

124. Solter D, Knowles BB. Monoclonal antibody defining a stage-specific mouse embryonic antigen (SSEA-1). Proc Natl Acad Sci USA 1978;75:5565–5569.

125. Kannagi R. Stage-specific embryonic antigens (SSEA-3 and -4) are epitopes of a unique globo-series ganglioside isolated from human teratocarcinoma cells. EMBO J 1983;2:2355–2361.

126. Bernirschke K, Kaufmann P, eds. Pathology of the Human Placenta. Springer-Verlag, New York, NY, 1990.

127. Luckett WP. The development of primordial and definitive amniotic cavities in early rhesus monkey and human embryos. Am J Anat 1975;144:149–168.

128. Luckett WP. Origin and differentiation of the yolk sac and extraembryonic mesoderm in presomite human and rhesus monkey embryos. Am J Anat 1978;152:59–98.

129. Hogan B, Beddington R, Costantini F, Lacey E, eds. Manipulating the Mouse Embryo: A Laboratory Manual. Cold Spring Harbor Laboratory Press, Plainview, NY, 1994.

130. Jones CW, Reynolds WA, Hoganson GE. Streptozotocin diabetes in the monkey: plasma levels of glucose, insulin, glucagon, and somatostatin, with corresponding morphometric analysis of islet endocrine cells. Diabetes 1980;29:536–546.

131. Burns RS, Chiueh CC, Markey SP, Ebert MH, Jacobowitz DM, Kopin IJ. A primate model of parkinsonism: selective destruction of dopaminergic neurons in the pars compacta of the substantia nigra by N-methyl-4-phenyl-1,2,3,6-tetrahydropyridine. Proc Natl Acad Sci USA 1983;80:4546–4550.

132. Collas P, Barnes FL. Nuclear transplantation by microinjection of inner cell mass and granulosa cell nuclei. Mol Reprod Dev 1994;38:264–267.

133. Meng L, Alexander M, Wolf DP. Developmental potential of rhesus monkey parthenotes. 52nd Annual Meeting of the American Society of Reproductive Medicine, Nov 2-6th, 1996, Boston, MA, Abstract S137.

134. Wilmut I, Schnieke AE, McWhir J, Kind AJ, Campbell KHS. Viable offspring derived from fetal and adult mammalian cells. Nature 1997;385:810–813.

135. Campbell KHS, McWhir J, Ritchie WA, Wilmut I. Sheep cloned by nuclear transfer from a cultured cell line. Nature 1996;380:24–25.

17

Cloning and Nuclear Transfer in Humans

Don P. Wolf, PHD

CONTENTS

INTRODUCTION

Public fascination with human cloning (reproduction of an existing human being, asexually, accomplished by transferring the nucleus from a diploid cell into an enucleated oocyte) dates back many years, preceding even the first report of successful cloning of mammals where embryonic cells were used as the nuclear donor source. Early animal studies, largely built on pioneering work in amphibians *(1)*, were done in mice, sheep, cattle, goats, and pigs *(see* Chapters 13, 14, and 15). The next notable technological development was cloning from more advanced embryos or cultured embryonic cells *(2, 3)*, and then, quite recently, our working assumptions on the impossibility of somatic cell cloning were completely rewritten with the announcement of Dolly *(4)* and subsequent success in cloning sheep, cattle, and mice from either fetal or adult somatic cells *(5–7)*. Cloning from adult cells is now perceived as so successful that pet cloning efforts were commissioned; for instance, Missy, a mixed border collie and husky involving scientists at Texas A&M, funded by a $2.3 million private grant *(8)*.

Fascination with cloning has not been focused so much on the ability to produce an identical twin or two by blastomere separation and culture, but on nuclear transfer from a cell line where very large numbers of nuclear donor cells are available, because individuals could in theory be cloned repeatedly creating large numbers of the same genotype; an

From: *Contemporary Endocrinology: Assisted Fertilization and Nuclear Transfer in Mammals*
Edited by: D. P. Wolf and M. Zelinski-Wooten © Humana Press Inc., Totowa, NJ

army, as it were. We have a number of fictional accounts that predict the probable outcome. Alvin Toffler, in his 1970 book "Future Shock," speculates that cloning would make it possible for people to see themselves anew, to fill the world with twins of themselves. Science writer David Rorvik, in his 1978 book entitled "In His Image: The Cloning of a Man," tells the story of a wealthy man who secretly has himself cloned; later uncovered as a hoax. In the movies, Woody Allen's "Sleeper," made in 1973, describes a futuristic world whose leader left behind his nose for cloning purposes. Allen's character was responsible with cloning to bring the leader back. A later movie, "Boys from Brazil," released in 1978, involves a Nazi scheme to clone multiple Hitlers; and in 1996, the Michael Keaton movie "Multiplicity," has Doug, in an effort to make his demanding life easier, with three clones of himself. Predictably, disaster ensues. As if this were not sufficient, further "benefits" from our newly developed ability to clone "at will" were portrayed dramatically in Stephen Spielberg's 1993 movie, "Jurassic Park", where cloning extinct animals led to an exciting, but predictable, doomsday outcome. With this rather biased cultural heritage, the present challenge is to question whether there are any acceptable uses of human cloning or nuclear-transfer technology in the treatment of human disease, including infertility.

HUMAN CLONING: A HISTORICAL OVERVIEW

The earliest study involving nuclear transfer in the human may be that of Shettles in 1979 (9), described in a manuscript entitled "Diploid nuclear replacement in mature human ova with cleavage." Glass micropipets were used to penetrate the vitelline membrane (oocyte plasma membrane), remove the nucleus by aspiration, and replace it with a diploid nucleus derived from spermatogonial cells. Many (unspecified number) attempted nuclear transfers resulted in only 3 "ova" that cleaved to the 2-cell stage in 30 h and into morula by the end of the third day of culture, at which time the experiment was discontinued. The author concluded that "there was every indication that each specimen was developing normally and could readily have been transferred in utero by the catheter technique cited in 1971." In retrospect, it is highly unlikely that these conclusions were accurate. First, the "living human ovum" depicted in this report by phase contrast microscopy, with a first polar body and a nucleus with a single nucleolus, is not a mature ovum or oocyte. If it were, it would not contain a nucleus; rather, the chromosomes would be aligned on a metaphase plate in the cortex underlying the polar body. Hence, the "human ovum" most probably had activated spontaneously but not abstricted a second polar body or, alternatively, one of the polar bodies had disintegrated. Furthermore, the subsequent "normal development" of these "ova" was probably fragmentation. In order to draw the conclusion that these were viable nuclear-transfer embryos, appropriate controls would be required to eliminate parthenogenetic activation or fragmentation and to confirm participation of the donor nucleus. Finally, it is interesting to note that this experimentation on human tissues was conducted before successful nuclear transfer had been reported in any mammalian species.

"Cloning" in the human was first reported to the scientific community by Hall and coworkers (10) at the annual meeting of the American Fertility Society (now the American Society of Reproductive Medicine) in 1993. The reason cloning appears in quotes is that the study did not involve nuclear transfer, but rather blastomere separation and culture. Indeed, if the word "clone" had been absent from the title, nobody would likely have noticed the abstract, let alone responded to it so dramatically. By way of explanation, clinical embryology laboratories (315 in the US alone) normally encounter significant numbers of nonviable gametes and abnormal embryos. Embryos that arrest during early development or embryos that result after penetration by more than one sperm (polypronuclear) are generally discarded because they would be sloughed or miscarried if returned to the uterus. The Hall study used polypronuclear embryos to assess whether individual cells (blastomeres) can develop after separation and in vitro culture. They also asked whether early development was different when separation occurred at the 2-cell, 4-cell, or later stages. Seventeen polypronuclear embryos underwent protease exposure to remove the surrounding casing (zona pellucida), and were then dissociated in divalent cation-free medium. A surrogate zona was created by coating individual blastomeres in a sodium alginate gel, and the blastomeres were cultured for several days before the maximum extent of growth was assessed. The authors concluded that blastomeres from earlier stages tended to undergo slightly more cell divisions than those from later stages; however, the data did not reach statistical significance. The question remains: what would it have meant if significance had been attained? After all, these are polypronuclear embryos with limited developmental potential. Does this have relevance to the developmental potential of normal blastomeres? It seems unlikely; nevertheless, it does represent experimentation on discarded, abnormal human embryos, and the press treated this announcement as if cloning technology was now perfected for the mass production of human beings (11). Despite the hysteria created by the popular press, a reasoned defense of the work was presented by Jones and co-authors (12), based on the fact that the study had been scrutinized and approved by a local institutional review board (IRB). The authors also argued that the study had medical and scientific merit and was ultimately directed towards the improvement of human reproduction.

Concerns created or stimulated by Hall and coworkers (10) over human cloning largely rested until the February 1997 announcement of adult somatic cell cloning in sheep (4). President Clinton, in recognizing the need for a rapid response to this new technological achievement, turned to a 15-member, preexisting (albeit inactive) group, the National Bioethics Advisory Commission (NBAC). The NBAC was formed in 1995 to assess the ethical problems that might arise in medical research involving human subjects and to look at genetic information and how it is handled by medical institutions. The President asked the NBAC to review the legal and ethical issues associated with cloning and to report back within 90 days with recommendations and possible federal actions to prevent abuse. The challenge of this assignment should not be underestimated, especially given the limited time frame imposed on the group. A week later, President Clinton stated that "no federal funds shall be allocated for cloning of human beings." This announcement was primarily symbolic, because a longstanding moratorium was already in place concerning the use of federal funds to conduct research on human embryos. The Commission addressed "a very specific aspect of cloning namely where genetic material would be transferred from the nucleus of a somatic cell of an existing human being to an enucleated human egg with the intention of creating a child."

The consensus of the NBAC was that efforts to clone a person would be unsafe, at least at present and in the near future, because of the likelihood of creating malformed fetuses. Interestingly, although there were many unresolved ethical concerns, there was not one compelling reason why cloning should be banned apart from the consensus on unacceptable risk to the fetus. The report, published in June of 1997 (13), recommended that "since it is morally unacceptable for anyone in the public or private sector, whether in a research or clinical setting to attempt to create a child using somatic cell nuclear transfer cloning," there should be a continuation of the current moratorium on the use of federal funding in support of any such attempt. An immediate request for everyone to comply voluntarily with the intent of the federal moratorium was also made. This request was directed to the private sector, which, without federal funding, was and still is without federal oversight. Further, it was recommended that federal legislation should be enacted to prohibit anyone from attempting, whether in a research or clinical setting, to create a child through somatic-cell nuclear transfer, and it was proposed that any such ban should contain a sunset clause with re-review suggested in 3–5 years. The Commission also recommended that close scrutiny be given to the possible effects of any regulatory actions on other important areas of scientific research, for instance, the cloning of human DNA sequences and cell lines. Finally, the Commission encouraged the federal government, and all interested and concerned parties to continue deliberation on these ethically difficult issues and to cooperate in educational efforts designed to enlighten the public.

At about the time the Commission issued its report, private ventures appeared, purportedly directed at providing cloning services. Of course, little, if any, evidence of competence accompanied the announcements. An Internet site called Breamtech advertised a commercial service to create either "custom clones" or "designer clones." The company would clone various celebrities for a range of licensing fees, depending on the anticipated value of the product. In another commercial sales effort, the Raelian Movement formed a Bahamas-based company named Vallant Venture offering a service called "Clonaid" to provide technical assistance to would-be parents wanting a cloned child. The service, at a nominal cost of $200,000, claims to offer "a fantastic opportunity to parents with fertility problems or homosexual couples to have a child cloned from one of them."

Richard Seed, a Chicago physicist, stunned the world the week of Jan 10th 1998 by announcing that he would open a cloning clinic *(14,15)*. Seed, while trained as a physicist, has experience in reproductive technology, because he founded a company 20 years ago to transfer embryos from prize cows to less valuable surrogates. Shortly thereafter, he established a company called Fertility and Genetics to apply this technique to people, using uterine lavage and embryo transfer to move blastocysts from healthy women inseminated several days before to those with fertility problems. This effort never gained prominence, perhaps reflecting extraordinary franchise fees. More recently, Dr. Seed not only suggested that his company may move to Mexico, but also offered himself as the guinea pig, to clone himself first and have his 69-yr-old wife carry the pregnancy!

New ground was again broken in December of 1998 when a research group associated with the infertility clinic at Kyunghee University Hospital in Seoul, South Korea announced that they had cloned a human cell from a consenting infertility patient *(16)*. The work, headed by Dr. Lee Bo-yeon, was stopped short of transferring the embryo to a recipient because of the ethical issues surrounding somatic cell cloning. (The question might be asked: then why was it started?) The team cultured 6 embryos produced by nuclear transfer on two different occasions with only one developing to the 4-cell stage within 2 d. These results are scientifically insignificant because of their preliminary nature and because of the lack of evidence that nuclear-transfer embryos were actually produced, but they represent a quantum jump conceptually in the application of cloning technology to human tissue.

CAN WE CLONE HUMANS?

Somatic-cell cloning in humans, on a routine basis, seems very unlikely in the fore-seeable future despite the dramatic progress made in nonhuman animals or the prediction of several "experts" in the field that success in humans is inevitable within five years *(17)*. As noted previously, cloning from fetal or adult cells is becoming a viable approach for propagating transgenic or commercially valuable nonhuman animals; thus far, in 3 different species by different research groups, including one report in cattle where the efficiency in term births was an amazing 80% *(7)*. The likelihood that this technology can be applied to the human with "acceptable risk" is increasing. However, ignoring feasibility, the unknown risks to the fetus or newborn remain daunting issues, making it highly unlikely that human cloning will occur, at least with any consistency, before greater insight is obtained about the fundamental processes involved in reprogramming the donor nucleus (*see* Chapter 14). Such experience is appropriately gained in animal models, including nonhuman primates.

To illustrate the magnitude of the methodological achievement required before somatic-cell cloning can be used to produce animals on demand, consider our efforts to clone rhesus monkeys (*see* also Chapter 16). In all, a colony of 80 adult, cycling females served both as egg/cytoplast donors and as embryo-transfer recipients. In the fourth quarter of 1998 alone, 50 animals underwent follicular stimulation, resulting in the recovery of 1000 oocytes, approx 750 of which were mature. Some oocytes were set aside for controls including the production of normal embryos by intracytoplasmic sperm injection (ICSI) and parthenotes by chemical activation. The balance was subjected to enucleation with a 95% efficiency. Following addition of a nuclear donor cell, electrofusion, chemical activation, and culture, 250 embryos were available for immediate transfer or cryopreservation. Most significantly, over 100 embryos were transferred without an ongoing pregnancy. Thus, although the equipment and expertise for micromanipulation, such as that required for ICSI, exists in many clinical embryology laboratories, the procedures of oocyte enucleation and nuclear transfer required for cloning—not to mention the fusion and activation steps in the process—are quite different and far from simple. Finally, and perhaps most importantly, there is no guarantee that the embryos produced by nuclear transfer have the developmental potential to result in viable pregnancies. Cloning humans would require a consistent and robust supply of gametes and embryos, involving hundreds of oocytes, as well as healthy women to serve as surrogates. Given these limitations, my expectation is that the first human clones will arise from twinning, either the splitting of an advanced embryo or blastomere separation and culture at the 2- or 4-cell stage, rather than from nuclear transfer. The National Bioethics Advisory Commission did not directly address the ethics of twinning, but did point out that twins occur in nature and that this process does not involve producing a copy of an existing individual. Having made the prediction, however, fertility clinics interested or active in twinning have not yet gone public.

SHOULD WE CLONE HUMANS?

The answer for adult somatic-cell cloning is an emphatic NO, because feasibility is low (*see* earlier), risk to the embryo/fetus is unacceptably high, and there is no persuasive reason to clone. Furthermore, human somatic-cell cloning is likely to result in societal

Table 1
Groups With a Theoretical Interest
in Asexual Reproduction by Somatic Cell Cloning

Patients who want to be biological parents, both infertile and fertile
    (could include individuals with no gametes)
Lesbians and gays
Heterosexuals
  Singles
  Couples where the women is older and does not want donor
    oocyte IVF
Grieving parents who want to reproduce a terminally ill child
Parents who want a match for a sibling for medical purposes
Parents/couples in which one member has a genetic disorder that
    the couple does not want to propagate
Parents who are carriers of a lethal recessive gene

objections in the form of jeopardized federal research funding, a fine, or incarceration. Having given an opinion against human cloning in its current context, I still would not describe cloning as immoral or intrinsically wrong or, for that matter, threatening to our society, excluding the repugnant and totally unacceptable possibility of using this technology to create humans as organ donors. Arguably, there are those with legitimate interests in human somatic-cell cloning (Table 1). For a more detailed consideration of the ethics of human cloning, the reader is referred to two recent articles in the New England Journal of Medicine *(18,19)* and an entire issue of Biomedical Ethics Reviews *(20)*.

ON THE REGULATION OF HUMAN CLONING

In the U.S., human cloning, as supported by federal research funds, has always been banned in so far as the work involves human embryos. As well, the Fertility Clinic Success Rate and Certification Act of 1992, provides oversight of clinic activities and thus represents a second tier of regulation *(21)*. In 1994, the legislative ban on the federal funding of human embryo research was removed and the opportunity to implement a new policy arose. Harold Varmus, Director of NIH, appointed a panel to consider such research. The panel's recommendations would limit research to the first 14 d of development after fertilization but included, with the use of special safeguards, the creation of human embryos for research *(22)*. However, President Clinton interceded and reinstated the federal ban on funding research involving human embryos.

After the President's Commission issued the report on human cloning in 1997, several bills were fashioned in the U.S. Congress. In Febuary of 1998, the U.S. Senate voted against bringing a rather Draconian anti-cloning bill directly to the floor for a vote. A second bill, sponsored by Senators Kennedy and Feinstein, more closely reflected the Commission's recommendations, but unfortunately has not seen the light of day and federal level legislation has not yet been passed. Partly in response to the bold announcements of Richard Seed, the FDA has reiterated its jurisdiction in cloning matters and has threatened to shut down anyone attempting human somatic-cell cloning without permission. The agency regulates products, drugs, and devices intended for human use and has broad authority to enforce compliance.

Legislative action at the state level includes a 5-yr moratorium in California on the cloning of an entire muman being *(23)*. The bill outlaws "the practice of creating or attempting to create a muman being by transferring the nucleus from a muman cell from whatever source into a muman egg cell from which the nucleus has been removed." It also provides for penalties for violations: $1,000,000 on a corporation, firm, clinic, hospital, laboratory, or research facility and $250,000 on an individual. Several experts *(24)* have identified potential loopholes in legislative efforts to regulate cloning, such as the possibility of substituting bovine cytoplasts (*see* Chapter 15) for the "muman egg cell from which the nucleus has been removed." Another example that bypasses the "cloning of a genetically identical person" involves a clone produced by nuclear transfer into a donor cytoplast with genetically different mitochondrial DNA, which would not, therefore, be identical genetically *(24)*.

Although there is widespread consensus that muman cloning should be banned, at least temporarily, the question remains, do we have adequate regulation in place? Certainly the vast majority of interested parties with the capability to begin muman cloning will be very strongly dissuaded by existing disincentives or regulation, notwithstanding the premature South Korea adventure *(16)*. On the other hand, no regulatory effort is 100% effective and individuals willing to push the envelope of progress in the name of technology development, financial gain, or potential patient benefit will always exist. If new policies are to be developed, coupling the regulation of muman somatic-cell cloning with federal funding for the assisted reproductive technologies (ARTs) might be attractive. In this way, legitimate research could be conducted while oversight is maintained. Approaches to regulate muman cloning might fall under the jurisdiction of existing agencies, similar to the Human Fertilization and Embryology Commission established in 1990 in England. Although muman cloning is currently in a disapproved category, this group has been progressive in its approach and effective for several years in regulating research involving muman embryos. Another, albeit restrictive approach, as outlined by Annas *(19)*, would serve as a paradigm for all "potentially dangerous boundary-crossing experiments." In this plan, a broad-based regulatory agency primarily composed of non-researchers and nonphysicians would consider proposals from the scientific community. The burden of proof for a proposed series of experiments would be placed on the shoulders of the experimenter; to establish overwhelming reasons why the experiments should be conducted with no clear evidence of harm.

NUCLEAR TRANSFER
IN THE TREATMENT OF HUMAN INFERTILITY

Although nuclear transfer is an integral step in somatic-cell cloning, the procedure need not be restricted to cloning. Four different applications of nuclear transfer in the treatment of muman disease will be considered that are clearly therapeutic in nature (Table 2). The first technique now widely practiced in the clinical ARTs for the treatment of male infertility is ICSI (*see* Chapter 7), in which nuclear transfer is used to place a haploid cell nucleus (usually an intact sperm) into an intact oocyte. ICSI typifies one of the ethical dilemmas created by the clinical ARTs, namely the application of technology before safety and efficacy is established in animal studies. The development of ICSI illustrates the "slippery slope effect" in creating new treatment options. This ethical dilemma is exacerbated by the infertile couple desperate to have a biological child, where risk or safety may well be defined in unique terms. ICSI with ejaculated sperm was adopted as

Table 2
Examples of Nuclear Transfer in the Treatment of Human Disease

ICSI for the treatment of male infertility
Germinal vesicle exchange for female-based infertility
Nuclear transfer for the treatment of mitochondrial-based disease
Polar body transfer for the treatment of female infertility

standard medical practice without extensive animal studies. In part, technical problems were limiting as only recently has it been possible to produce live young in mice, arguably the most appropriate model, using the ICSI procedure *(25)*. No sooner had ICSI been established for the treatment of asthenozoospermia or oligozoospermia, then it was extended to cases of obstructive and nonobstructive azoospermia involving epididymal and testicular sperm (*see* Chapter 7). Moreover, ICSI with testicular sperm quickly progressed from injecting a viable, differentiated cell to inserting an immature, partially differentiated, round spermatid *(26)* without even first establishing protocols to reliably isolate and identify the round cell to be injected. In many ways, the development of new treatment options for infertile couples is a significant achievement in and by itself. However, it is important to recognize that although thousands of infants have been born as a direct result of ART technologies, questions concerning safety continue to plague us. For instance, little detail exists with regards to ICSI specifically, in the incidence of genetic abnormalities in offspring *(27,28)*, in the propagation of genetic disease *(29)*, and in the creation of children who underperform compared to their matched cohorts *(30)*. Therefore, it is important to reiterate that the adoption of a new therapeutic procedure as standard medical practice should ideally involve extensive animal studies, followed by IRB approved clinical trials in much the same manner as would be dictated by the FDA in any attempt to bring a new medication or device to market. These same issues are operative in any consideration of somatic-cell cloning in humans (*see* earlier).

The second entry in Table 2, germinal vesicle (GV) transfer, addresses the alleviation of infertility secondary to advanced maternal age in which an increase in aneuploidy is seen. This increase is owing to cytoplasmic incompetence in spindle formation, resulting in errors in chromosome segregation during meiosis, which, it can be hypothesized, could be overcome by allowing maturation of the nucleus from an older oocyte to occur in the presence of the cytoplasmic machinery of a younger oocyte. GV transfer as envisioned by Zhang and coworkers *(31,32)* involves the use of nuclear transfer to move the immature nucleus from a patient, 38-yr-old or older to a young immature donor cytoplast. The reconstructed oocyte is then allowed to mature in vitro before sperm exposure. One major disadvantage to this approach is the relatively low pregnancy rates currently seen after the in vitro maturation of nonmanipulated human oocytes (*see* Chapter 4). In preliminary studies using micromanipulation, GVs were moved from oocytes to cytoplasts with subsequent completion of maturation to MII in the reconstructed oocytes at control, unmanipulated oocyte rates. Such reconstructed oocytes, in a very small series, also showed a lower rate of chromosomal abnormality when compared with the rate in control oocytes from older patients. At the October 1998 annual meeting of the American Society of Reproductive Medicine, an ongoing clinical trial at NYU was described involving immature nucleus transfer in infertility patients. This procedure would be unlawful in California, but apparently is perfectly legal in New York.

A third application of nuclear transfer is in the treatment of patients at risk for transmitting genetically based mitochrondrial disease (33). Mitochondria, as double-membrane cellular organelles devoted to energy production, are unique in that they contain DNA; a 16,569 base-pair-long, circular chromosome composed of double-stranded DNA encoding several subunits of the respiratory chain, among other components. Molecular lesions of mitochondrial DNA (mtDNA) have been reported with increasing frequency as a source of human disorders (33). Clinical manifestations of mtDNA abnormalities are heterogeneous, but have been linked to early fetal demise. MtDNA is maternally transmitted because the few mitochondria that accompany the sperm are rapidly eliminated (34). Consequently the use of nuclear transfer, to place an immature nucleus, a polar body (see later) or a blastomere from an affected patient into the cytoplast from an unaffected egg donor with normal mitochondria, could circumvent disease transmission from mother to offspring. This application would require an enucleated donor egg containing normal mitochondria, and it need not involve the production of genetically identical individuals, although it may raise ethical problems of its own.

The fourth application cited in Table 2, polar body transfer, focuses on increasing the number and perhaps the quality of embryos available for embryo transfer, especially for the patient of advanced maternal age. Because this approach may be new to some readers and represents an active research interest for our group at OHSU, a detailed presentation of the concept follows. The production of mature germ cells, oogenesis, involves one round of DNA replication transforming a diploid precursor cell with 2N copies of DNA into a cell with 4N copies. Two reductive divisions reduce the amount of DNA from 4N to a single copy or 1N. In the male, each precursor 4N cell undergoes 2 equal reductive cell divisions, resulting in 4 mature sperm each with 1N copy of DNA. In the female, the first reductive division is unequal resulting in a large oocyte with 2N and the formation of a small vesicle, also 2N, called the first polar body (PB1). The second reductive division at fertilization is also unequal creating an egg or oocyte with 1 copy of maternal chromosomes (1N) and a second polar body (PB2) with 1N. Neither PB1 nor PB2 participate in embryo development and they can be removed without consequence to the egg or embryo (35). Thus, in the normal process of meiosis, three of the four haploid sets of maternal chromosomes produced are discarded in polar bodies that degenerate shortly after ovulation.

Experimentation in the mouse has shown that chromosomal DNA within the first and second polar bodies can be used to produce embryos, making it possible theoretically to produce four offspring from a single oocyte (Fig. 1). In order to demonstrate that the second polar body is capable of supporting full embryonic development in mice, Wakayama and coworkers (36) transferred second PBs into zygotes (pronuclear, 1-cell stage) from which the female pronuclei had been removed. The ability of these reconstructed embryos to develop to blastocysts in vitro was monitored as one outcome measure and embryos were transferred to host mothers to evaluate in vivo developmental potential. In the latter experiment, 30 embryos were transferred into 6 females, all of which became pregnant, and 18 pups were delivered. One pup was dead at birth, three failed to be raised by foster mothers and 14 (47%) were weaned and grew normally with subsequent proven fertility. Recently, a second study in mice has confirmed these results using the same approach (37). Eleven of 23 reconstructed embryos developed to blastocysts and were transferred to host females with the birth of 4 pups.

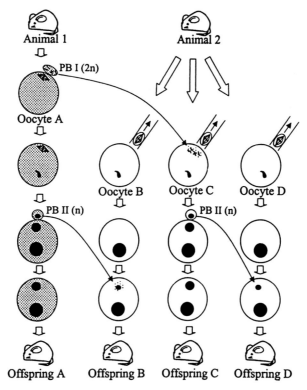

Fig. 1. The use of polar-body transfer strategies in mice to expand the number of viable embryos from 1 to 4. Animal 1 serves as the source of an unfertilized oocyte and a first polar body. Animal 2 serves as the source of oocytes that are enucleated and then injected with a first polar body and a sperm (Oocyte C). Oocytes B and D receive a second polar body from zygotes A and C respectively, along with a sperm, in the process of completing the production of 4 embryos for transfer. Reproduced with permission from Wakayama and Yanagamachi *(38)*.

Use of the first polar body has also been demonstrated in mice *(38)*. A total of 171 enucleated oocytes was injected with first polar bodies, resulting in the recovery of 92 intact oocytes. Next a sperm was injected and 79 of 92 oocytes fertilized normally. Seventy-four of the 79 were transferred to host mothers, producing 37 live offspring (50%) who subsequently grew into fertile adults.

Expression of the maternal DNA in the first and second polar bodies would, in the context of the clinical ARTs, allow a fourfold increase in the number of embryos available. For a 40-yr-old patient who produces only 5 oocytes per stimulation cycle, this amplification to 20 would be highly significant if it reduces the financial and medical costs associated with repeat stimulation cycles and increases the chances of becoming pregnant. A major attraction to PB transfer and the production of reconstructed embryos is conservation of a maternal genetic contribution. The current alternative for women in this age category is to participate in an egg-donor program where a "young" egg donor is selected and subjected to ovarian stimulation and egg harvest. The recovered eggs are fertilized with husband/partner sperm and the resultant embryos are transferred to the wife. Unfortunately, although highly successful, such oocyte donation does not allow a genetic contribution from the female member of the infertility couple.

THE FUTURE

Human Cloning

This brief review leads us toward the conclusion that with the rapid pace of technological development tempered by the considerable ethical and moral problems surrounding cloning, a human clone will be produced somewhere in the world in the next few years. Four points are worthy of reiteration:

1. A significant shift in the cultural and medical attitude towards human cloning has occurred and is continuing to occur from outright, knee-jerk rejection to consideration of the potential benefits of cloning;
2. Regulatory efforts to control human cloning have usually contained a sunset clause, thereby conferring legitimacy to the process sometime in the future;
3. The unacceptable risk argument against human cloning has weakened substantially with the repeated cloning successes in nonhuman species and the production of cloned cattle in high efficiency; and
4. The first clones may result from twinning and not somatic-cell nuclear transfer.

Given the inevitable, if our culture can only attribute all the basic human rights to a clone, then the impact on our society could be limited, if not negligible. Certainly the expense and availability of the technology will affect its use and dictate, for better or worse, its highly selective application. Finally, somatic-cell cloning will not serve to improve the human species; to wit, the comment of Eisenberg *(39)* "To improve our species, no biologic sleight of hand is needed. Had we the moral commitment to provide every child with what we desire for our own, what a flowering of humankind there would be."

Nuclear Transfer

The importance of nuclear transfer is more likely to be felt in other biomedical applications as, for instance, in the creation of embryonic stem (ES) cell lines. Immortalized human embryonic stem cell lines were recently established by isolating and growing cells from the inner cell mass of IVF-produced embryos *(40)*. However, if you or I wanted to create our own ES-cell lines, nuclear transfer of our fibroblast nuclei (or similar cells) into donor cytoplasts with subsequent growth to blastocysts would be required before ES cells could be isolated. The cytoplasts would originate presumably from an oocyte donor, although the possibility has been offered that bovine oocytes could act as universal recipients *(see* Chapter 15). In any event, these ES cells could be preserved at low temperature and might eventually be used for relatively mundane purposes like personalized drug screening or, more importantly, for the provision of an endless supply of matched cells, tissues, and organs for transplant. Thus, an adult fibroblast would be dedifferentiated by passage through a cytoplast, immortalized as a totipotent precurser cell, and then induced to differentiate as needed, in the laboratory, into a specific cell lineage. Of course, the best part is that such cells, tissues, or organs would be our own and should, therefore, circumvent any problems of immune rejection.

Genetic Engineering

We next consider germ line genetic engineering, a concept that only a few short years ago was considered unthinkable, but that has recently been discussed in the context of treating incurable disorders caused by relatively simple genetic defects *(41,42)*. Cloning technology has also been extrapolated by Lee Silver in his book, "Remaking Eden" *(43)*, to the creation of two species of human, the genetic haves and the have-nots, that is, one engineered to "perfection" and one not. This is a far reaching treatment of the subject.

In conclusion, although it may be impossible to predict how and where technology will take us in the future, take us it will, as we seem incapable of effectively regulating anything but its pace of development. Hopefully, any analogy to the creation and use of mass weapons of destruction is simply unfortunate and we, in the scientific community that bring the public these wonderful technologies, will focus attention only on their application to the enhancement of human health and welfare.

REFERENCES

1. DiBerardino MA. Genomic Potential of Differentiated Cells. Columbia University Press, New York, NY, 1997.
2. Campbell KHS, McWhir J, Ritchie WA, Wilmut I. Sheep cloned by nuclear transfer from a cultured cell line. Nature 1996;380:6466.
3. Wells DN, Misica PM, Day AM, Tervit HR. Production of cloned lambs from an established embryonic cell line: A comparison between in vivo- and in vitro-matured cytoplasts. Biol Reprod 1997;57:385–393.
4. Wilmut I, Schniede AE, McWhir J, Kind AJ, Campbell KHS. Viable offspring derived from fetal and adult mammalian cells. Nature 1997;385:810–813.
5. Wakayama T, Perry ACF, Zuccotti M, Johnson KR, Yanagimachi R. Full term development of mice from enucleated oocytes injected with cumulus cell nuclei. Nature 1998;394:369–374.
6. Cibelli JB, Stice SL, Golueke PJ, Kane JJ, Jerry J, Blackwell C, et al. Cloned transgenic calves produced from nonquiescent fetal fibroblasts. Science 1998;280:1256–1258.
7. Kato Y, Tani T, Sotomaru Y, Kurokawa K, Kato J, Doguchi H, et al. Eight calves cloned from somatic cells of a single adult. Science 1998;282:2095–2098.
8. Turner A, Ackerman T. Scientists hope to teach old dog new trick:cloning. Portland Oregonian, August 26, 1998, p. D10.
9. Shettles LB. Diploid nuclear replacement in mature human ova with cleavage. Am J Ob Gyn 1979;133: 222–225.
10. Hall JL, Engel D, Mottla GL, Gindoff PR, Stillman RJ. Experimental cloning of human polyploid embryos using an artificial zona pellucida. Conjoint Meeting of the American Fertility Society and the Canadian Fertility and Andrology Society, Oct. 11–14, 1993, Montreal, Quebec, Canada, Abstract 001, p. S1.
11. Kolata G. Scientist clones human embryos and creates an ethical challenge. New York Times, Oct 24, 1993.
12. Jones HW Jr, Edwards RG, Seidel GE Jr. On attempts at cloning in the human. Fertil Steril 1994;61: 423–426.
13. National Bioethics Advisory Commisssion. Cloning Human Beings: Report and Recommendations of the National Advisory Commission. National Bioethics Advisory Commission, Rockville, MD, 1997.
14. Weiss, R. Scientist will try to clone humans. Washington Post, January 7, 1998, p. A03.
15. Cole W. Seed of controversy. Time, January 11, 1999. p. 77.
16. S.Korea claims cloning advance. New York Times on the Web, Dec 16, 1998.
17. Kolata G. Human Cloning: Yesterday's Never Is Today's Why Not? New York Times, 12-2-1997.
18. Robertson JA. Human cloning and the challenge of regulation. NEJM 1998;339:119–121.
19. Annas GJ. Why we should ban human cloning. NEJM 1998;339:122–125.
20. Humber JM, Almeder RF, eds. Human Cloning Biomedical Ethics Reviews. Humana Press, Totowa, NJ, 1998.
21. Andrews L. The current and future legal status of cloning. NBAC report pg 87–105, 1997.
22. NIH Advisory Committee. Report of the Human Embryo Research Panel. September 27, Bethesda, MD, 1994.
23. California Senate Bill No. 1344. 1997.
24. Boyce N. You want to clone: go ahead. New Scientist, 9 May 1998, p. 6.
25. Kimura Y, Yanagimachi R. Intracytoplasmic sperm injection in the mouse. Biol Reprod 1995;52: 709–720.

26. Tesarik J, Rolet F, Brami C, Sedbon E, Thorel J, Tibi C, Thebault A. Sermatid injection into human oocytes. II. Clinical application in the treatment of infertility due to non-obstructive azoospermia. Hum Reprod 1996;11:780–783.
27. Pauer HU, Hinney B, Michelmann HW, Krasemann EW, Zoll B, Engel W. Relevance of genetic counselling in couples prior to intracytoplasmic sperm injection. Human Reprod 1997;12:1909–1912.
28. In't Veld PA, Halley DJJ, van Helmel JO, Niermeijer MF, Dohle G, Weber RFA. Genetic counselling before intracytoplasmic sperm injection. The Lancet 1997;350:190.
29. te Velde ER, van Baar AL, van Kooij RJ. Concerns about assisted reproduction. The Lancet 1998;351: 1524–1525.
30. Bowen JR, Gibson FL, Leslie GI, Saunders DM. Medical and developmental outcome at 1 year for children conceived by intracytoplasmic sperm injection. Lancet 1998;351:1529.
31. Zhang J, Grifo J, Blaszcyzk A, Meng L, Adler A, Chin A, Krey L. In vitro maturation of human preovulatory oocytes reconstructed by germinal vesicle transfer. 53rd Annual Meeting of the American Society for Reproductive Medicine, 1997, Abstract O-001, p. S1.
32. Zhang J, Wang C-W, Krey L, Liu H, Meng L, Blaszczyk A, et al. In vitro maturation (IVM) of human preovulatory oocytes reconstructed by germinal vesicle (GV) transfer. In: Kempers RD, Cohen J, Haney AF, Younger JB, eds. Fertility and Reproductive Medicine. Elsevier Science, Amsterdam, The Netherlands, 1998, pp. 629–635.
33. Zeviani M, Antozzi C. Mitochondrial disorders. Mol Human Reprod 1997;3(2):133–148.
34. Sukosky P, Moreno R, Schatten G. Sperm mitochondrial ubiquitination and a model explaining the strictly maternal mtDNA inheritance in mammals. Mol Biol Cell 1998;9:309a.
35. Verlinsky Y, Cieslak J, Rechitsky S, Ivakhnenko V, Lifchez A, Kuliev A, and the Preimplantation Genetics Group. Polar body biopsy. In: Kempers RD, Cohen J, Haney AF, Younger JB, eds. Fertility and Reproductive Medicine. Elsevier Science, Amsterdam, The Netherlands, 1998, pp. 213–222.
36. Wakayama T, Hayashi Y, Ogura A. Participation of the female pronulceus derived from the second polar body in full embryonic development of mice J Reprod Fertil 1997;110:263–266.
37. Feng JL, Hall JL. Birth of normal mice after electrofusion of the second polar body with the male pronucleus: a possible treatment for oocyte-factor infertility. 53rd Annual Meeting of the American Society of Reproductive Medicine. 1997, Abstract P-050, p. S116.
38. Wakayama T, Yanagamachi R. The first polar body can be used for the production of normal offspring. Biol Reprod 1998;59:100–104.
39. Eisenberg L. Would cloned humans really be like sheep? N Engl J Med 1999;340:471–475.
40. Thomson JA, Itskovitz-Eldor J, Shapiro SS, Waknitz MA, Swiergiel JJ, Marshall VS, Jones JM. Embryonic stem cell lines derived from human blastocysts. Science 1998;282:1145–1147.
41. Superhuman, Cloning special report. New Scientist, Oct 3, 1998.
42. Lemonick MD. Designer Babies. Time, January 11, 1999, pp. 64–66.
43. Silver L. Remaking Eden: Cloning and Beyond in a Brave New World. Avon Books, Avon, NY, 1997.

INDEX

DATE DUE